The English Catholic Church
in the Nineteenth Century

The English Catholic Church in the Nineteenth Century

Edward Norman

CLARENDON PRESS · OXFORD

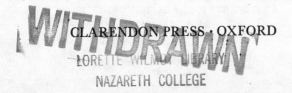

Oxford University Press, Walton Street, Oxford OX2 6DP
London New York Toronto
Delhi Bombay Calcutta Madras Karachi
Kuala Lumpur Singapore Hong Kong Tokyo
Nairobi Dar es Salaam Cape Town
Melbourne Auckland
and associated companies
Beirut Berlin Ibadan Mexico City Nicosia

Oxford is a trade mark of Oxford University Press

Published in the United States
by Oxford University Press, New York

First published 1984
Reprinted (New as Paperback) 1985

British Library Cataloguing in Publication Data

Norman, E.R.
The English Catholic Church in the nineteenth
century.
1. Catholic Church—England—History—19th
century
I. Title
282'.42   BX1493
ISBN 0–19–822955–0

Library of Congress Cataloging in Publication Data
Norman, Edward R.
The English Catholic Church in the nineteenth
century.
Bibliography: p.
Includes index.
1. Catholic Church — England — History — 19th century.
2. England — Church history — 19th century.   I. Title.
BX1493.N67 1984   282'.42   83-17313
ISBN 0–19–822689–6
ISBN 0–19–822955–0 (pbk)

Printed in Great Britain
by Billing & Sons
Worcester

Preface

The present study was written with the intention of providing the general reader with an account of the central events in the history of the Catholic Church in England during the last century. It is an analysis of the character and ideas of the leaders, and an assessment of their achievements. In that sense this is a study in ecclesiastical history, and not a history of religious ideas or theological learning. Nor is it social history—there are no detailed accounts of local Catholic congregations or of their social composition, and no resort to regional studies: these constitute an expanding area of scholarly enquiry, which has attracted increasing attention in recent years, but which, because of its still relatively undeveloped condition (at least as it relates to the English Catholics), and because of its quite different emphases and issues, is best left for separate treatment by others. My hope has been to provide the general reader with a critical assessment of the sort of questions raised by most writers of English Catholic history since the formative works of Mgr. Bernard Ward—the sort of questions discussed most recently by Dr Derek Holmes in his book *More Roman than Rome*, published in 1978—and to provide a reference work for those seeking information about the general nature of the Catholic achievement in the nineteenth century. It is based upon a comprehensive use of available sources, archival and published; and I am grateful to all those, in England and in Rome, who have generously assisted in making manuscript materials available. I am especially indebted to Mgr. D. Simon Lourdusamy, Secretary of the Congregation for the Evangelization of the Nations, for permission to work in the archives of Propaganda; and to Mgr. George Hay, Rector of the Venerable English College in Rome, as also to Mr David Manson, seminarist of the College, for assisting my use of the College's archives; and to Miss Elizabeth Poyser, archivist to the Archdiocese of Westminster. I have received especial assistance in England from Dr Sheridan Gilley at Durham, from

Dr Dominic Bellenger at Downside, and from Hazel Dunn and David Hole here in Cambridge. It would also be ungenerous not to mention those whose kindness has enabled me to work in English archives: Dom Philip Jebb at Downside; Sisters Cecily and Jude at St. Dominic's Convent, Stone; Fr. F. J. Turner, SJ, at Stonyhurst; Fr. Michael Sharratt at Ushaw; Fr. T. G. Holt, SJ and Fr. F. Edwards, SJ at Farm Street in London; Miss Judith Close at the Bristol Record Office; and Fr. Peter Dennison at the Birmingham Diocesan archives. I should also like to record my gratitude for much encouragement to Ivon Asquith of Oxford University Press.

Edward Norman
September 1982

Contents

Introduction

It should never be forgotten that beneath the official religious leadership of the Catholic Church in the nineteenth century—of the authorities and institutions whose activities are related in a study like the present one—there existed a sub-structure of rich spiritual enterprise and astonishing personal heroism. The lives of bishops and scholars are rightly valued for shaping the course of events, but the substance, the largely unrecorded and forgotten labours and prayers of the local clergy and religious, provided the presence of Christianity visible to the sight of most ordinary people throughout the land. The Catholic Church in nineteenth-century England was a Church of poverty: poor in the material resources of the world. It was the local clergy, the 'missionary priests' as they were properly known (since parishes as understood by canon law did not exist until 1918) whose efforts and whose inspiration of the laity provided the places of worship, the schools, and the clergy houses, the Catholic orphanages and conventual institutions, which became the external manifestations of the great revival and expansion of the Church in England. Their main contribution, however, was spiritual. It was seen in devotion to the care of their people in conditions of considerable cultural and personal hostility. The robust Protestantism of English public life was not happy about the signs of new growth and confidence. The priests also faced the harrowing and, at times no doubt, dispiriting conditions of the industrial cities and, like their Protestant counterparts, recognized in them a Christian work for the salvation of the huge unchurched masses. Many sacrificed themselves in the pursuit of their calling. Ten priests died in Liverpool alone, during the great cholera epidemic of 1847, as they attended to the sick and brought the consolations of religion to the dying.[1] Behind the impressive statistics of Catholic expansion was the mission

[1] David Milburn, *A History of Ushaw College*, Ushaw 1964, 153.

priest, gently advancing his beliefs against the strong currents of public and sometimes official opposition and disapproval. There exists, in the archives of Propaganda in Rome, a detailed account of the English Mission, compiled around 1834: it recorded new buildings, and the increasing numbers of priests and people. Of the construction of St. Mary Moorfields, the pro-Cathedral of London, in 1820, 'a magnificent Catholic Church', it was observed that the completion of the building was 'without opposition from the Government'.[2] That had not always been the case: Catholic expansion occurred within living memory of the penal laws, and periodic resurgences of traditional English anti-Catholicism reminded the clergy that they operated on a knife's edge, or so they thought. Two of what Cardinal Wiseman once called the 'three epochs', each marking 'the date of a step in the progress of English Catholicism'[3]—Catholic Emancipation in 1829, the enlarged episcopate of 1840, and the Restoration of the Hierarchy in 1850 —were accompanied by public displays of hostility to indications of Catholic growth. Still the priests persisted in their obligations. 'It was charity that moved him to become a pastor', Cardinal Manning wrote of the Catholic priest in 1883, 'and charity binds him to give his life for his flock.'[4]

At the top end of the Church, however, within the leadership, charity at times did not seem, at least to some observers, especially well distributed. From certain perspectives, the history of the English Catholic Church in the nineteenth century can appear as an accumulation of disputes—of Milner with Douglas and with Poynter, of Wiseman with Errington and with Grant, of Baines with the monks of Downside, of Manning with Searle and with Capel, and of Vaughan with Gallwey. There were also some clearly recognized personal animosities which usually fell short of open disputation— of Faber for Newman, of Clifford for Manning, of Manning for Newman, and of Talbot for Errington. 'Ought we not if

    [2] Propaganda Archives, *Scritture Riferite nei Congressi, Anglia* 9 (1834–41), 1, Missioni di Europa: Inghilterra' [in Italian].
    [3] *The Religious and Social Position of Catholics in England. An Address Delivered to the Catholic Congress of Malines, August 21, 1863, by H.E. Cardinal Wiseman*, London 1864,|7.
    [4] H. E. Manning, *The Eternal Priesthood*, London 1883, 59.

possible to do something to stop this constant discussion of matters of Church discipline by ecclesiastics in news-papers', Bishop Ullathorne wrote to Wiseman in 1848 from Birmingham; 'It is giving great scandal.'[5] And so it did. Officials in Rome tended to attribute the English internal strife to qualities of native character rather than to breaches of charity.[6] Mgr. George Talbot in Rome, whose own contributions to the difficulties were not exactly minimal, kindly remarked, in this regard, that 'prejudice and jealousy are the failings of good men', and added that 'the religious orders have them in high degree'.[7] In some measure the strength of the personalities involved explained the discords; Graham Greene has noted that 'Roman Catholicism in this country has been a great breeder of eccentrics.'[8] In much larger measure, however, the disputes and the personal incompatibilities are to be attributed to the scale of events and the seriousness with which the various issues were regarded. Considering the relatively small numbers of Catholics, the sheer size of the expansion was very dramatic, especially when it was inflated by the Irish immigration of the mid-century: Catholic leaders encountered problems and needed adaptations quite new to their experience, and the body of beliefs and practices they sought to guarantee within the Church as it developed were both closely-defined and exactly stated by them. At the centre of most of the disputes lay the differences between the 'Roman' party within the Church, the Ultramontanes whose vision of the styles and claims of the triumphalist Rome which emerged from the humiliation of the French Revolutionary period was heightened (though not actually introduced to England) by the appointment of Wiseman as head of the new hierarchy in 1850, and the 'Old Catholics', conscious of their quiet English spirituality, their rootedness in the virtues of common English notions of liberty, and their

[5] Westminster Diocesan Archives, Wiseman Papers (Bishops' Letters) R.79/3, Ullathorne to Wiseman, 10 Oct. 1848.

[6] Shane Leslie, *Henry Edward Manning. His Life and Labours*, London 1921, 133.

[7] E. S. Purcell, *The Life of Cardinal Manning, Archbishop of Westminster*, London 1895, II. 101 (Dec. 1860).

[8] Graham Greene, *Collected Essays*, London (Penguin books) 1970, 260 (actually written of Eric Gill).

antipathy to centralized authority. The expansion of the Church produced pressing issues which were only too readily converted into symbols of this greater divergence. But the issues in themselves *were* important—for those who took their convictions seriously. To the extent that the history of the Catholic Church of the nineteenth century was a history of disputes—and it is a summary which is anyway exaggerated— it is to be interpreted as an unhappy side-effect of resolute activity rather than as a mere descent, by petty minds, into unnecessary minutiae of disagreement. When he published his great and seminal studies of the nineteenth-century Catholic Church, early in the present century, Bishop Bernard Ward was thought by some to have erred in 'opening up', as Dom Cuthbert Butler put it, 'long-ago controversies and quarrels, long since dead and buried'. Butler added: 'But for better or for worse, Church History is in great measure made up of the differences and quarrels of good men.'[9] It is necessary to secure a balanced perspective, and to appreciate how enormous was the achievement of those whose enterprise sometimes involved competition with the endeavours of others. Religious professionals often lack the required perspective themselves. 'I am not a theologian,' Duchesne once said, 'that is why I can praise God with joy.'[10]

The Church which emerged from the penal laws was not quite so retiring or decimated as subsequent interpreters have sometimes imagined. The nineteenth-century Ultramontanes had an interest in representing its devotional life as at a particularly low ebb—just as their High Church counterparts in the Church of England depicted eighteenth-century Anglicanism as a slumbering inconsequence. It threw their own achievements into a sharper light; it justified the decisiveness of the changes they sought to accomplish. The penal laws themselves had often remained unenforced, and though an encumbrance when it came to professional qualifications and advancement of landed and financial transactions, they rarely interfered with the performance of public worship. Catholics of the eighteenth century spoke discreetly of 'going to prayers'

[9] Cuthbert Butler, *The Life and Times of Bishop Ullathorne, 1806–1889*, London 1926, I. v.
[10] John J. Heaney, *The Modernist Crisis: von Hügel*, London 1969, 49.

rather than of 'going to mass', in order to avoid offending their Protestant neighbours, but the Church did not really strive 'to make herself invisible'.[11] In London the Embassy chapels were plainly open for public worship, with the acquiescence of the authorities, and provided the splendour of the liturgy in its most adorned form. 'Secret' Catholic services in taverns or halls were known to the magistrates who chose to take no action: they were, indeed, distinctly put out when William Payne, a common informer, began to force prosecutions in the 1760s against a number of Catholic priests and schoolteachers for violations of the penal code.[12] The Church of the second half of the eighteenth century was in the open. In the 1770s there were around four hundred priests serving the English mission, most of them in the private chapels of the gentry or in churches on their estates; some were in chapels established through their influence in the towns. The Church was still dominated by the laity—it was they who appointed the clergy to their positions and who provided their stipends. But it was a situation in transition. Missions were becoming independent of the families who had set them up; lay patrons everywhere were losing their control. One of the most important features of the nineteenth-century Catholic Church, the rise of clerical authority, was already coming into existence—long before the Ultramontanes put their stamp upon the process. Anglican patrons retained their powers throughout the nineteenth century; Catholic ones did not. It was a key difference in developments which otherwise sometimes showed surprising similarities. There were odd exceptions to the Catholic experience. As late as 1857 the Abbot of Mount St. Bernard's monastery in Leicestershire, a Cistercian house founded by Ambrose Phillipps de Lisle, most prominent of Catholic laymen, was complaining to Rome about his patron's interference, even in small things apparently. 'The Vicar General ordered curtains to be fixed or nailed between the secular and monastic Church *at all times*',

[11] Paul Thureau-Dangin, *The English Catholic Revival in the Nineteenth Century*, London 1914, I. xxiii.

[12] Eamon Duffy, 'Richard Challoner, 1691–1781: A Memoir', in Eamon Duffy ed., *Challoner and his Church, A Catholic Bishop in Georgian England*, London 1981, 22.

he reported; 'this regulation so much displeased Mr. Phillipps our Patron and Founder that he threatened never to enter the Church again.'[13]

Received opinions about the church of the eighteenth century perhaps relied too much on Joseph Berington's *State and Behaviour of English Catholics from the Revolution to the Year 1780* (published in 1780). It represented a Church in decline, and considerably underestimated both the actual numbers of Catholics and the existing signs of advance. For by that time the Church had in fact enjoyed a 'modest growth' and was certainly, according to Professor Bossy, 'in a condition to face the future with reasonable confidence'.[14] The first half of the nineteenth century was for the Catholics, as for the other Dissenting Churches in England, a time of growth. Before the great tide of Anglican conversions in the mid-century, and the Irish influx—stimulated though not begun by the Famine—Catholic advance was steady if unspectacular. The Parliamentary 'Papist Returns' of 1767 had yielded a Catholic population in England and Wales of 69,376. Those returns, Lesourd remarked, 'constituent un document d'une telle importance qu'il nous permet de décrire la minorité catholique en la saisissant à un moment où il ne reste qu'un noyau de gens décides et convaincus mais peu nombreux'.[15] The figures were in fact higher than the returns showed: there were perhaps 80,000 Catholics when all the rural communities are included. By the time of the general religious census of 1851, there were an estimated three-quarters of a million Catholics; about three and a half per cent of the total population.[16] The Irish immigrants gave the Catholics a large working-class membership—something which the other churches, and especially the Anglicans, notably lacked.[17] The

[13] Propaganda, *Scritture* 14 (1855-7), 1082, Abbot of Mt. St. Bernard's to the Cardinal Prefect, 29 May 1857.

[14] John Bossy, *The English Catholic Community, 1570–1850*, London 1975, 287.

[15] Jean Alain Lesourd, *Les Catholiques dans la société anglaise, 1765–1865*, Lille 1978, I. 4.

[16] Philip Hughes, 'The English Catholics in 1850', in *The English Catholics 1850–1950*, ed. G. A. Beck, London 1950, 44. For a discussion of the census returns, see chapter 5 following.

[17] J. Derek Holmes, *More Roman than Rome: English Catholicism in the Nineteenth Century*, London 1978, 163.

Irish moved to the cities, altering the distribution pattern
of Catholicism; but the traditional Catholic centres, where
groups had survived since the Reformation—Lancashire, the
West Midlands, and parts of the north-east—continued to provide the basis of Catholic organization. The leadership of the
Church was never taken over by the Irish, as it was in the
United States or the British overseas territories: most bishops
continued to come from traditional Catholic families and from
the convert elements. It has been convincingly argued, by
Professor Bossy, that existing developments within English
Catholicism already presaged expansion, and that the notion
that English Catholicism grew, in the nineteenth century, in
a form largely dictated by the Irish influx, requires severe
modification.[18] Nevertheless, by the 1850s, something like
eighty per cent of the congregations were Irish and working-
class. It gave the Catholic Church a huge impetus to missionary zeal. The missionary nature of the Church at the end of
the eighteenth century had, anyway, well adapted it to face
the social dislocations of the new industrial concentrations. It
had no ancient structure of parochial administration or out-
moded diocesan finance, as the State Church had, to encum-
ber its approach to the new population. All the English
churches became critically conscious of the problem of
'Church Extension' in the first decades of the nineteenth century, and all rushed to build new churches for the overflowing
masses of the crowded cities. In extending their ministry,
therefore, the Catholics were responding to a common movement: the remarkable thing is that they were able to do so in
the hostile climate of anti-Catholic feeling, and so soon after
the atmosphere of the penal laws had inhibited their public
activities within society. In the first decade of the century,
there were thirty new chapels in the Northern District. Expansion was noted in most of the places where traditional
Catholic strength provided a basis. In Bath, with its still-
fashionable entertainments, which attracted Catholics along
with others, and with its proximity to the Benedictine house
at Downside, the first decade of the century saw the construction of four chapels of increasing size, with a Catholic

[18] Bossy, 297.

school.[19] Bishop Baines, who resided at Bath, in order to administer the Western District, abolished pew rents in 1830.[20] This, too, was a sign of the general expansion—the Protestant Churches, also, were abolishing payment for seats in church during the century, as the churches all moved away, or tried to, from social exclusivity. The Second Provincial Synod of Westminster, in 1866, required all Catholic churches to provide a quota of free seats sufficient in each place to accommodate all who came. Despite the continuing legal difficulties about testated possessions and charitable trusts, Catholic property expanded too. In 1829, for example, the monks of Downside told Propaganda in Rome that their property was 'now wonderfully increased'. Within the preceding sixteen years, they declared, 'we have acquired almost a hundred acres of very fertile land, paying the price;' they had 'built a Church in the old English style;' and they had 'established a flourishing college where some fifty young gentlemen devote themselves to study and moral discipline'.[21] Throughout the country, Catholic chapels and churches were being built; schools, charitable institutions, and the houses of the religious orders were being established in a visible advance of the faith which, reinforced by the concession of Emancipation in 1829, elevated the expectations of the English Catholics and gave them that sense of what Newman, in his famous sermon before the assembled prelates at the First Provincial Synod of Westminster, at Oscott in 1852, called 'The Second Spring'.

More important even than buildings and facilities, Catholic worship began to be transformed. Until after Emancipation, Catholic chapels rarely had any external sign of their religious use, in order to avoid giving offence to the Protestants. Wiseman related how, on his English tour of 1832, he had been told of a priest who was warned by the police that a cross on the façade of his church would probably lead to its destruction by a mob.[22] The new churches of the mid-century

[19] J. Anthony Williams, *Bath and Rome: the Living Link*, Bath 1963, 44.

[20] Bernard Ward, *The Sequel to Catholic Emancipation*, London 1915, I. 38.

[21] Downside Archives, I.A, Allanson Records, III. 89, Petition by the Prior and Convent of St. Gregory's, Downside, to Cardinal Capellari, (n.d., but 1829; in Latin).

[22] Wilfrid Ward, *The Life and Times of Cardinal Wiseman*, London 1897, I. 220.

changed all that—the neo-classical Italianate structures favoured by the Ultramontanists, or the gothic buildings put up by Pugin, were triumphant expressions of the new confidence of the Church. The styles of worship within were different, too. It was in the interests both of the 'Romans' and of the 'English' parties within the Church to depict the services of traditional English Catholicism as in a sorry state: both were advocates of change, though they differed hugely over what those changes should be like. Yet, in all truth, the traditional worship of the 'Old Catholics', with its rejection of 'continental' devotional practices—a rejection which extended to images of the Virgin, votive candles, processions, and so forth—was, like Anglican worship at the start of the nineteenth century, extremely plain and subdued in tone. The standard of preaching, already low, was not assisted by the arrival of the *émigré* clergy from France. Archbishop Ullathorne recalled how the priest at his home chapel in Yorkshire, when he was a boy, had four sermons only, and how 'when he had read the first line of his discourse the little flock knew all the rest by heart'.[23] Things were sometimes worse: W. G. Ward was shocked by the styles of preaching he encountered in the church of his conversion. One priest, 'of the old school', he once said, 'habitually read translations from the old Court sermons of Bourdaloue, without any regard to the nature of his congregation, which consisted of the poorest of the poor'. In consequence, 'the subtle temptations of wealth and titles and wordliness were earnestly dwelt on, and exhortations to curb the love of the excitements of the Court, and of the delicacies of sumptuous living, were pressed on the attention of blacksmiths and carpenters.'[24] Services at the major churches in London were characterized as 'florid', 'theatrical', and 'operatic', rather than devotional. Those in the 'Roman' party who disliked this style overlooked its general prevalence in continental Catholic practice. At the funeral for Cardinal Weld in Rome, the Italians hissed Wiseman because of the length of his oration: they were impatient to

---

[23] *From Cabin-Boy to Archbishop. The Autobiography of Archbishop Ulla-thorne*, London, 1941 edn. [1891], 4.
[24] Wilfrid Ward, *William George Ward and the Catholic Revival*, London, second edn. 1912, 75.

hear the music of Mozart's *Requiem*. English Catholic worship before the nineteenth century revival wrought its transformation had more vitality and more beauty even—thanks to Challoner's translations of traditional Catholic works, and his attempts to encourage 'English' piety—than was later allowed to appear. Bishop Milner introduced public devotions to the Sacred Heart in 1814. He also read the Epistle and the Gospel at mass in English, though there were problems in this: 'the consequence was that from his translating the Latin extempore, one heard considerable variations from the usual version'.[25]

The quiet style of English Catholicism at the start of the nineteenth century was fashioned in order to respect Protestant sensibilities; but it had something of a reverse effect. Precisely because Catholic practices were hidden and unknown, they were popularly imagined to be purposefully secretive, and because secret, in some way disgraceful. Public ignorance of Catholicism was very profound. Wiseman, who knew continental conditions well—perhaps better than he knew the condition of England—remarked that Catholicism was so little visible that foreigners supposed it existed only in Ireland.[26] Newman, in his 'Second Spring' sermon, misrepresented the Catholicism of the period before the conversions as 'a mere handful of individuals, who might be counted, like the pebbles and detritus of the great deluge'; but he more accurately caught the atmosphere of general belief when he spoke of 'An old fashioned house of gloomy appearance, closed in with high walls, and with an iron gate, and yews, and the report attaching to it that "Roman Catholics" lived there; but who they were, or what they did or what was meant by calling them Roman Catholics, no one could tell—though it had an unpleasant sound, and told of form and superstition.'[27] At the time of the Catholic Relief Bill of 1791, Pitt had been seen to enter Coghlan's, the London Catholic bookshop, in order to acquaint himself with what Catholics actually

[25] F. C. Husenbeth, *The Life of the Right Rev. John Milner, D.D.*, Dublin 1862, 555.
[26] *Recollections of the Last Four Popes and of Rome in their times, by H. E. Cardinal Wiseman*, London, revised edn. 1859, 248.
[27] J. H. Newman, *Sermons Preached on Various Occasions*, London 1857, 200.

believed, so little did he know of them.[28] The paucity of Catholic literature was another cause of public misunderstanding. The market for Catholic books was so small, in 1800, that very few could get published.[29] This also resulted in a cultural as well as a religious gap in Catholic life. Manning, remarking in 1863 on the absence of a Catholic literature, wrote 'The Catholics of England have been compelled either to read foreign Catholic works, which are accessible only to a few, or the books of anti-Catholic writers, or, as with the great majority, to be deprived of the wholesome culture and information on which the development of the intelligence depends.'[30] For a society as preoccupied with literacy as Victorian England, this was a serious matter. Unlike the Protestants, the Catholics did not even have the popular culture of the open Bible: Ullathorne recorded his doubt that his parents were even aware that an English translation of the Bible for Catholics existed.[31] The public controversy over Emancipation helped to stimulate a popular Catholic polemical literature. In Liverpool, for example, the 'Catholic Defence Association', founded in 1826, spent £50 in its first six months on the distribution of cheap Catholic tracts.[32] The writings of Charles Butler and John Lingard presented Catholic ideas to a wide public. But the widest public was undoubtedly achieved by a non-Catholic apologist of Catholicism: William Cobbett in his *History of the Protestant "Reformation"*, published in parts between 1824 and 1825. His thesis was simple and directly expressed: 'the "Reformation", as it is called, was engendered in beastly lust, brought forth in hypocrisy and perfidy, and cherished and fed by plunder, devastation, and by rivers of innocent English and Irish blood'.[33] The book sold 60,000 copies in its first year, an astonishing figure for the time. Pope Leo XII read it in translation. 'With what information, and

[28] Husenbeth, op. cit. 36.

[29] Joseph Gillow, *A Literary and Biographical History of the English Catholics*, London 1885, I. xiii.

[30] H. E. Manning, *Miscellanies*, London 1877, I. 63, 'The Work and Wants of the Catholic Church in England' (*Dublin Review*, July 1863).

[31] *From Cabin-Boy to Archbishop*, 5.

[32] Thomas Burke, *Catholic History of Liverpool*, Liverpool 1910, 43.

[33] William Cobbett, *A History of the Protestant "Reformation" in England and Ireland*, Dublin 1826, 2.

with what deep sense of force does that man write,' he said; 'surely such a man cannot be a Protestant.'[34] But he was; and his influence was with Protestants, too. It helped to renovate something of a Catholic past, with an emphasis on the charitable works done before the Dissolution of the Monasteries. English Protestants were accustomed to thinking of monastic institutions as hotbeds of depravity. Cobbett's picture, no less inaccurate in its way, helped Catholic respectability.

A change in the public climate was seen in the adoption of clerical dress. At the start of the nineteenth century, Catholic priests and religious never appeared in public except in the guise of laymen. That, however, was the custom of the Protestant clergy, too, at the time. Regulars did not even wear habits within the conventual walls. Bishop Poynter, in the London District, actually, 'endeavoured to strip the nuns of Newhall' (—it should be added, 'of their religious habit'—) in what a hostile Catholic observer called the 'spirit of appeasing Protestant fanaticism'.[35] Ullathorne, though he was a Benedictine monk, had never seen a monastic habit till he first visited Rome.[36] Father Luigi Gentili, arriving as a missioner from Italy in 1835, was the first priest in England to wear clerical dress in public—in his case, a Rosminian habit.[37] Blessed Dominic Barberi, travelling to England in 1841, felt obliged to change out of his Passionist habit at Boulogne and wear ordinary secular clothes.[38] Even Cardinal Consalvi, on a diplomatic mission to England in 1814, had to wear a black coat and white tie, in the English clerical manner, to avoid giving offence.[39] A crowd objecting to Newman wearing his Oratorian habit in the streets once emptied a sack of flour over him.[40]

The quality as well as the numbers of priests improved in the first half of the century—and so did their professional self-consciousness, another feature common to Protestantism as well, and related, of course, to general developments within

[34] Westminster Dioc. Archives, Gradwell's *Journal*, E.8.II (26 May 1825).

[35] Stonyhurst Archives, Glover's *Excerpts* III, MS B.I.17, 246.

[36] Bernard Ward, *Sequel*, II. 19.

[37] Denis Gwynn, *Father Luigi Gentili and his Mission (1801–1848)*, Dublin 1951, 10.

[38] Denis Gwynn, *The Second Spring, 1818–1852. A Study of the Catholic Revival in England*, London 1942, 116.

[39] Wilfrid Ward, *Wiseman*, I. 11.

[40] Ronald Chapman, *Father Faber*, London 1961, 221.

the secular professions. The increase in vocations derived from the expansion of Catholic education, both because of the creation of an educated Catholic class and because of the example and encouragement given to schoolboys in Catholic schools to regard the priesthood as the highest calling. There survives, in Wiseman's papers at Ushaw College, a memoir by a former pupil at Oscott in which there is a description of Wiseman's manner of procuring vocations among the boys— 'with what heavenly gush of soul-saving charity he would make you promise to devote yourself to the priesthood, and, as the diffident answer came, he would exclaim with prophetic joy: "Dear, my dear child, I know you will become a priest."'[41] The older clergy were sometimes thought not to be of high intellectual quality—as indeed became a matter of some public comment after the Anglican converts in the mid-century (in their journal the *Rambler*) began to criticize the low educational levels of the Old Catholics. Döllinger testified to this as well. When Herbert Vaughan called on him in Munich in 1855, he found Döllinger 'much pained by the unpolished manner in writing and general ignorance of our old English Catholic clergy'.[42] The priests of the 'Second Spring' were an enormous improvement in this respect. Successive heads of the English Church—Wiseman, Manning, and Vaughan—placed clerical training as first among their priorities for the furtherance of religion in England. Financial difficulties imposed some restraints, however, and certainly helped to perpetuate the system (despite widespread criticism) whereby clerical and lay students were educated in the same colleges. The reopening of the English College in Rome, in 1818, helped to elevate standards, as well as to acquaint generations of students with the new Ultramontanism. Training in England was, early in the century, a constant worry to the Vicars Apostolic. 'Your Eminence probably knows that I have no means of educating Priests for the sixteen counties which the Holy see has committed to my care except the little College and Seminary at Oscott', Milner wrote to the Cardinal Prefect of Propaganda, in 1818; and

---

[41] Ushaw College Archives, Wiseman Papers, 420, J. P. Stapletone's MS memoir (n.d.)

[42] J. G. Snead-Cox, *The Life of Cardinal Vaughan*, London 1910, I. 63.

this college, he continued 'having no funds, nor other support, except what I myself can procure for it, is incapable of raising more than half the number of priests who are wanted in the Midland District.'[43] In 1836 Poynter began holding annual retreats for the clergy, a practice which was greatly encouraged by most of the bishops thereafter and which must have considerably assisted the rise in clerical standards—as did the periodic convening, after the restoration of the Hierarchy in 1850, of diocesan synods and conferences. What they were acquiring, through such means, was a sense of distinct Catholic practice in the conduct of institutions; and that was new. Catholic priests had before shared common English assumptions, which some supposed amounted to a version of Gallicanism. 'Trained as all Englishmen are in the principles of the British Constitution and imbibing its elements daily from the Newspapers, those principles form as it were the atmosphere of English life, and the standard of measure in questions of social right and wrong,' Ullathorne, that most English of bishops, observed to Propaganda in 1859; 'But whilst all breathe equally the atmosphere of English Constitutionalism, very few even of the clergy have had any training in the laws and principles of Ecclesiastical government and discipline.'[44] In some areas the regular clergy, as the President of the English Congregation of the Benedictines put it, 'leave the monastery for supplementary ministries in the missions on account of their poor health or absence of an incumbent'.[45] These arrangements led to friction with the Vicars Apostolic over questions of jurisdiction, but the effects must, in the wider perspective, have been tremendously beneficial to the Church in its constant attempts to meet the shortage of priests and the lack of means for supporting them. The regulars must also have given an example of just the sort of disciplined life, while serving the missions, which assisted the general cultivation of professionalism among the secular clergy. The Catholics were not unaffected by that moral seriousness which helped to produce

[43] Propaganda, *Scritture* 7 (1818–22), 41, Milner to the Cardinal Prefect, 22 Jan. 1818 [in English].

[44] Birmingham Dioc. Archives, B.3915, Draft Letter by Ullathorne to Propaganda (n.d., but 1859).

[45] Downside Archives, I.A. Allanson Records, III. 86, President Birdsall to Cardinal Capellari, of Propaganda, 18 June 1829 [in Latin].

the sober earnestness of Protestant ministers in Victorian England. In 1869, at the Low Week meeting, the Catholic Hierarchy agreed to forbid the clergy 'to sing at concerts, to be present at dances, or to allow their names to be printed in any other than ecclesiastical or literary advertisements'.[46] In 1895 Propaganda repeated the ruling.[47] It was a small indication, but a telling one, of clericalization. The laity and the clergy were no longer able to enjoy the same recreations and, to some extent, the same life-styles as they had done in the preceding century.

Throughout the nineteenth century, the Catholic advance was achieved against the persistent background of Protestant antipathy, both popular and intellectual in style and appeal. The true heroism of the clergy has to be appreciated in this perspective. At any time, so it seemed, opinion could be aroused, or the mob turned out, against 'Popery'.[48] As Cobbett accurately observed, in his *History*, 'In books of all sizes, and from the pulpit of every church, we have been taught, from our infancy, that the "*beast*, the *man of sin*, and the *scarlet whore*," mentioned in the *Revelation*, were names which *God himself* had given to the Pope.'[49] Ignorance of Catholic doctrines, a sensationalized popular literature about Catholic practices, a political tradition of civil liberty which associated Catholicism with autocracy, treason, and intellectual enslavement: all tended to foster a widespread dislike—some would even express it as loathing—of the Roman Church. 'I solemnly believe blue and red baboons to be more popular here than Catholics and Presbyterians' Sydney Smith wrote in 1807; 'they are more understood, and there is a greater disposition to do something for them.'[50] The passage of relief legislation to mitigate, and eventually to abolish, most of the penal enactments in the last decades of the eighteenth century, and the achievement of Catholic Emancipation

[46] Westminster Dioc. Archives, ACTA, Meeting of the Bishops in Low Week, 1869, 23 (9 Apr.).
[47] Ibid., 1895, II (23 Apr.), 'Connection of the Clergy with Dances'.
[48] For a recent account of this sentiment and agitation, see Walter L. Arnstein, *Protestant versus Catholic in Mid-Victorian England. Mr. Newdegate and the Nuns*, Columbia 1982.
[49] Cobbett, 5.
[50] Sydney Smith, *Peter Plymley's Lettters*, London, 1886 edn., 57.

itself, in 1829, were accompanied by threats of popular mob
disturbances. It is actually surprising that the Gordon Riots of
1780—themselves prompted by the Relief measure attempted
in 1778—were not repeated throughout the years of the
Emancipation debate. Anti-Catholic rioting was to reappear
in England in the years between 1840 and 1870. Surviving
civil disabilities also indicated the strength of Protestant feeling, and were, in their way, a much greater hazard for Catholics, affecting, as they did, the security of legal inheritance
and the conditions upon which property might be held. Property bequeathed for what the law continued to regard as
'superstitious uses'—which might mean anything from the
endowment of masses to the building of conventual establishments—was liable to confiscation. Most property escaped legal
interference, but the threat remained, and introduced uncertainty and extra difficulty. So did the threat of popular
disturbances. When St. Edmund's College, Ware, the seminary
of the London District, rented an adjacent farm, in 1813, the
lease contained a provision obliging liabilities should it be
'damaged by any riot in consequence of the same premises
being attached to a Catholic College, or occupied by a tenant
of the Catholic persuasion'.[51] The shadow of the penal laws
lay still across English Catholic life long after they had been
abolished. Emancipation stimulated nationalism in Ireland,
and O'Connell captured first local government institutions
and then the core of the parliamentary representation—in
1841, as a symbol of this, he became Lord Mayor of Dublin.
In England, the fruits of Emancipation were gathered with
more hesitancy. 'The penal laws have been abolished for half
a century', Manning wrote in 1880, 'but as yet Catholics are
only entering slowly into civil careers, and no Catholic holds
any political office of importance.'[52]

First among Protestant suspicions of the Catholics was the
belief that the Papacy was historically dedicated to the subversion of the Crown. Sequences of Reformation history, and
subsequent evidences of Catholic disloyalty—particularly the

---

[51] Bernard Ward, *History of St. Edmund's College, Old Hall*, London 1893,
217.
[52] H. E. Manning, *The Catholic Church in Modern Society*, London 1880,
19.

Jesuit mission under Elizabeth I, and Jacobite insurgency—
were spoken of as though of contemporary validity. In 1852,
under the title 'Propery Absolving Murders', the *Reformation
Journal* declared: 'Britain, ever since the Reformation, has
been the especial object of Jesuitical craft and recklessness,
and perhaps never more than at the present moment, and we
may rest assured that no means, foul or fair, will be left un-
tried to subvert the Protestantism of this country.'[53] To
nineteenth-century Protestants, it still seemed axiomatic that
those who held to a 'double allegiance', to Pope and Crown,
were more likely to obey the former; and they supposed, also,
that the testing of the allegiance was always a possibility. Nor
was this only a popular belief. It extended well into the
common assumptions of educated opinion. The burden of
Gladstone's case against the Decrees of the Vatican Council,
which he delivered in a pamphlet of 1874, was precisely that
the civil loyalty of the English Catholics was compromised by
their 'double allegiance'. Many of those who argued against
Catholic Emancipation in the first three decades of the century did so because they genuinely believed that Catholic
participation in parliamentary government would constitute
an actual threat to free institutions. Thus Blanco White, a
respected Irish-Spanish convert from Rome who lived in
England, wrote in 1826: 'A Roman Catholic cannot, without
guilt, lend his support to a Protestant establishment, but is
bound, as he wishes to save his soul, to miss no opportunity
of checking the progress of heresy.' He added, 'Murder itself
is less sinful.'[54] In defending Catholics at the time of the
national uproar over the restoration of the Hierarchy in 1850,
Cardinal Wiseman went to some lengths to explain that they
were not alone in rejecting the Royal Supremacy in religion—
the English Dissenters also rejected it, and they were no longer
considered disloyal.[55] 'The danger to the religious and civil
liberties of Englishmen is not from any infringement on them
by the Pope,' he argued, 'but from those who are taking

---

[53] *The Bulwark or Reformation Journal*, London, I (1851–2), 212.
[54] Joseph Blanco White, *Practical and Internal Evidence Against Catholicism*,
London 1826 (revised edn.), 49.
[55] *An Appeal to the Reason and Good Feeling of the English People on the
subject of the Catholic Hierarchy*, by Cardinal Wiseman, London 1850, 10.

advantage of the occurrences to go back a step, if they can, in the legislation of toleration.'[56]

After the question of civil allegiance, it was the superstition of Catholicism, as it was supposed, which most inflamed Protestants, and England in the nineteenth century produced a rich texture of anti-Catholic literature to demonstrate it. It was a multi-class literature; the arguments and illustrations against Rome were the same in books and pamphlets written both by academic writers and by the popular preachers. Archbishop Richard Whately's *Essays on the Errors of Romanism*, which went into three series, was perhaps characteristic of educated opinion, even if more distinguished than most. All the traditional polemics about superstitious practices, from 'pious frauds' to 'idolatry', were reproduced in his pages. Of the mass, when 'a Romanist adores the true God under the form of bread', he wrote: 'he is clearly as much guilty of idolatry as the Israelites in worshipping the golden calf'.[57] All the literature emphasised the apparent lack of respect paid to the authority of the Bible in the Catholic Church, and the exaltation of ecclesiastical authority—'priestcraft'. This seemed especially outrageous to English Protestants, immersed as the popular culture was in Biblical knowledge. 'Great dislike to the Bible was shown by those who conversed with me about it', as *Maria Monk* recorded, of her (largely fictional) experiences at the Hôtel Dieu convent in Montreal.[58] Her *Awful Disclosures*, published in 1836, became a popular classic of the literature; so did *Fifty Years in the Church of Rome* by Father Charles Chiniquy, a priest from Quebec who defected to Protestantism (at St. Anne, Illinois) in 1858, and published his account in 1885. This book was full of the horrors of the confessional, of instruments of self-mortification, of moral improprieties by monks and nuns, and—especially shocking for contemporary sensibilities—of 'the girl in the garb of a man in the service of the curates of Quebec'.[59] These publications,

[56] Ibid. 13.

[57] Richard Whately, *Essays on the Errors of Romanism* (Third Series), London 1856, 7.

[58] *The Awful Disclosures of Maria Monk* [1836], London, 1965 edn., 31.

[59] Charles Chiniquy, *Fifty Years in the Church of Rome*, London, 1948 edn., 226.

both of which went through numerous editions, were of international reputation. The domestic products relied on Irish,
rather than on Canadian, illustration, though the literature
was not, as such, anti-Irish. Patrick Murphy's *Popery in Ireland*
(1865) was actually written by G. H. Whalley, the Member of
Parliament for Peterborough.[60] Like many roused English
Protestants, he looked to the Italian *Risorgimento* for inspiration—and especially to the Piedmontese 'Law of Convents'
in 1854, which had suppressed many religious houses. 'What
English bosom or Irish Protestant heart did not heave and
swell with emotion as we read of the undisguised joy expressed by those pale-faced Italian ladies [the expelled nuns]
the morning their doors were unlocked, and they stepped
outside their prisons', he wrote; 'I thanked my God for
Garibaldi.'[61] The book describes the 'rescue' of a young girl
from a convent where she had been 'imprisoned' for reading
the Bible. Encompassing the literature was an emphatic sense
of the moral unhealthiness of Catholicism. Questions asked
by priests of women in the confessional were thought to be
'often of the most improper and revolting nature, naming
crimes both unthought of and inhuman'.[62] The staple text here
was *The Confessional Unmasked*, a scurrilous commentary on
the moral theology of St. Alfonso di Liguori and Peter Dens,
which circulated widely in the 1860s, and was much employed in illustration by such 'No Popery' lecturers as William
Murphy. An unshakeable belief in the blasphemous nature of
Marian devotions and in the corrupt lives of the Papal Court—
supported by evidence drawn from centuries past but asserted
as if of contemporary reality—were also part of general depiction of Catholicism as 'a sink of iniquity'.[63] Those who faintly
discerned that the lives of the English Catholic clergy of the
day seemed to be blameless also had an explanation to hand.
'We do not ask what Romish priests are when surrounded by
Protestantism, but what, where the system develops itself

[60] E. R. Norman, *Anti-Catholicism in Victorian England*, London 1968, 14.
[61] *Patrick Murphy on Popery in Ireland, or Confessionals, Abductions, Nunneries, Fenians and Orangemen*, London 1865, 191.
[62] *Awful Disclosures of Maria Monk*, 25.
[63] William Elfe Tayler, *Popery: Its Character and Its Crimes*, London 1847,
327.

without restraint:' thus the explanation of the author of *Popery: Its Character and Its Crimes*.[64] Very many, however, were not so enlightened; for them, the English Catholic Church represented an outpost of the vileness of Rome as depicted in the literature—the English clergy, too, needed to be watched, for they were enemies of decency. It was an astonishing achievement that the Catholic Church in nineteenth-century England was able to make such advances in the face of such a culture of antipathy.

The popular manifestation of the culture took different forms. In opposition to Catholic Emancipation in the first decades of the century there was the organization of opinion —the Brunswick Clubs. Public disturbances were rare, but the issue frequently inspired what George Brown, the Vice-President of Ushaw College, on returning to England from a visit to Rome in 1826, called 'No Popery phrenzy'.[65] In the mid-century, fired by public anger at the government's decision in 1845 to place the state endowment of Maynooth (the Irish seminary for the training of Catholic priests) as a permanent charge on the consolidated fund, and by the restoration of the Catholic Hierarchy in 1850, there was a growth of anti-Catholic literature. By the 1860s, there was rioting: localized, small in scale, and usually produced by the presence of itinerant preachers and lecturers. Most celebrated of these were Giacinto Achilli, an ex-Dominican from Rome, who became a national figure as a result of the legal action he brought against Newman in 1851; Alessandro Gavazzi, a lapsed monk from Naples, who had, according to the *Reformation Journal*, 'all the grace and majesty of a Julius Caesar, and declaims with all the fervour and power of a Demosthenes';[66] and William Murphy, a Protestant convert from Co. Limerick who came to England, after the failure of his shoe shop in Dublin, with the prediction—which to some extent he fulfilled—that 'I'll blaze England yet!'[67] The sort of petty rioting

[64] Ibid. 332.

[65] Ushaw College Archives, Wiseman Papers, 29, Brown to Wiseman, 7 Apr. 1826.   [66] *The Bulwark or Reformation Journal*, I (1851–2), 83.

[67] Walter L. Arnstein, 'The Murphy Riots: A Victorian Dilemma', in *Victorian Studies*, XIX, no. 1 (1975), 52. For a comprehensive view of the subject, see Sheridan Gilley, 'The Garibaldi Riots of 1862', in *Historical Journal*, XVI. 4 (1973), 697–732.

the preachers generated was not really serious, in that there was no real risk of a sustained or national movement. But to Catholics it was often terrifying, as well as involving risk to property. Wiseman believed, in 1862, that there was no doubt 'that Government connived at the disturbances'.[68] But that cannot have been the case. The annual celebration of Guy Fawkes night on 5 November—which was still allocated special prayers in the Anglican Prayer Book—was a sort of national day of anti-Catholicism. Blessed Dominic Barberi, arriving in England for the first time in 1841, was surprised at the intensity of the Protestant tone: in fact he had crossed the Channel on 5 November and witnessed the burning of the Pope in effigy in virtually every place he had passed through on the journey between Folkestone and London.[69] Children began their hatreds early: it was the practice of Protestant schoolboys to stick pins through the eyes of Queen Mary in the illustrations of history books.[70] Phobias once acquired were developed and sustained. Pugin once crossed himself while engaged in private prayers on a railway journey—to the horror of a lady, alone with him in the compartment, who cried out: 'You are a Catholic, Sir;—Guard, Guard, let me out.'[71] Doubtless the popular disturbances against Catholics were stimulated by the arrival of large-scale Irish immigration to the English cities during the Famine years of the mid-century, but the English anti-Catholic tradition was by then already in a very advanced and developed condition, and the Irish provided illustrative evidence of established attitudes, not causes of them.[72] The Old Catholic gentry of England had also, long before the immigration, settled their opinions about Irish Catholicism. 'The religion of the low Irish', Sir John Throckmorton wrote in 1806, 'forms a strange assemblage of strong faith and much superstition.' It was 'not changed by a free intercourse with other people, nor the

[68] English College Archives, Talbot Papers, 1102, Wiseman to Talbot, 15 Nov. 1862.

[69] Bernard Ward, *Sequel*, London 1915, II. 22.

[70] *From Cabin-Boy to Archbishop*, 10.

[71] Michael Trappes-Lomax, *Pugin. A Medieval Victorian*, London 1932, 76.

[72] Sheridan Gilley, 'Protestant London, No-Popery and the Irish Poor, 1830–60', in *Recusant History*, 10 (1969–70), 212.

ordinary operations of arts, of sciences, or the general progress of social improvements'.[73]

As yet unperceived by all but the most acute of Catholic Victorians, however, the 'No Popery' tradition of England was actually losing ground within educated opinion, as notions of liberal government and free institutions spread within the nineteenth century intelligentsia and the governing groups. Its decline within the working classes had still to await the general decline of all religious feeling. But educated opinion was becoming less hostile—not to Rome, as such, as Gladstone's outburst in 1874 showed, but to the attachment of civil and social disabilities to religious belief.[74] The 'pro-Catholic' side in the Emancipation debates had demonstrated this. Speakers who entertained the strongest traditional antipathies to Catholic practices were yet anxious to uphold the principles of civil liberty. The Protestant Bishop of St. David's, for example, speaking in the House of Lords on the Relief Bill of 1791, said he had 'an abhorrence of penal legislation'.[75] It was a characteristic Whig view, which in the succeeding century developed into a general set of references in relation to constitutional qualifications. 'We have the satisfaction to find', Charles Butler said in 1813, in an address directed to Protestants, 'that the prejudice against us decreases rapidly.'[76] The arrival of the French *émigré* clergy, in 1791, escaping the Revolution, assisted good feelings: within a few years there were around five and a half thousand of them in England.[77] Most returned to France in 1802, but nearly a thousand remained, as tutors and chaplains, making a lasting impression upon the progress of Catholicism. The French clergy were well treated—and that within a few years of the Gordon Riots—many receiving state pensions, and the

[73] Sir John Throckmorton, *Considerations arising from the Debates in Parliament on the Petition of the Irish Catholics*, London 1806, 29.

[74] Norman, 20.

[75] Bernard and Margaret Pawley, *Rome and Canterbury through Four Centuries. A Study of the Relations between the Church of Rome and the Anglican Churches, 1530–1981*, London 1981, 66.

[76] Charles Butler, *Historical Memoirs Respecting the English, Irish, and Scottish Catholics from the Reformation to the Present Time*, London 1819, III. 243.

[77] J. Derek Holmes, *More Roman Than Rome: English Catholicism in the Nineteenth Century*, London 1978, 20.

Univeristy of Oxford, bastion of Protestantism, printed an edition of the Vulgate for their use. Collections for the *émigrés* were held in many Protestant churches. In some places the exiles were especially heavily concentrated, as in Winchester and Farnham—there were actually two hundred priests in the small town of Farnham between 1793 and 1802.[78] The welcome they received was in general good everywhere. The greatest disruption they seem to have caused was within the English Catholic Church itself: French opponents of the concordat between Pius VII and Napoleon, in 1801, formed the Blanchardist schism, and their activities in England elicited differing responses from the Vicars Apostolic. Milner, in the Midland District, was hostile to them; Poynter, in London, avoided an open condemnation to preserve the peace, and in consequence his 'long connivance' (as a Jesuit source put it)[79] attracted hostility and suspicion. At a crucial period in Catholic recovery, however, the arrival of the French clergy imparted a new respectability to the Catholic priesthood, as it appeared in Protestant perspective, and a useful auxiliary for the mission.[80]

In some small things, significant changes in official attitudes to Catholicism could be noticed throughout the century. In 1808 a British naval ship was dispatched to take the Pope to safe exile in Naples should it be needed; in 1848 the government offered the Pope refuge in Malta (he chose Gaeta instead)—an offer repeated in 1863; and in 1870 a British frigate was sent to Civita Vecchia to evacuate the Pope should the assault upon Rome send him fleeing from the city. The Queen's Speech at the opening of Parliament in November, 1867, contained a reference to 'the Sovereign Pontiff'—'a decided gain', as Bishop Grant said, 'on the older phrases'[81] before used in demonstration of Protestant antipathy to the Bishop of Rome. In 1887 Queen Victoria received a Papal

[78] Étienne Robo, *The Story of a Catholic Parish: St. Joan's, Farnham*, Farnham, 1938, 23.

[79] Stonyhurst Archives, Glover's *Excerpts* III, MS B.I.17, 247.

[80] For an excellent account, see D. T. J. Bellenger, 'The French Ecclesiastical Exiles in England, 1789–1815' (Cambridge Ph.D. thesis, 1978; Cambridge University Library).

[81] Kathleen O'Meara, *Thomas Grant, First Bishop of Southwark*, London (2nd edn.) 1886, 198.

envoy at her Jubilee, and the Duke of Norfolk was sent to Rome in reciprocation: it was not a formal diplomatic exchange, but it showed a softening of attitudes. 'There is still much hostility and much ignorance,' Manning said of Catholic progress in England, in 1866, 'but the hostility is more civilized, and the ignorance is breached on all sides.'[82]

Despite the antipathy of the social and political environment, the Catholics had not, by the end of the eighteenth century, become a 'sect'. Though in the most literal sense disinherited, they had not become what Troeltsch and later sociologists of religion have characterized as a 'church of the disinherited'. They had not become exclusivist, had not developed millennial hopes of apocalyptic messianism, and had not embraced radicalized politics. A strong traditional sense of community had survived, but the internal loyalties were highly localized and unaffected by external English influence. Preserved from potential clericalism by the domination of the Catholic gentry, the Church was more nearly 'a branch of the English nonconforming tradition', as Professor Bossy has observed,[83] than it was a version of sectarianism. The statistical insignificance of the Catholic middle class, at the start of the nineteenth century,[84] kept the Catholic traditional landed group and the newly self-conscious priesthood as the major influences in English Catholic development—a crucial difference from Irish Catholicism, with its buoyant connection between radical and nationalist politics, based upon O'Connell's appeal to the emergent Irish middle class. In England, the professionalization of the clergy, and the successful control of the central leadership of the Church by the Ultramontanes, effectively eclipsed the lay element in ecclesiastical management—leading, by the mid-century, to Mgr. George Talbot's famous observation to Manning: 'What is the province of the laity? To hunt, to shoot, to entertain? These matters they understand, but to meddle with ecclesiastical matters they have no right at all.'[85] The Voluntary System of religious endowments, of which the expansion of Catholicism was a notably successful example, did not produce the evidences of

---

[82] Purcell, II. 286.   [83] Bossy, 7, 296.

[84] Lesourd, I. 560, 'Le Prêtre catholique dans la société'.

[85] Purcell, II. 318 (Apr. 1867).

lay participation which the opponents of the system, in the Protestant Church of England, usually feared (—in defending their own possession of the state religious endowments). But nor did the Catholics adopt an ideology of 'Voluntaryism' the way the English Dissenters of the nineteenth century did; they never regarded 'a free church in a free state'—a phrase tainted because of its origin among Italian liberal opponents of the Papal Temporal Sovereignty—as an ideal. Ireland, again, was different. There the campaign for the disestablishment of the Protestant Church placed nearly all of the Catholic bishops, during the 1860s, on the side of a quite theoretically expressed voluntaryism. The support of religious institutions by independent offerings was usually, among English Catholic leaders, regarded as a necessary condition of things, not an ideal. 'The Churches on the Continent have all some kind of endowment,' Ullathorne wrote in a draft on the question, which survives among his papers; 'either from the state or from endowments, independent of the offertory.'[86] The failure of the Catholics to embrace the sort of view of the Church, and its place in society, which 'Voluntaryism' supplied for so many of the English Dissenters in the nineteenth century, must modify the contention that their history relates closely to that of general religious Nonconformity. Yet the Catholic Church was, in some things, 'denominationalized' during the century. As a Church (rather than a sect) it sought a kind of relationship to government and society, and not a rejection of either. It sought, in fact, in such questions as educational finance and the provision of institutional chaplains, a place in the sun: it aspired to participate in the emerging pluralism of religious associations, to benefit from the broadening of the constitution as the exclusive support of the State for the Anglican establishment was progressively abandoned by piecemeal reforms. In aspiring to a share in the national life in such matters, the Catholics did act like 'Nonconformists'.

Perhaps the greatest influence in preserving the Church from sectarianism or complete denominational identification,

---

[86] St. Dominic's Convent, Stone, Ullathorne Papers, Box X (8), Draft on the Church (n.d.).

however, was the authority of Rome itself. However much the eighteenth-century gentry, or the later Cisalpines, or the 'Old Catholic' clergy, might resist some features of Roman control, or extravagant notions of Papal authority in any other than spiritualities, self-conscious adhesion to a source of authority beyond their immediate circumstances always operated to foster ecclesiastical regularity. The English mission was conducted according to the Bull of 1743, *Apostolicum Ministerium*, which, by 1800, was clearly out of date—it assumed, still, the existence of a Church under penal legislation with no open institutions. Yet it still represented Roman authority, and linked the English clergy to Roman discipline. The actual conduct of the English Church was in the hands of the Sacred Congregation of Propaganda in Rome. Knowledge of English conditions, though influenced by partisan reporting, was good, as examination of the archives makes clear. By the start of the nineteenth century, it was plain to Rome that England was worth special attention—not so much because of its tiny Catholic population, but because of Ireland, united to England by legislation in 1800, and, even more, because of British overseas government of Catholic territories like Quebec or parts of the West Indies. Propaganda's own activities expanded during the century, as Catholicism extended itself over vast new areas of the world, and over the churches of the former colonial empire of Spain, now (though imperfectly) freed, by the wars of independence, from governmental control. The personal authority of the Pope was enhanced in the process, and so was the centralizing tendency in the Church: the English mission began to expand just at this moment, and it was absorbed into the general pattern of Ultramontanism which Propaganda established throughout the areas of its responsibility. Propaganda even made occasional financial contributions—in 1879, for example, full travelling expenses were paid to Catholic chaplains serving with the British Army in Afghanistan. In 1830, Pius VIII made Thomas Weld a cardinal partly, as Wiseman said, in response to 'a desire of seeing an Englishman among the highest dignitaries of the Church'.[87] English bishops—Vicars

---

[87] Wiseman, *Recollections of the Last Four Popes*, 242.

Apostolic until formal sees were restored in 1850—were expected to make regular *ad limina* visits to Rome to report on the progress of the areas under their jurisdiction. Manning made twenty-two visits.

Rome, it is true, tended to complain of lack of respect by the English prelates, but this usually indicated ignorance of correct forms of protocol in dealings with the Curia by those who, educated in the 'Old Catholic' tradition of Douai, were simply inadequately informed about procedures. As more of the bishops came to receive at least some training in Roman institutions during the nineteenth century, the difficulties, at least on that score, diminished—but did not completely disappear, as the dealings of both Errington and Newman with Rome were to show. The agent of the English bishops in Rome, the Rector of the English College after its reopening in 1818, maintained some sort of liaison. Leo XII, Robert Gradwell recorded during his tenure, 'desired me to come from time to time to talk about English matters'.[88] On every issue of disputed opinion or jurisdiction, on every aspect of policy in relation to education or relations with the civil government, Propaganda required the bishops to send in reports, both individually and collectively. An enormous amount of information became available. Yet Newman was possessed of 'a feeling that they *cannot* understand England' at Propaganda.[89] His gloom partly reflected unhappiness that they did not understand him; but it also contained some truth. For however well informed Rome may have been, the interpretation of the data often lacked sympathetic appraisal of local sensibilities. It was, perhaps, unavoidable. The bureaucracy was also slow. 'Rome is properly called the Eternal City, because they never decide a question before they have heard all the *pros* and *cons*, which sometimes occupies much time,' Talbot once remarked.[90] Rome also tended to misunderstand the extent of support for the Anglican establishment, reading the lack of popular respect, which was undoubted, and the Oxford Movement defections, as

[88] Westminster Dioc. Archives, Gradwell's Journal, E.8. II, 16 May 1825.

[89] *John Henry Newman, Autobiographical Works*, ed. Henry Tristram, New York 1957, 260 (Journal, Feb. 1865).

[90] Purcell, II. 123 (Jan. 1860).

indications that the entire edifice was about to disintegrate. Wiseman's and Manning's teachings about the impossibility of a 'national' church producing authentic fruits of spiritual growth further encouraged the belief in Rome that the whole thing was liable to wither away once the Catholic Church was able to make a fair presentation of its doctrines. Hence the later incomprehension of the Vatican when the 'Anglo-Catholics' adopted the language and ritual practices of Catholicism without the structure of doctrinal authority. When Gasquet explained this to Leo XIII in 1895, at the time of the controversy over the invalidity of Anglican orders, the Pope 'held up his hands in surprise and said "Ma questo è una questione di dottrina!" '[91] Not a sect, nor properly a denomination, nor a branch of the powerful Irish Church, the English Catholic Church occupied an unusual position, which itself—not fitting the conventional models furnished by the anti-Catholic tradition—puzzled men in English public life. From time to time, it was reported, the government opened letters on ecclesiastical subjects sent to Rome by the bishops—a practice which annoyed Cardinal Barnabò at Propaganda.[92] But it is doubtful if the government learned anything surprising, and least of all anything sensational. The Catholic Church of the nineteenth century was engaged in a steady and confident expansion: it avoided, where it was able to, offending Protestant feelings, and it promoted, as far as its resources would allow, a full pastoral presence for its adherents. In the unpromising circumstances of popular suspicion and traditional national hostility, its achievements were extraordinary—even for a century of general religious vitality.

[91] Downside Archives, Gasquet Papers, 873, Diary, 31 Jan. 1895.
[92] Claude Leetham, *Luigi Gentili. A Sower for the Second Spring*, London 1965, 280.

1
Emancipation

It was not only the achievement of civil liberties as such—important though they were—which made Emancipation in 1829 a crucial point in Catholic history: the advance into public life came just as much from the experience of organization gained during the agitation of the question in the preceding half century, from contact with political leaders in the national life, and from acquaintance with the developing attitudes of their Protestant neighbours, as the matter disturbed or interested the localities. 'The year 1829 was to us', as Cardinal Wiseman once said, 'what the egress from the catacombs was to the early Christians.'[1] The long years of debate over the Catholic claims, from the 1770s, and the piecemeal concessions made in periodic Relief Acts, also stimulated a *denominational* self-identity, as many Catholics, emerging from the sub-society of those whose civil freedoms had been severely circumscribed, joined the buoyant religious nonconformity of the nineteenth century. The matter must be viewed with careful balance, however. Considering the extent to which many lay claims for concession had emphasized the detachment of English Catholicism from Papal dominion, a paradoxical outcome of the Emancipation debate was an enhancement of Roman influence. The English Catholics divided in a number of ways about the extent and nature of the compromises they could entertain to acquire civil liberties, and this resulted in a number of appeals to Rome, whose authority was accordingly increased, and in an area—political and civil obligations—from which its voice had been rigorously excluded for a couple of centuries. It was, at the time, 'Columbanus' who saw this most clearly: the Rev. Dr O'Conor, a rancorous polemicist of immoderate style and tone whose assaults upon the leadership of his Church, for showing undue

[1] Wiseman, *The Religious and Social Position of Catholics in England*, 9.

deference to Rome, should not disguise the fact that in one thing, at least, he had detected an important tendency. 'Rome has outwitted our government,' he wrote in 1816, rather inaccurately—for Rome took no initiatives in the Emancipation question. Her authority was the authority of one to whom appeal was made; as he continued, 'she has established an alarming precedent of *reference to her power*'.[2] In this sense, the Emancipation debate prepared the ground for the Ultramontanes. Whatever the conflict between clerical and lay interests, furthermore, the agitation showed that in the end the Vicars Apostolic *were* able to control the Church. On the questions of the Veto and the Oath it was their reservations and objections which prevailed with the politicians actually involved in the formulation of legislation, rather than the civil latitudinarianism of the lay leaders of Catholic opinion.

In one important matter the laity showed great sensitivity as well as political realism. They appreciated the difficulties in which Protestants were placed by the Emancipation question. Subsequent Catholic writers have sometimes seemed to imply that objections to the Catholic claims were a compound of ancient fears and modern bigotry, that opposition to Emancipation was a matter of ignorant prejudice and verbal self-interest. But it was not so—or, at least, it was not so for the leaders of political society. Parliament was the governing body of the State Church of England; corporations and civil institutions were the guarantors of national Protestantism. To admit Catholics to a voice in the government of the Church of England seemed to them both illogical and dangerous. For unlike the Protestant Dissenters, whose religious convictions could not be thought to convey a threat to the settlement of religion—a belief which had to be considerably modified as the century progressed and militant Nonconformity bared its teeth—the Catholics were regarded as bound in allegiance to a foreign authority. In view of the disturbed state of Ireland, the notion that Catholic loyalty could not be relied upon, though absurd in relation to England, still carried enough substance to make men halt in their tracks on the

[2] *Columbanus No. VII. The Gallican Liberties. Indispensable Securities for the Constitutional Government of the Irish Catholic Church*, London 1816, 56–7.

road to concessions. Almost no one could as yet envisage the emergence of the liberal state, with its privileges opened up to all citizens without reference to their religious opinions. The union of throne and altar, the settlement of property, the stability of institutions, the very political freedoms which Englishmen so cherished, seemed all to be related to the maintenance of the Protestant Constitution. Now the lay Catholics whose 'toadying' to the politicians for concessions has seemed so distasteful to some later observers had actually some perception of all this. In part, they shared the prevalent phobia about Papal power: they were 'good Englishmen', that is to say. But in part they saw also the dilemma before their fellow-countrymen—the difficulty of broadening the basis of the constitution without weakening just those institutions upon which the national liberties were thought to rest. Lay Catholic emphasis on loyalty, and on their rejection of all but the most refined 'spiritual' authority of the Pope, derived from this appreciation. The higher clergy were not without some of these perceptions either—in 1826, for example, the bishops issued a Declaration showing that Catholics held no principles incompatible with civil allegiance—but their priorities were different. Their major concern was the preservation, uncompromised, of Roman authority, of the English Catholic Church as the Church, and not as a national entity in the Gallican tradition. For them, therefore, the Emancipation question was sometimes merely an irritant with the horrendous liability to foster division and even schism. They could not, after all, be expected to be enormously committed to a cause—the right of entry into political life—from which they would themselves be excluded. The fear of the State remained: the lay Catholics were seeking admission to a structure of government which no one yet envisaged as likely to become transformed. There were movements to widen the basis of the system of representation, and some radicals had advanced ideas about changing the nature of institutions: but in the years of the Emancipation debate these did not seem so far-reaching as to project a wholly different kind of state. The Catholic bishops could only see what their contemporaries saw—a compulsive desire by the laity to join in the existing Protestant Constitution. This conflict of clerical and lay

interests in the Emancipation question was present throughout, operating to confirm other causes of internal Catholic
division.

The loyalty issue was debated at a time when—after the
French Revolution, the Jacobin scare, the growth of the
radical clubs—the union of throne and altar and the general
stability of institutions seemed particularly under threat. There
were French *émigré* clergy in many parts of the country, bearing personal and vocal witness to the consequences of revolution. The Emancipation debate took place in just those years
when the threat to political stability seemed most imminent:
during the periods of cyclical depression following the end of
the Napoleonic Wars. It was not surprising, both that the
Protestant politicians, and the Catholic lay leaders, should be
concerned about loyalty. It was a national preoccupation.
'The only argument which has any appearance of weight', as
Sydney Smith observed in 1827, about the Catholic claims,
'is the question of divided allegiance; and, generally speaking,
we should say it is the argument which produces the greatest
effect in the country at large.' In his own Whiggish view, of
course, the threat was without substance: the Papal Court
lacked real power; there was 'a wax-work Pope'.[3]

Social rather than political shifts produced a greater immediate effect. The agitation of the Emancipation question
elicited an organized and articulate Catholic middle class. This
was more noticeable in Ireland than in England; for there
O'Connell's various associations for Emancipation gave Catholicism a public expression and a national unity it had not
known before—he inspired ordinary Catholics with a confidence in themselves and in the national destiny of their
religion which was to have a lasting importance in Irish development. In England, to some extent in direct emulation of the
Irish example, a small middle-class Catholic element emerged
as a distinct force in the Emancipation agitation. Their views
and interests were sometimes rather different from those of
the Catholic nobility and gentry who had, until then, been
exclusive spokesmen for the laity. The middle-class men were
more inclined to set stricter terms for concessions to the

---

[3] *The Works of Sydney Smith*, London, third edn. 1845, II. 246–7.

politicians; they tended to be more liberal in political out-look; they were more deferential to the higher clergy than the old gentry. Their expectations for the future were also greater. It was a matter of degree, but like the Irish who followed O'Connell—rather than the Old Catholic leader of the Irish laity, the Earl of Fingall—the English middle-class Catholics saw Emancipation as only a first step to some wider changes in their position in society. They lacked a leader, and to some extent looked to O'Connell. But his Irish nationalism and his radical politics were not universally acceptable, and the English Catholic middle class remained without an effective national spokesman during the Emancipation debate.

The Irish dimension of the question was, of course, at times predominant. It is barren to speculate, as some have done, on whether Emancipation would have been delayed still further had there not been the pressure of events in Ireland: the evidence would probably suggest that, like the Reform of Parliament, it might be said to have been 'irresistible' by some point around the later 1820s. The Irish dimension probably also extended both ways. It held back concessions because many in England (and some in Ireland) feared for stability if the massed peasantry got up by O'Connell were given a political voice; it promoted concessions, however, by force of numbers—five million subjects of the Crown who were Catholics. The English and the Irish Catholic leaders were usually divided, and that operated to delay concessions. The higher clergy of the two countries were often in disagreement about the terms of compromise with the politicians, and O'Connell's Irish middle-class political agitators were held in considerable suspicion by the English lay leaders. There was, above all, a suspicion in England that events in Ireland would pass out of control and get Catholicism a bad name everywhere. There was a suspicion, also, that under O'Connell's leadership the Catholic agitation in Ireland would pass into some very radical politics. These fears were undiminished by Emancipation when it came. 'How mistaken men are who suppose that the history of the world will be over as soon as we are emancipated!' O'Connell declared in 1829;

'Oh! *that* will be the time *to commence* the struggle for popular rights.'[4]

The penal code excluding Catholics from public life had been consolidated in the last quarter of the seventeenth century. The Test Acts of 1673 and 1678 required office-holders under the Crown to make a declaration against the doctrine of Transubstantiation, and this remained, by the start of the nineteenth century, one of the most solid barriers to the entry of Catholics into public life. The Oath of Supremacy had the same effect: it denied the spiritual as well as the temporal authority of the Papacy. Catholic bequests for 'superstitious uses' could be, and sometimes were, held to be illegal, and this was a very real difficulty for those charged with the maintenance of Catholic ecclesiastical property. There was a supplementary land tax for Catholic proprietors. There was no legal form of Catholic marriage. Catholics in the armed forces were obliged to attend Protestant worship. Yet an Act of 1793 had extended the parliamentary franchise to Catholics in Ireland who qualified in the counties as forty-shilling freeholders. The penal sections of the old code were, by the end of the eighteenth century, largely in abeyance—though as recently as 1769 James Talbot, one of the Vicars Apostolic, had been prosecuted for saying mass. The laws remained in formal existence, however, and as the Gordon Riots had shown in 1780, attempts to modify them could still stimulate a violent reaction. Their existence, *ad terrorem*, even in so residual a form, remained a symbol of the Catholics' civil inferiority, an indication of their separation from the national life; and those who argued for reform, such as Charles Butler, were able to show how comprehensive the Code still was.[5] Butler, the leading figure in the Catholic Committee of 1782, had been educated at Douai: a layman of serious disposition and ascetic life, who became the first Catholic barrister in England since the end of the seventeenth century. His expert knowledge of the law in relation to Catholics was invaluable

---

[4] *Correspondence of Daniel O'Connell*, ed. W. J. Fitzpatrick, London 1888, I. 176.

[5] See his *Historical Account of the Laws Respecting Roman Catholics, and of the Laws passed for their Relief; with Observations on the Laws remaining in force against them*, London 1795.

to the various lay agitations for relief which were got up in the last two decades of the eighteenth century, and he acquired, indeed, a national reputation.

Relief measures passed by Parliament from the 1770s gave a practical exemption to the Catholics from the formal severities of the penal code.[6] In 1778 the first significant measure enabled Catholics to conduct schools, and it removed most of the legal hindrances to the acquisition and transmission of property. The Act of 1791 was more comprehensive, and to its provisions, in fact, Mgr. Bernard Ward attributed the real attainment of Catholic religious—as opposed to civil—liberties.[7] Many of its benefits were actually formal: it legalized practices which had anyway gone on for years. Some restrictions persisted even in these areas. Catholic chapels were now sanctioned, provided they registered; but mass was forbidden in any building with a bell or steeple. The habits of religious orders were not to be worn in public. Catholics were admitted to the professions. Legislation to concede civil liberties was pressed forward by the Catholic lay organizations, but it was the Irish dimension of the issue which held out the prospect of success here. The old Irish Parliament had itself passed a number of important measures of relief, and the movement towards a full emancipation was enhanced by general Catholic support for the Act of Union in 1800. Pitt's undertaking to raise the Emancipation question at the time of the Union was widely supposed to presage actual legislation, and Pitt resigned in 1801 when George III, who regarded the concession of the Catholic claims as a violation of his Coronation Oath to preserve the Protestant Constitution, refused to countenance 'putting Papists and Presbyterians in a state of equality with the Church of England'.[8] Milner wrote a pamphlet to ease the King's mind. The Coronation Oath, he argued, contained provisions which were inapplicable to the actual state of things—or, as he put it, 'is purely ideal, and the apprehension of it a mere scruple'.[9] Although Pitt wrote to assure Milner

---

[6] There is a historical survey of the various measures in Charles Butler, *A Memoir of the Catholic Relief Bill Passed in 1829*, London 1829.

[7] Bernard Ward, *The Eve of Catholic Emancipation*, London 1911, I. viii.

[8] W. G. Addison, *Religious Equality in Modern England, 1714–1914*, London 1944, 44.

[9] J. Milner, *The Case of Conscience Solved; or The Catholic Claims proved*

that the King had read the pamphlet and satisfied his mind,[10] the Coronation Oath remained a substantial obstacle to civil concessions.

John Milner was one of the great ecclesiastics of modern English Catholic history. It could be said that he left a 'lasting impress of his work upon English Catholicism in his day;'[11] the first quarter of the nineteenth century was 'dominated' by him.[12] Born in London in 1752, the son of a tailor from Lancashire, Milner was educated at Sedgley Park School, and then, from 1766, at Douai. It was probably when he first went to Sedgley Park that he changed his family name—which was Miller—to that by which he was always known. As a youth he enjoyed the support of Bishop Challoner, and it was under his patronage that he got to Douai. There he was known to some of his fellow students as 'Jupiter', in virtue of his scholarly application, and to some others, for reasons more opaque, as 'Apollo'. Ordained as a priest in 1777, he served first in London, and then, after two years, he left for Winchester to act as pastor to the French Catholic prisoners detained in the city. This move also enabled him to develop his antiquarian interests, and he wrote a history of the city.[13] In 1803—the year which also saw Poynter's consecration as Coadjutor of the London District—Milner became Vicar Apostolic of the Midland District, with the titular bishopric of Castabala. From Wolverhampton he directed the affairs of the region until his death in 1826 at the age of 73.

To the first judgement of the external world, Milner cannot have seemed especially remarkable. He had a slight lisp, and execrable taste—which extended to a *penchant* for corned beef. He had his bedroom fitted with stained-glass windows. His life was generally austere, especially in personal dress; but his custom of staying in the rooms allocated to commercial travellers at hotels may have derived as much from the dictates of his financial resources as it did a desire to shun

to be compatible with The Coronation Oath [1801], London, second edn. 1807, 7.

[10] Husenbeth, *The Life of the Right Rev. John Milner D.D.*, 81.
[11] Bernard Ward, *Eve*, I. xi.
[12] David Mathew, *Catholicism in England, 1535–1935*, London 1936, 149.
[13] Husenbeth, 53.

ostentation. He was a competent scholar rather than a brilliant one; an excellent administrator and an attractive and sympathetic counsellor and guide to the clergy under his charge. He had no interest in public life as such—a consideration much to be borne in mind by those who evaluate him in the light of his polemical writings (which were often drawn from him against his natural inclinations)—and eschewed political concerns. 'Religion is all my politics', he used to say.[14] During the Queen Caroline affair, in 1820, when the clergy appealed to him about the highly charged issue of whether or not the Queen should be prayed for in church, he ruled that it was a mere political matter, best left to the judgement of each priest.[15] His national outlook was typical of the rest of English political society. He was loyal to the Crown, and argued the conventional case that there was a close alliance between revolutionary politics and infidelity.

Milner is best remembered, however, as a divisive figure, especially for his quarrels with Bishop Douglass—who 'for a time refused to receive any more letters from him'[16]—with Bishop Poynter—whom he once delated to Rome for financial irregularity[17]—and with Charles Butler—characterized as among 'false brethren'.[18] A report in the archives of Propaganda, on the state of his District, describes Milner as 'combative and zealous, but he is not very prudent; he is ardent, variable, open to the criticisms made against him by Mgr. Poynter'.[19] His biographer attributed this history of disputation to the isolation those must endure who elect to stand by the truth: 'It will surprise no one conversant with Church history', wrote the Provost of Northampton in 1862, 'that a Prelate so vigilant, zealous, and intrepid, as Dr Milner, should find himself opposed and surrounded by enemies.'[20] In an age of virulence, however, Milner used virulent language in the exercise of his literary accomplishments on behalf of truth—a

[14] Husenbeth, 548; Mathew, 149.
[15] Husenbeth, 549.
[16] Bernard Ward, *Eve*, I. 27.
[17] Ibid. II. 104.
[18] Charles Butler, *Historical Memoirs Respecting the English, Irish and Scottish Catholics from the Reformation to the Present Time*, London 1821, IV. 423.
[19] Propaganda, *Scritture* 9 (1834-41), 4, *Missioni di Europea: Inghilterra* (n.d.).
[20] Husenbeth, 196.

fact mentioned even in his funeral oration. 'If, in thus assert-
ing the cause of God, and of his Church, some few expressions
escaped his pen, which appeared to savour of over harshness
and severity', the Revd. Francis Martyn then observed, 'it was
not that his pen was dipped in the gall of uncharitableness or
malignity, but that his zeal for the glorious cause which he
advocated, in its ardour outstepped the kinder feelings of a
heart ever alive to the impulse of charity'.[21] Pruned of florid
excess, these sentiments are actually quite correct. Milner was
not a mere polemicist, or a man of inherent perversity: he
believed Catholicism was under a real internal threat—that his
brother Vicars Apostolic and the lay leaders were preparing
to compromise its spiritual integrity in order to secure temporal advantages, that the Catholic Emancipation question
was drawing the English Church towards the hidden reefs of
Gallicanism. They, in turn, regarded Milner as inflexible and
unlettered in the statesmanlike arts of sensible compromise.
There was a genuine failure of communication between the
two positions, which Milner's sharpness of tone unhappily
helped to exacerbate. Yet he often had the ear of the Catholic populace. His instincts and prejudices were as English as
theirs; he had a natural sympathy with the middle social sections and with the poor—it was the nobility and the gentry,
with their aspirations to public life, that he found alien.
Although the emergent Catholic middle class lacked a leader
in those years, Milner came near to being it: 'he realised
vaguely the great future of Catholicism in the towns'.[22] His
differences with the other bishops were also sharpened by his
support of the Jesuits. 'His uniform defence of the Society,
during so many years of unrelenting opposition from the
other Vicars Apostolic', as Glover noticed in his unpublished
Excerpts—now in the library at Stonyhurst—'drew down upon
him a persecution from some in England, which was most
cruelly carried on by others in Rome, even so far as to traduce
his character there in a manner most unworthy and most
unwarrantable'.[23] Even accounting for Glover's language,

[21] Husenbeth, 526.   [22] Mathew, 151.
[23] Stonyhurst Archives, MS B.I.17, Glover's *Excerpts* III, 241. 'A Collection
of notes, memoirs, and Documents, respecting the re-establishment of the English
Province of the Society of Jesus,' [by the Revd. J. T. Glover].

which was often as exaggerated as Milner's own, there is much truth in this, especially in view of the anti-Jesuit intriguing practised in Rome by Robert Gradwell. But Milner's personal style did not diminish the impressions fostered by his opponents. After receiving him in 1814, Pius VII referred to Milner as 'a firebrand';[24] others in the city, with whom he seems to have enjoyed more *rapport*, advised him to moderate his language.[25] Again, a balance of judgement must be carefully constructed: Milner's strength of expression was not particularly remarkable, but the extent of his polemical writing was. He simply placed more of his sentiments before the public; more of it was noticed, including what one of his victims called 'the vulgar illiberalities of Dr. Milner's personal abuse.'[26]

Milner used to say that he 'should like to live in a house of glass, open to all beholders.'[27] In fact he actually did so. No leader of Catholicism was scrutinized by his co-religionists the way he was. He stood at the centre of controversy over Catholic Emancipation. He saw no compromise, either in the concessions the Catholics should make to the state, or in the position the state should adopt in relation to the Catholic claims—'it appears to me there is no middle way', he wrote in 1801.[28] It was precisely his attachment to immovable principles that led, over the Veto question, to charges of inconsistency. Indeed, his change of mind here was the turning point of his life; it was the completion of opposition to compromise, a position from which he never again departed. Like the Irish bishops, whose agent in England he was, he had originally accepted the idea of a Crown veto on Catholic episcopal appointments as a reasonable security for civil concessions. In 1808, furthermore, in his *Letter to a Parish Priest*, he explained his preparedness to accept the Veto in theoretical language. This tract was originally intended for private circulation, but it was in fact greatly publicized and this made Milner's later retraction of its contents—'his own folly', as he

---

[24] Ward, *Eve*, II. 100.
[25] Husenbeth, 275.
[26] *Columbanus No. VII. The Gallican Liberties*, London 1816, 55.
[27] Husenbeth, 539.
[28] Milner, *The Case of Conscience Solved*, 34.

came to call it[29]—a public event. Through this difficulty, as through the other episodes of his controversial dealings with the other leaders of English Catholicism, he retained the loyalty of his own clergy in the Midland District—which often, in appearance, must have seemed like a church within a church. The clergy, as Ward wrote, 'carried this feeling to such lengths that they sometimes even refused a priest from the South permission to say Mass in their churches unless he would first promise to take no part in persecuting their bishop'.[30] Milner can hardly have approved of that; the essential element of his apparent intransigence was the preservation of proper spiritual jurisdiction in the Church. That is what is so frequently overlooked in subsequent rather harsh judgements of his life and accomplishments. His priority was the integrity of the faith; the purity of the system of authority by which truth was preserved inviolate. His forcefulness of expression is to be set within this context of the seriousness of the dangers he perceived. While others sought to conciliate those straining for a place in public life, Milner's preoccupation was with spiritual integrity. He pursued his eternal priorities with great singleness of purpose.

Milner's connection with the Irish bishops added to his isolation within the leadership of the English Church. The 'old Catholic' elements who had floated the Emancipation agitation shared many of the current reservations about Irish Catholicism and Irish popular politics, and rather lamented the way in which, after the Union, the Emancipation issue became 'mainly an Irish question'.[31] The leadership passed to Irishmen, such as the Protestant Emancipationists Henry Grattan and William Plunket, and the Catholic Daniel O'Connell. Burdett's Bill, in 1825, was formed almost exclusively according to Irish requirements. But there was, as Denis Gwynn remarked, a 'fundamental difference between the position of Catholics in the two countries'.[32] In Ireland

[29] Husenbeth, 154.

[30] Ward, *Eve*, II. 181.

[31] G. I. T. Machin, *The Catholic Question in English Politics, 1820 to 1830*, Oxford 1964, 10.

[32] Denis Gwynn, *The Struggle for Catholic Emancipation (1750–1829)*, London 1928, 3.

Catholicism was the religion of the people, and of the rising middle class of the South; its buoyancy in the post-penal days preceded that of England's modest 'Second Spring' of the mid-nineteenth century; its network of institutions for social welfare and education was enormous; its financial resources, even in so poor a country, were considerable. In England, it is true, the pre-Emancipation Church was not so deeply buried within the catacombs as subsequent propagandists of Ultra-montanism like to suppose—the years of the Emancipation debate coincided with a revival which would have continued whether or not Emancipation itself was conceded—but Catholicism was, numerically, insignificant compared with the national Protestantism. The emphasis of the leaders of the two countries was accordingly rather different. Irish Catholics were at first led by the Old Catholic aristocrats, like the Earl of Fingall: O'Connell's rise to prominence symptomized the emergence of the new classes. O'Connell's political outlook was radical—Emancipation was a matter of political rights. English Catholics continued to be led by traditional groups; their version of Emancipation fitted into the politics of deference, and they looked for accommodations and concessions as the means whereby they could integrate with the existing political order. For many Irish Catholics, Emancipation was the gateway to a new political and national landscape; for the English it was an entry to the old world of place and patronage. The Irish were therefore to become more intransigent about the question of 'securities', to be conceded to Protestant sentiment, as the price of Emancipation. In 1729, ten of the Irish bishops had supported the idea of a Crown Veto of episcopal appointments, and in 1808 they had agreed that it should be included in a Whig bill. But in that year also, as a sign that the old influences in Ireland were being overtaken by the political forces called into existence by O'Connellite radicalism, the laity revolted against episcopal concessions and rejected the Veto. The bishops, following their initiative, then rejected it also; and so did Milner, their English agent. In 1808 'the attack upon the Veto', as Butler recorded, 'commenced in the public prints'.[33] The contrast

---

[33] Charles Butler, *Historical Memoirs*, II. 188.

with England could not have been greater: there Milner was
alone among the bishops in eschewing the Veto. He did have
a counterpart—an Irish prelate who was prepared to negotiate
upon the matter. Dr Doyle ('J. K. L.'), the Bishop of Kildare
and Leighlin, was willing to accept moderate 'securities' in
any Emancipation legislation, provided the conditions were
honourable. In 1825, most notably, he was prepared to accept
state payments of the Catholic clergy—a device sometimes
suggested as a 'security' since it was supposed that by detach-
ing the priests from financial dependence on their flocks it
diminished their liability to political sympathy with the
masses, who in Ireland were thought to be potentially disloyal. Yet Doyle was very cautious about the conditions on
which financial subvention could be received. There must be
no question of Court favour or payment for spiritual services
as such: 'if my hand were to be stained with Government
money, it should never grasp a crozier'.[34] O'Connell criticized
him for even so limited a concession. Despite his later acceptance of 'securities'—including the drastic one of the forty-
shilling disfranchisement—O'Connell's ideological rejection of
such accommodations was, again, in huge contrast to the
temper of the English leaders. As he wrote to Doyle in 1829:
'We are ardently desirous of Emancipation, but we would not
attain it by any species of condition which could in any, the
remotest, degree infringe upon the discipline of the Catholic
Church in Ireland, or upon its independence of the State or
of temporal authority.'[35] While the Emancipation debate continued in Parliament and in public life, the English and Irish
Catholics worked together in uneasy alliance. With the passing
of the Act of 1829 their divergent political and social sympathies were allowed to reveal themselves, and links between
the Catholics of the two countries, during most of the rest of
the nineteenth century, became personal and local rather
than national.

The predominance of the Irish dimension in the Emancipation question after 1800 also had an ambiguous effect
upon English public opinion. The apparent threat to order in

---

[34] W. J. Fitzpatrick, *The Life, Times, and Correspondence of the Right Rev.
Dr. Doyle, Bishop of Kildare and Leighlin*, Dublin 1861, I. 442.
[35] *Correspondence of Daniel O'Connell*, ed. W. J. Fitzpatrick, I. 171.

Ireland—not really a fear of revolution, but that a major disruption of the system of influence was imminent, through O'Connellite capture of constituency organization—persuaded some within the political groups in England that Emancipation should be conceded. Yet with public opinion in general, the reverse was probably the case. Since the Gordon Riots there had been those who, like Butler, sensed 'a regular increase of public favour towards the Catholics, but it was slow'.[36] Fear of Irish excesses tended to arrest this development from time to time; and there was, apparently indelibly, the pervasive influence of traditional English 'No-Popery' sentiment as a barrier to concessions which many thought insuperable. Anti-Catholic agitation was not successfully organized in these years, however. The Orange Lodges in England, the Pitt Clubs, and the Brunswick Clubs set up in 1828, were predominantly upper-class and rural, an agitation inspired by the landed gentry.[37] The clergy of the Church of England were active in getting up petitions against the Catholic claims.[38] In the propaganda disseminated by these groups, it was political fears that most obviously obtruded—the belief that once he had his Catholic subjects within the legislature of Great Britain, the Pope would seek to further his traditional designs upon the Realm itself. And as Bishop Poynter remarked in a letter of 1821, 'the idea of the exercise of any temporal power by the Pope in England is a frightful thing to John Bull'.[39] Catholics were increasingly impatient of the narrow confines of traditional English anti-Catholicism, seeing a wider context of revolutionary threat to stability in which ancient fears of Rome seemed simply irrelevant. 'Whatever may be the prejudices of many in this country against what is called Popery,' Bishop Thomas Smith wrote, 'it is strange that many persons of observation should not see that the clamour raised in France against Jesuits etc. etc. is the work of men who are enemies of all Religion whether Catholic or Protestant, and the object of whose unwearied pestilential zeal has

---

[36] Charles Butler, *A Memoir of the Catholic Relief Bill*, 27.
[37] Machin, 8, 132, 140.
[38] Ibid. 145.
[39] Westminster Dioc. Archives, Gradwell Papers, Letter Books, B3, Poynter to Gradwell, 6 March 1821.

always been and still is as much as ever the subversion of the altar and the throne in every country.'[40]

Whatever difficulties the laity may have made for the Irish bishops over the Veto in 1808, it was in England that the Emancipation debate fostered substantial divergences between the laity and the clerical leaders of Catholicism. In England, the laity had a well-established tradition of leadership, and were quite prepared to act independently of the Vicars Apostolic if they deemed it necessary. Their interests and priorities were different. 'It is inconceivable', Poynter reported to Rome in 1821, 'how eager our Catholic noblemen and Gentlemen are to possess their seats in Parliament. It is impossible to stop them.'[41] Poynter was more sympathetic to this desire than the other Vicars Apostolic—indeed he was criticized in 1815 by Cardinal Litta, when on a visit to Rome, for being led by the laity.[42] But even Poynter recognized that their preparedness to make too far-reaching concessions to the Protestant temper was a characteristic of the lay leaders that needed curbing.

Something must be said of this great rival of Milner's, for William Poynter was the other ecclesiastic whose opinions and accomplishments dominated the early years of the nineteenth century. Educated at Douai, where he was a noted linguist, he first taught theology at Ware. As Vice-President, and then President of St. Edmund's College, he established lasting links and sympathies with the Old Catholic families whose sons he educated. In 1803 he became coadjutor of the London District, and was then Vicar Apostolic until his death in 1828. His clergy were as loyal to him and his opinions as were those of Milner to his. But his coolness towards the religious orders, and especially towards the Jesuits, made him enemies in Rome—enemies whose effectiveness was blunted by his success, in 1818, in securing Gradwell's appointment as agent of the English bishops, for Gradwell shared his suspicions both of Milner and of the orders. In Glover's view,

---

[40] Stonyhurst Archives, MS A II, 28 (57), Thomas Smith to T. Glover, 19 March 1829.

[41] Westminister Dioc. Archives, Gradwell Papers, Letter Books, B3, Poynter to Gradwell, 28 March 1821.

[42] Bernard Ward, *Eve*, II. 122.

which naturally was dominated by his own support of the Jesuits, Poynter's influence in the Church was almost wholly baneful. 'Disappointment and disgust probably hastened his death,' he recorded of the prelate. 'It cannot be denied', he continued, 'that during the whole course of his episcopal career he servilely courted the successive ministers who ruled England, the worst enemies of the Catholic name: in the vain hope of emancipation he was ever ready to yield to them.'[43] But this was an excessively pejorative manner of describing Poynter's actual attempt, undertaken with impressive skill, to balance the divergent interests of lay and clerical over the question of 'securities'. He was as critical of the extremes of the anti-Roman party as he was of the intransigence, as he saw it, of Milner. In public controversy with Dr O'Conor in 1812 he castigated this priest for inattention to the canons of the Council of Trent and for too great an acceptance of temporal views.[44] His balanced and moderate opinions, in fact, were successful in securing some important changes to the legislation proposed for Emancipation in 1821. He had a clear understanding of the benefits to religion that would accrue if there was a good representation of Catholicism in public life; realistic adaptations of Roman discipline to the tone and condition of English political society seemed the right course, provided nothing of substance was conceded. Poynter's own devotional life offered an example of the balance he advocated. Though not successful, at least with Emancipation, in his own lifetime, his contribution to the development of Catholic interests in the first quarter of the nineteenth century was very impressive.

Some of the English laity were prepared to make extensive denials of Papal authority as an indication of their loyalty to the English Crown and Constitution, and of their suitability for entry into political society. A number even supposed that Catholics could take the existing Oath of Supremacy, with its rejection of Papal temporal and spiritual authority, without violating religious integrity.[45] Sir John Throckmorton, a

---

[43] Stonyhurst Archives, MS B.I.17, Glover's *Excerpts* III, 245–6.
[44] *Columbanus No. VI. Unpublished Correspondence between the Rt. Rev. Dr. Poynter and the Rev. Dr. O'Conor*, London 1813, xviii.
[45] Bernard Ward, *Eve*, III. 57.

member of the Catholic Committee and of the 'Protesting Catholic Dissenters', was among them. In 1790 he published three pamphlets on the appointment of bishops, arguing for a lay voice in the procedure. These drew a hostile counterblast from Milner. Throckmorton later contended that Papal action had in the past justified Protestant fears, because of 'the immoderate extent to which the papal power always dominated the *spiritual*'. Then Catholic loyalty could well have been 'divided and incomplete'. But that was no longer the case, he argued. He also held, on the other hand, that if the Oath of Supremacy really was intended to deny *any* spiritual authority of the Pope, rather than seek to oblige acknowledgement of 'the independent sovereignty of the state', Catholics would refuse it.[46] Others were less guarded. A pamphlet widely circulated in the first decade of the century, entitled *Roman Catholic Principles with Regard to God and the King*, denied both Papal Infallibility (which was anyway not a dogma of the Church until 1870), and the claims of the Papacy to any temporal authority over princes.[47] Milner still found it necessary to denounce the pamphlet as late as 1823, citing, as he complained to Propaganda, its 'heretical doctrines'.[48] The very title adopted by those members of the Catholic Committee who constituted the 'Protesting Catholic Dissenters' indicated their desire to associate the Catholic claims with the views of civil liberty characteristic of the Protestant Dissenters. Milner, in a memorial addressed to Propaganda in November 1802, did not hesitate to categorize them and their 'irregular' opinions as 'erroneous and schismatical'.[49] In 1788 they drew up a *Protestation* which denied Papal temporal powers. To these extremes, the Vicars Apostolic eventually brought condemnation. Their last concession to the lay spirit in its fulness came in 1788, when three of the Vicars Apostolic and 240 priests signed the *Protestation*; in the following year the Vicars Apostolic condemned the new oath proposed by its authors as part of an Emancipation settlement. This

---

[46] Sir John Throckmorton, Bart., *Considerations Arising from the Debates in Parliament on the Petition of the Irish Catholics*, 45–6.
[47] A second edition was published in 1813 with the title *The Faith of Catholics*.
[48] Propaganda, *Scritture* 8 (1823–33), 11, 21 Jan. 1823.
[49] Propaganda, *Scritture* 6 (1801–17), 102 [in Latin].

decision, at a meeting in Hammersmith, was arrived at by the unanimous decision of the four Vicars Apostolic. An important change had been made; an era of tension opened with the assertion of independence by the ecclesiastical leaders in an area previously left to the laity—the question of concessions to secure civil advantages. 'None of the faithful, clergy or laity,' the Vicars Apostolic declared at Hammersmith in their Encyclical Letter (October 1787) 'ought to take any new oath, or sign any new declaration in doctrinal matters, or subscribe any new instrument, wherein the interests of religion are concerned, without the previous approbation of their respective bishops.' The words of the proposed oath to which they objected, denied 'any spiritual authority, power, or jurisdiction whatsoever, that can directly or indirectly affect or interfere with the independence, sovereignty, laws or constitution of this kingdom'.[50] The laity in the Catholic Committee ignored the condemnation and continued to work for the passage of the Bill which included the oath—the Bill of 1791. The Vicars Apostolic used their influence with several peers when the Bill got to the House of Lords, and the oath was replaced by the acceptable oath in the Irish Act of 1778. The whole episode indicated the differences between lay and clerical which the Emancipation question was opening up. The quarrels between Milner and Butler represented the polarization of opinion with clarity and publicity. Milner had anyway been sceptical of the Catholic Committee, later writing that from its formation in 1782 there began 'that system of lay interference and domination in the ecclesiastical affairs of English Catholics which has perpetuated divisions and irreligion among too many of them for near the last forty years'.[51] In fact it was the higher clergy who were the innovators in the matter of influence. Milner could not see it. To his vision 'many Catholics have been led into a foolish and dangerous confidence in their great political friends'.[52] 'Be

[50] Charles Butler, *Historical Memoirs*, II. 124–5.
[51] Gwynn, *Catholic Emancipation*, 47. See also Eamon Duffy, 'Ecclesiastical Democracy Detected', I (1779–87), II (1787–96), *Recusant History* 10 (Jan. and Oct. 1970), 193–209, 309–31.
[52] John Milner, *An Elucidation of the Veto, in a threefold Address to the Public, the Catholics, and the Advocates of Catholics in Parliament*, London 1810, 16.

assured that it is for those pastors exclusively to judge of its faith and discipline with whom Christ has deposited his divine authority', he continued; 'All the claims of others, whether Catholics or not Catholics, to judge and still more to act in these matters, however high, powerful or numerous they may be, are vain and schismatical.'[53] In his *Instructions Addressed to the Catholics of the Midland Counties of England* (1811), he again questioned the propriety of lay Catholics pronouncing on matters of religious discipline—such as deciding about the limits of Papal authority. In 1813 he objected to the Pastoral Letter issued by the other Vicars Apostolic on the Emancipation Question on the grounds—among others—that it praised the part taken by the laity.[54] He was convinced it was the laity who had persuaded two of the other Vicars Apostolic to accept the Veto in 1810.[55] All these suspicions were concentrated in the disputes with Butler. In 1813 an accommodation between the two men was attempted, at a meeting in Lord Clifford's House in Portman Square—of which there is a manuscript account in the Stonyhurst archives—which was intended by Clifford as part of a more ambitious plan to reconcile lay and clerical interests. Milner generously retracted five particular allegations 'wholly founded in mistake'.[56] The effects were not enduring. In 1822 Butler presented a memorial to Cardinal Fontana, the Prefect of Propaganda, complaining that Milner had 'incessantly, and in contumelious and low language, calumniated and reviled him'.[57] The Cardinal took no action.

The successive organizations established to press the Catholic claims to relief showed a steady increase in clerical participation and control.[58] The first Irish Catholic Association had been set up as long ago as 1756, but it was not until 1778 that the first Catholic Committee, of five leading laymen, was formed. In 1782 it was re-established, and again, in 1787, it reconstituted itself. Charles Butler, the Committee's

[53] Ibid. 48.
[54] Husenbeth, 246.
[55] Bernard Ward, *Eve*, I. 132.
[56] Stonyhurst Archives, M.S. A. II, 24 (21), Meeting of 19 Feb. 1813. See also Husenbeth, 222.
[57] Husenbeth, 450–1
[58] Holmes, *More Roman than Rome*, 24.

Secretary, was the leading figure of the new organization. According to the first Resolution of the Catholic Committee, it was 'commissioned to watch over, and promote the public interest of the English roman-catholics'.[59] In 1788 they presented a memorial to Pitt, noting that a 'doctrine of general toleration universally prevails',[60] and seeking its benefits. In the following year, and in order to influence the Vicars Apostolic at their Hammersmith meeting, Butler produced a *Red Book*—its title derived from the colour of the binding— detailing the background for relief measures as understood by the laity. When the assembled bishops condemned the oath endorsed by the Committee, they, in turn, issued a rejection of the bishops' judgement. This became the first of the *Blue Books*, collections of papers on the Catholic claims, published by the Committee.[61] In substance and tone these papers, like the general outlook of the Committee, tended to a sort of Gallicanism. 'Eagerness to convince an intensely prejudiced public that Catholics could be as loyal and sensible as their fellows, that they were not Jacobites, nor minions of the Pope, nor Jesuitical equivocators, nor slaves to superstition,' as Wilfrid Ward put it, 'became their one absorbing desire.'[62] This assessment is rather highly coloured by subsequent Ultramontanist criticism but is in essence a correct understanding of the atmosphere in which the lay leaders worked for Emancipation. That atmosphere was most authentically represented in the Cisalpine Club, formed by senior members of the Catholic Committee in 1792—by Lord Petre, Sir Henry Englefield, and Mr (later Sir John) Throckmorton. 'In theory,' Archbishop Mathew wrote, 'they accepted the dogmatic teaching of the Holy See; but they regarded all other forms of Papal action with chill reserve.'[63] The Club emphasized civil obedience and the virtues of the English Constitution, loyalty to the Crown, and disavowal of foreign—including papal—influence. By about the end of the first decade of the

---

[59] Charles Butler, *Historical Memoirs*, II. 103.

[60] Ibid. II. 104.

[61] James MacCaffrey, *History of the Catholic Church in the Nineteenth Century*, Dublin and St. Louis (Mo.), 2nd edn. 1910, II. 7.

[62] Wilfrid Ward, *The Life and Times of Cardinal Wiseman*, I. 202.

[63] Mathew, 146.

nineteenth century, however, the Club became more social than theological or political: it was a gathering of upper-class lay Catholics. It was, indeed, upper-class antipathy to O'Connell's middle-class manners and following which probably accounted for his being blackballed for membership in 1829, after the passing of Emancipation. The Liberator had expressed a wish to join.[64] The Club lasted to 1830, when it transformed itself into the Emancipation Club, and continued for a further fifteen years.

In 1808 the Catholic Board had been established. Its purpose was originally literary and propagandist: to monitor anti-Catholic publications and produce replies. The Board demonstrated the increasing clerical participation—in contrast to the Catholic Committee. All four of the Vicars Apostolic were members (although Milner entertained grave reservations); so were the Presidents of Ushaw, Oscott, St. Edmund's, Stonyhurst, Sedgley Park, and Acton Burnell, and the subscription lists also included 'nobility and gentry', and priests. It was a fairly balanced vehicle for clerical and lay opinion. The Secretary was a lawyer, Edward Jerningham. A weakness of the Board was Milner's developing hostility to the lay spirit he sensed was still too strong within its counsels. In 1809, when it was approached by leading Catholic families in the North of England to draw up a petition for Emancipation, and did so, Milner objected to what he called 'a mere matter of politics in which religion was not concerned'.[65] In the end he signed the petition, but the divergences of attitude remained, and in 1813, after fundamental differences with the policy of the Board over Emancipation 'securities', Milner was expelled from its Executive Committee—the Board would actually have liked to have removed his membership altogether, but found it had no procedure to do so. At least, Milner told the Board as he withdrew, 'You cannot exclude me from the kingdom of heaven'.[66]

The last of the great organizations for Emancipation was founded under the influence of O'Connell's Irish agency, the

---

[64] Bernard Ward, *Eve*, III. 267.

[65] Bernard Ward, *Eve*, I. 106.

[66] Gwynn, *Catholic Emancipation*, 175. See Charles Butler, *Historical Memoirs*, IV. 423.

Catholic Association. It was intended to foster good relations and co-operation between the Irish and the English agitations, and to some extent did so during the final crucial years of the campaign. The British Catholic Association was formed in 1823 with the explicit purpose of bringing the new middle classes and 'the people' into the movement for Emancipation —in contrast to the upper-class Catholic Board. The first meeting, in June 1823, was held, inappropriately enough, at the Freemasons' Tavern in London, and was presided over, equally inappropriately, by the Duke of Norfolk. All the clergy were, as in Ireland, *ipso facto* constituted members, and the Committee included all the Vicars Apostolic and fifty elected persons. The Association was financed by public subscription, since the Irish device of the 'Catholic Rent' could hardly operate successfully in so small a Catholic population as England's. Provincial branches were set up, particularly in Lancashire, during 1824, largely through the enterprise of the Catholic barrister, John Rosson.[67] Edward Blount, the Secretary, was, in Butler's words, 'the soul of all the proceedings of the British Catholic Association'.[68] Blount was actually a member of the old Catholic gentry, but the Association really did indicate the entry of the middle class Catholics to a voice in the public affairs of their Church. With the passage of the Act of 1829 the Association wound itself up.

Discussion of Emancipation, both in Parliament and within the Catholic Church, turned on the question of the 'securities'. There were of course those—often a majority—who were opposed to the principle of concession at all; but within the political classes the drift to acceptance of some sort of change in the civil status of English and Irish Catholics, stimulated by the Union of 1800, led to a sense of inevitability. The question was: what was the price to be exacted? Since the centre of the Emancipation issue resided in the unacceptable words of the parliamentary and office-holders' oaths, the wording of the amended oath was the leading item; the difficulty was how to accommodate Catholic consciences whilst still safeguarding the Protestant Constitution. For many

[67] Machin, 46.
[68] Charles Butler, *A Memoir*, 31.

Protestants, the declaration against Transubstantiation and the Oath of Supremacy were still 'the bulwarks' of English liberty. According to the Oath, subscription had to be made in the following words—'I AB do swear that I do from my heart detest and abjure as impious and heretical that damnable doctrine and position, that Princes excommunicated or deprived by the Pope or any authority of the See of Rome, may be deposed or murdered by their subjects or any other whatsoever; and I do declare that no foreign prince, prelate, state or potentate hath or ought to have any jurisdiction, power, superiority, pre-eminence or authority, Ecclesiastical or Spiritual, within this realm.' The first part of the text could be liberally interpreted as merely a protection of the national sovereignty, but the last clause, denying the 'Ecclesiastical' and 'Spiritual' authority of the Pope raised really substantial difficulties for Catholics. After the Oath, it was the Veto question which dominated the Emancipation debate: whether the Crown should acquire the right—which the sovereigns of many other countries exercised—to delete the names of candidates submitted by Rome for vacant sees. Another 'security' suggested in these years was the *Exequatur*, the right of the state to scrutinize documents arriving from Rome and to have an exclusive decision as to whether or not they could be received in the country. Both the Veto and the *Exequatur*, as it happened, were in these same years the subject of enormous controversy in South America, where the new republics, following the rejection of Spanish colonial rule early in the nineteenth century, were claiming the same powers of control over the Catholic Church formerly granted to the Crown by the Papacy.[69] From the viewpoint of Rome, therefore, the British debate constituted the fringe area of a very wide problem, and the attitude of Rome should be evaluated accordingly. The question of the payment of state stipends to Catholic priests—raised in relation to Ireland rather than England— was one of the proposed 'securities' which had least possibility of success, both on grounds of parliamentary retrenchment, in an era when the civil list was coming under increasingly

[69] See E. R. Norman, *Christianity in the Southern Hemisphere*, Oxford 1981, 4–7.

close scrutiny from Economical Reformers, and on the grounds that it was bad in principle to create a financial link between government and the Catholic Church. Burdett's Bill, in 1825, was the last occasion on which the idea was seriously entertained. It was denounced by many leading Whigs as a tax on Protestants to pay for the Catholic religion.[70] Wellington favoured it in 1829, but it was opposed by almost all his Cabinet colleagues.[71]

The first mention of the Veto in Parliament came with Sir John Cox-Hippisley's speech on Grattan's motion in 1808. In 1810 his own Bill proposed both a Veto and the *Exequatur*, and also a state financial provision for clergy. This aroused strong opposition in Ireland, but two of the English Vicars Apostolic supported the Bill and the Veto. This prompted Milner to pen a public criticism of the proposals—*An Elucidation of the Veto*—which, in turn, drew a public reply from Butler (*Letter to an Irish Catholic Gentleman*), to which Milner wrote two replies in pamphlet form. In 1810, therefore, the contending parties over the Veto arrayed their arguments in full for the first time. 'Now would it not be a palpable absurdity for a person who, like His Majesty, strongly protests against the supposed heterodoxy and even the idolatory of Catholics in general, to vouch for the orthodoxy of their very teachers?' Milner asked.[72] It was an 'attempt to deprive the successor of St. Peter in the See of Rome . . . of his right to give investiture to our bishops'; an attempt, furthermore, liable 'to drive the Catholics into a downright schism'.[73] An undeclared schism actually came quite near. On 1 February 1810, meeting in St. Alban's Tavern in London, the Catholic Board passed a *Fifth Resolution* which endorsed the devices of a state provision and, in veiled language, a Veto. For Milner, this was, as he put it, 'the Veto in its most hideous form'.[74] The other two bishops present, Poynter of London and Collingridge of the Western District, at first declared that they could not subscribe the Resolution (—Douglass, the fourth Vicar General, was absent due to illness—); but when

---

[70] Machin, 57.   [71] Ibid. 160.

[72] J. Milner, *An Elucidation of the Veto, in a threefold Address to the Public, the Catholics, and the Advocates of Catholics in Parliament*, London 1810, 6.

[73] Ibid. 19.   [74] Husenbeth, 174.

Milner was in another part of the room they both signed it.
To Milner it seemed the worst betrayal, particularly in view
of the strength of feeling in Ireland against the Veto. In his
later argument, the *Fifth Resolution* 'separated the Irish from
the English Catholics'; it 'caused more dissension and mischief
among the Catholics of England, than any other measure
since the divorce of Henry VIII'.[75] At a Synod held in London
on 20 February, at which Poynter's view prevailed, the *Fifth
Resolution* was upheld. Milner's *Explanation with the Rev.
Dr. Poynter*, written and privately circulated in 1812, attacked the decision with characteristic vehemence. The legacy
of controversy was so important that the text of the *Fifth
Resolution* ought itself to be recorded: it was 'That the
English Roman Catholics . . . are firmly persuaded that adequate provision for the maintenance of the civil and religious
establishments of this kingdom may be made consistently
with the strictest adherence on their part to the tenets and
discipline of the Roman Catholic religion; and that any
arrangement on this basis of mutual satisfaction and security
and extending to them the full enjoyment of the civil constitution of their country, will meet with their grateful concurrence.'[76] Cox-Hippisley's original Bill, the occasion of all
the difficulty, was easily defeated in Parliament.

An attempt was made in 1812 to repair some of the damage done to relations between the Irish and the English
Catholics, when the Bishop of Cork, Dr Francis Moylan, in
England to take the waters at Bath, sought to conciliate.
Meetings were arranged with the Vicars Apostolic, but the
'Moylan Mission' was not successful. The Emancipation debate returned to Parliament in 1813, when Grattan managed
to carry several resolutions in favour of Catholic relief, and
then introduced a Bill containing a Veto. Poynter sent a long
account of the Bill to Propaganda, with an Italian translation
of the clauses, drawing attention to what he called 'the penal
clauses' in it.[77] The bishops divided again, three of the four
accepting both the Veto and the Oath. Milner attributed the
Bill to 'the spirits of wickedness in high places mentioned by

[75] Ibid. 184.
[76] Bernard Ward, *Eve*, I. 129.
[77] Propaganda, *Scritture* 6 (1801–17), 378 [in Italian].

St. Paul';[78] Butler, in his support of the proposals, saw the
Bill as a simple act of toleration—'in the true sense of that
much abused word'.[79] But he had reservations about the form
of the Veto, and met Cox-Hippisley (whose speeches in its
favour had been particularly strong) in London to discuss the
matter. He found, as he explained in a letter to John Weld at
Stonyhurst, that Cox-Hippisley answered 'the description of
a Jansenist', and that he was persisting in a belief that the
Jesuits and the other Religious Orders 'should be brought
under restrictions' by the state.[80] This was the first appearance of an idea which was suddenly to surface again in 1829.
Milner circulated a *Brief Memorial on the Catholic Bill* among
members of Parliament, after a vain appeal to Poynter to join
his opposition to it. 'I am ready to encounter the white bears
of Hudson's Bay, and the Kangaroos of Botany Bay, rather
than yield,' he said.[81] But these expedients proved unnecessary: the Bill was abandoned in May 1813.

In October of the same year the Vicars Apostolic met in
Durham, at the suggestion of the Catholic Board, to arrive at
an agreed policy in the light of these events and in order to
prepare for a joint approach to fresh legislation. Milner was
not invited. They drew up a carefully balanced statement—
issued as a Pastoral Letter in each of the Districts (but not,
of course, in Milner's Midland District)—in which *some* of the
provisions of the 1813 Bill were declared to be 'inconsistent
with the duty of Catholics',[82] but which accepted the principle of a Veto by confirming the *Fifth Resolution* of 1810.
This endorsement was not unconditional, however. They
eschewed 'restrictions which control the exercise of the
power of the Pope in spiritual matters, particularly in the
appointment of his own Vicars'.[83] Milner's public reply, an
Encyclical Letter addressed to the Catholics of the Midland
District, was made the subject of a complaint by Poynter
when he was in Rome in 1815.

[78] Bernard Ward, *Eve*, II. 41; Husenbeth, 231.
[79] Charles Butler, *Historical Memoirs*, II. 229.
[80] Stonyhurst Archives, MS A II, 24 (22), Charles Butler to Revd. John Weld,
16 March 1814.
[81] Husenbeth, 231.
[82] Bernard Ward, *Eve*, II. 62.
[83] Bernard Ward, *Eve*, II. 65.

Rome delivered its view—or, as it turned out, *a* view—on the Veto question in 1814. During the absence in France of Pius VII, and with the dispersal of the Papal Court, the Secretary of Propaganda, Mgr. Jean Baptiste Quarantotti, delivered judgment. He was, as he wrote in his formal letter to Poynter in February 1814, 'invested with full pontifical powers'; and having 'taken the advice of the most learned prelates and divines', having read all the relevant letters and papers from England, and having discussed the matter at a special Congregation, 'it is decreed that Catholics may, with satisfaction and gratitude, accept and embrace the bill which was last year presented for their emancipation'.[84] The arrival of Quarantotti's *Rescript* in England caused jubilation to the Vetoists and to the Catholic Board, some embarrassment to Poynter, and great alarm to Milner—who at once set off for Rome, in such haste that he crossed the English Channel in a small open boat rather than await the regular packet. His salutation to the Pope, who had just returned from exile, might be described as fulsome: 'As the hart panteth after the fountains of waters, so my soul hath panted to see your Holiness and kiss your feet.'[85] The Pope, in reply, suggested that Quarantotti—whom he disliked for having taken an oath of allegiance to Napoleon—did not have the authority of the Holy See for the *Rescript*. Cardinal Laurence Litta, whom Milner also saw, announced that the conditions for Emancipation would be reconsidered: a statement which was received as meaning that the *Rescript* was in practice revoked. The victory was not Milner's, however. When Poynter met the Pope in Rome, in January 1815, 'His Holiness expressed his wish to satisfy the English Government as far as religion would permit, and his desire that the clergy should be well thought of by the Government, and not meddle in politics.'[86] In April, he heard from Litta ('with great satisfaction and pleasure') that the Pope hoped for 'a more perfect union between the Catholics and the Government'.[87] The upshot was Cardinal Litta's letter from Genoa, of April 1815, which

---

[84] The text is in Butler, *Historical Memoirs*, II. 399.

[85] Husenbeth, 273.

[86] Bernard Ward, *Eve*, II. 121.

[87] Propaganda, *Scritture* 6 (1801–17), 602 [in French].

disallowed the *Exequatur*, approved three forms of oath
which might without hazard to the Pope's *spiritual* authority
be allowed in an Emancipation Bill, and endorsed a limited
Veto for Irish episcopal appointments. The day had gone to
Poynter rather than to Milner. He asked Lingard to deploy
his historical talents in producing an examination of the way
in which the civil power exercised some control in the nomination of Catholic bishops in other countries, and where
the Catholics received a measure of 'civil establishment' in
return.[88] In the same year, 1817, a measure of Catholic relief
was passed: commissions in the Army and Navy, opened to
Irish Catholics since 1793, could now be held by English
Catholics. Another stone in the wall of exclusion had fallen
away.

The last occasion on which the Veto question took a
prominent place in discussions about Emancipation was in
1821.[89] Early in March of that year a parliamentary committee proposed two bills: both because of their importance
in the Veto controversy, and because of the oath question and
the Catholic leaders' successful dealings with political groups
over it, the fate of the bills requires close analysis. The first
bill consisted of a general relief measure and included the
Oath of Supremacy—but it was to be taken together with an
explanatory declaration implying that no essential tenets of
Catholicism were thereby denied. The second bill proposed
two 'securities': there were to be two permanent royal commissions, one to scrutinize Catholic episcopal appointments—
the Veto—and the other to examine communications from
Rome—the *Exequatur*. Both pieces of legislation were introduced by Plunket. In Ireland there were some divisions of
opinion. A meeting of the Dublin clergy welcomed the proposals; most clerical meetings in the provinces disclosed a
substantial hostility. Bishop Doyle was friendly, and so was
O'Connell, despite his objections to the 'securities'. In England
the lay Catholics welcomed the proposals, Milner was deeply
opposed, and Poynter went for a compromise.

---

[88] [John Lingard], *Observations on the Laws and Ordinances, which exist in
Foreign States, relative to the religious concerns of their Roman Catholic Subjects.
By a British Roman Catholic*, London 1817.
[89] Machin, 31.

Poynter acted in close co-ordination with Rome, and an examination of the correspondence which passed between himself and the agent of the English bishops, Gradwell, shows just how effectively he managed to secure the compromise he sought. Robert Gradwell was himself an old friend: his appointment to the Rectorship of the Venerabile in Rome, and his agency of the bishops, in 1818—in succession to Robert Smelt—were due to Poynter's and to Lingard's influence. At that time he had never actually been to Rome. Educated at Douai, he had suffered imprisonment, together with Poynter, when the French Militia occupied the College. He then taught at Ushaw before the appointment in Rome was made. His influence there was directed against the Jesuits and in support of Poynter's understanding of English Catholicism. In 1828 he returned to England as Bishop Bramston's coadjutor in the London District. The Papal Court, according to Glover, regarded him as 'their oracle for everything regarding England'.[90] Bishop Baines, unsuccessfully seeking to prevent his elevation to the episcopacy in 1828, described Gradwell as 'a man of artful and crooked policy, who never can go openly and honestly about any business', who was also 'a dissipated man, ever to be found in all the parties and conversations of Rome'.[91] It was not a particularly fair view. Gradwell was a good and conscientious agent. But his opponents among the religious orders—Baines was a Benedictine —could rightly point to his undoubted prejudice against their interests. Before appointing him as a bishop, the Pope gave him 'a severe lecture'.[92]

Poynter was from the start convinced that Plunket's proposals could be turned into a satisfactory settlement of the Catholic claims. He thought the introductory motion in Parliament, as he wrote to Gradwell, was 'one of the most eloquent and powerful speeches that was ever heard in the House'.[93] His optimism was soon tempered. On 6 March he reported to Rome that the Oath of Supremacy was to be modified by a

[90] Stonyhurst Archives, MS B.I.17, Glover's *Excerpts* III, 250.
[91] Ibid. 251.
[92] Ibid. 252.
[93] Westminster Dioc. Archives, Gradwell Papers, Letter Books B3, Poynter to Gradwell, 2 March 1821.

'legislative interpretation' while the old form of words was actually to be retained. He doubted if that was enough of a concession; that 'any explanation could justify a Catholic in taking the Oath of Supremacy in its present terms'.[94] This opinion was transmitted to Plunket, who regarded the retention of the Oath as a necessary condition for satisfying Protestant feelings. The result was a meeting arranged by the Duke of Norfolk, between Poynter and Plunket—and also attended by Sir John Newport, Sir James Macintosh, Sir Henry Parnell, and some others—at which Poynter explained that the words of the existing Oath explicitly denied the Pope's spiritual authority, and that, in his judgement, no 'legislative declaration' could enable Catholics to overcome their scruples. Poynter had also drawn up a paper on the question, which he presented to the meeting.[95] Its burden was to show that Papal authority over English Catholics 'is *purely ecclesiastical* and spiritual; it has not the least mixture of any portion of civil or temporal authority annexed to it'. His suggestion was to alter the Oath by the simple addition of the word 'civil' before 'allegiance', so making it clear that Papal *spiritual* authority was not in question, and retaining the 'legislative declaration' as explanation, to be read to Catholics before subscribing the Oath. Plunket and his supporters accepted the amendment—the majority on the first-reading of the bills in the Commons had been uncomfortably small. It was a very impressive success for Poynter's skill in the presentation of his case. As he explained to Gradwell, the amended oath required Catholics 'only to deny such foreign jurisdictions ecclesiastical or spiritual as interfere with civil duty and allegiance'.[96] The Relief Bill, as proposed in this form, was approved in Rome by Cardinal Fontana, despite representation against it made to Propaganda by Archbishop Troy of Dublin.[97] Milner's opposition was also proving a difficulty to the promoters of compromise. He called the Oath an apostasy

[94] Westminster Dioc. Archives, Gradwell Papers, Letter Books B3, Poynter to Gradwell, 6 March 1821.

[95] There is a copy in the Gradwell Papers, Letter Books B3, appended to the letter of 6 March to Gradwell. The paper is dated 5 March 1821.

[96] Ibid., Poynter to Gradwell, 8 March 1821.

[97] Westminster Dioc. Archives, Gradwell Papers, Letter Books B3, Gradwell to Poynter, 22 March 1821.

and declared that any Catholic taking it would be 'schismatic'. Poynter sought advice in Rome as to whether the other Vicars Apostolic ought to publish a Pastoral Letter to offset his opinion.[98] Milner's hope was to organize opinion against the bills and to get more satisfactory measures of relief introduced in the following year. Together with the Franciscan Father Richard Hayes, agent of the Irish lay Catholics in Rome (whom Cardinal Fontana called 'a great hypocrite and scoundrel'[99]) he campaigned openly against Poynter's acceptance of the amended oath. Milner and the Irish prelates, as Gradwell told Cardinal Consalvi, were 'ready to assail the least unguarded expression'; Consalvi, for his part, supported Poynter's actions—he was, he said 'a man of solid judgment'.[100] He asked Gradwell to write him a memorandum on the oath question for the guidance of the Curia.[101] Milner's petition against the legislation was presented to Parliament by William Wilberforce, a pro-Emancipationist who said that 'all the religious people are on the other side'[102]—meaning the national Protestant spirit. The petition was signed by all Catholic clergy and laity of the Midland District, and was duly translated into Italian so that Cardinal Consalvi could read it.[103] Gradwell also received a copy of Milner's published letter to Wilberforce—setting out opposition to the terms of Emancipation. 'This rubbish I did not translate', he wrote to Poynter;[104] but a few days later Consalvi showed him an Italian version that was already circulating in Rome. Both sides in the disputes had their friends at court.

There were, of course, even among Catholic friends of the Plunket proposals, grave reservations about the 'securities' in the second bill. Gradwell regarded it as 'impossible to submit' to the *Exequatur*: 'it is an act to enslave and degrade the clergy'.[105] Yet he modified the view as the debates proceeded, being, as he told Consalvi, 'sensible that it was necessary to

[98] Ibid., Poynter to Gradwell, 28 March 1821.
[99] Ibid., Gradwell to Poynter, 21 April 1821.
[100] Ibid., Gradwell's *Journal*, E.7.I, 29 March 1821.
[101] Ibid., 31 March 1821.
[102] W. G. Addison, *Religious Equality in Modern England*, 46.
[103] Gradwell Papers, Letter Books B3, Gradwell to Poynter, 21 April 1821.
[104] Ibid.
[105] Gradwell Papers, *Journal*, E.7.I, 2 April 1821.

make some sacrifice to the fears and prejudices of Protestants'.[106] On 13 April the terms of both bills were explained
to the Pope,[107] although shortly afterwards, to the incredulity
of Gradwell, there were reports that the Pope 'approves of
all that Dr. Milner has done and written on the subject'.[108]
Poynter, in London, had meanwhile been working with
Castlereagh to get more amendments both to the Oath and to
the 'restrictive clauses', the 'securities'. The two bills were
then consolidated into one and passed the Commons by 19
votes on 2 April. 'We have gained wonderfully in having the
explanation of the Oath of Supremacy incorporated into the
Oath itself,' Poynter wrote; 'It now simply amounts to a
denial that the Pope has any civil or temporal authority
here.'[109] The 'securities', however, remained in the legislation.
The Catholic nobility memorialized the House of Commons
with their gratitude. But the Bill was defeated in the Lords
by 39 votes.[110]

The next attempt at legislation, in 1825, was very different.
Sir Francis Burdett, the London Radical, drew his Bill up in
co-operation with Plunket and O'Connell, the first draft actually being made by O'Connell alone. The measure represented
Irish rather than English interests, and the English Catholics,
indeed, took no part in any of the negotiations.[111] They were
unprepared for action on the Emancipation question at that
time, and Clifford wondered whether an extraordinary meeting of the Catholic Board ought to be convened in order to
consider a common policy.[112] Burdett's motion for a Committee to consider the Catholic claims passed in the Commons
by 13 votes in February. This was followed by a relief bill,
which contained a moderate oath and two 'securities'—the
Veto and the *Exequatur*. A standing advisory commission of
Irish bishops was to operate the 'securities', however. No

---

[106] Ibid., Letter Books B3, Gradwell to Poynter, 21 April 1821.
[107] Gradwell's *Journal*, E.7.I, 13 April 1821.
[108] Ibid., 21 April 1821.
[109] Gradwell Papers, Letter Books B3, Poynter to Gradwell, 3 April 1821.
[110] Machin, 31.
[111] Bernard Ward, *Eve*, III. 124.
[112] Stonyhurst Archives, MS A II, 24 (26) H. Clifford to London Arundel, 9 Jan.
1825 (the letter is actually dated 1824 by the writer, but the postmark is quite
clear).

English Commission was provided for: 'O'Connell', as Ward wrote, 'seems to have drafted the whole bill as if it were to operate only in Ireland.'[113] Protestant fears about the insecure nature of the 'securities' were to some extent allayed by the two 'wings' of the bill. Separate measures were introduced providing for the disfranchisement of the 40-shilling freehold voters in Ireland, and state allowances for the Catholic clergy. O'Connell accepted both, despite the strong opposition of some Radicals, like Cobbett, to the disfranchisement—a measure anathema to those who were pledged to parliamentary reform. Milner was opposed to the whole scheme as embodying the Veto. Four hundred petitions against it were received by Parliament: an indication of the surviving popular antipathy of Protestants to Emancipation. Poynter and the other Vicars Apostolic gave cautious support to the bill, and when they met at Wolverhampton, on 1 May, for the consecration of Dr Walsh as coadjutor of the Midland District, even the 'ferocity and hostility' of Milner had subsided, and there was peace among them.[114] The Relief bill, and the 'wings', had passed the Commons by the end of April, and passed to the Lords. Here the proceedings were most remarkable for the Duke of York's declaration, on 25 April, that the Coronation Oath forbade the Royal Assent being given to any Relief bill— in words which *John Bull* said should be printed in letters of gold. But Gradwell, in Rome, believed that 'the Duke of York's imprudent declaration will not do much harm',[115] and this was the view generally taken by the Catholic leaders. The Vice-President of Ushaw, George Brown, wrote to Wiseman (in Rome) that neither the Duke's 'drunken oath' nor the 'bigotted exertions' of the Protestant spokesmen was likely to rouse the nation, and he expected the measure to pass 'silently'.[116] But the bill was rejected in the House of Lords by 48 votes. Charles Butler deployed his legal skills in writing a tract which showed that the Coronation Oath was not incompatible with changes in the will of Parliament. 'His Majesty

---

[113] Bernard Ward, *Eve*, III. 125.
[114] Westminster Dioc. Archives, Gradwell Papers, *Journal*, II, 26 May 1825.
[115] Ibid.
[116] Ushaw College Archives, Wiseman Papers, 29, George Brown to Wiseman, 7 April 1826; (the letter is also wrongly dated; it clearly belongs to 1825).

has no subjects more attached to his sacred person and government', he added, in Cisalpine style.[117]

The immediate prelude to Emancipation was the repeal of the Test and Corporation Acts in 1828: it was a clear precedent for alterations to the Constitution in the interests of religious toleration, a milestone on the way to establishing that religious opinion should not affect civil liberties. The Protestant Dissenters, of course, had anyway been exempted from the penalties of the Acts by the passage of annual measures of indemnity through Parliament; but their formal removal was seen by many to be a crucial preparation for the Catholic claims. Burdett's motion for a committee to consider them passed by 6 votes in May 1828. It was, thereafter, events in Ireland which dictated the chronology of Emancipation—the Clare election of July, and O'Connell's victory at the polls; the conversions of Wellington and Peel. In January 1829 the Cabinet began discussing a Catholic bill, and the King agreed. Most of the old 'securities' were considered and abandoned, only the disfranchisement of the 40-shilling freeholders in Ireland finding its way into the final measures.[118] These consisted of a Relief Bill, and two separate 'wings'—the Catholic Association was disbanded in Ireland in addition to the disfranchisement. The oath in the Act, as passed, contained a denial of the Pope's deposing powers and of any 'temporal or civil jurisdiction' in the United Kingdom. There was also a new clause in the oath, similar to one inserted as a 'security' to the Established Church in the Act repealing the Test and Corporation Acts: Catholics were to swear to 'disclaim, disavow and solemnly abjure any intention to subvert the present Church Establishment as settled by law'.[119] The Act contained no Veto or *Exequatur*, no payment of the Clergy. There was some feeling that a system of licensing should be introduced 'under some measure and degree of control from the British government', as Henry Phillpotts (Bishop of Exeter from 1830) put

---

[117] Charles Butler, *A Letter on the Coronation Oath*, London [1825], 2nd edn. 1827, 14.

[118] Machin, 216.

[119] X Geo. IV, cap. VII, *An Act for the Relief of His Majesty's Roman Catholic Subjects* (13 April 1829), II.

it,[120] to safeguard against potential disloyalty among the Catholic prelates. But this came to nothing.

The other provisions of the Act were simple and straight-forward. No Catholic priest was to sit in the House of Commons.[121] Most offices under the Crown were opened to Catholics—those reserved being the Lord Chancellor, the Keeper of the Great Seal, the Lord Lieutenant of Ireland, and the High Commissioner of the Church of Scotland.[122] Catholics were to be eligible to serve as members of lay corporations, though to take no part in the corporate exercise of ecclesiastical patronage.[123] No Catholic prelate was to assume any territorial title used by members of the Established Church.[124] No insignia of public office were to be worn in Catholic Churches.[125] The Catholic clergy were only to officiate in their usual places of worship and were not to wear ecclesiastical dress in public places.[126] And then came a very extraordinary provision: the banning of the religious orders, an additional 'security' that no one had expected. When the Bull *Sollicitudo omnium Ecclesiarum* had restored the Jesuits, in 1814, three of the English Vicars Apostolic had successfully resisted its formal application in England on the grounds, accepted in Rome, that explicit permission of the civil power was not forthcoming. But in 1828 Bishop Collingridge had shifted his position and had successfully petitioned the Holy See for a full restoration. The decree for this arrived in England during January 1829, just as the Emancipation Bill was being discussed in Cabinet. It elicited characteristic hostility from the Protestant public, and hence clauses XXVIII to XXXVII in the Act: all 'Jesuits and Members of Other Religious Orders, Communities, or Societies of the Church of Rome, bound by Monastic or Religious vows' were to register when the Act came into effect, 'to make a provision' for their 'gradual Suppression'.[127] No members of religious orders were to be allowed into the country after the

---

[120] Olive Brose, *Church and Parliament. The Reshaping of the Church of England 1828–1860*, Stanford 1959, 18.
[121] X Geo. IV, cap. VII, IX.
[122] Ibid. X, XII.   [123] Ibid. XIV.
[124] Ibid. XXIV.   [125] Ibid. XXV.
[126] Ibid. XXVI.
[127] Ibid. XXVIII.

passing of the Act—and any who arrived would be banished.[128]
'Orders of Females' were excluded:[129] women could not exercise the franchise and so were not considered a political
threat.

The Bill was introduced to the Commons by Peel on 10
March 1829, in a speech of four and a half hours' length
which, according to Butler, 'at times was accompanied with
cheers that were heard even in Westminster Hall'.[130] It successfully passed the House of Lords on 10 April, with a
majority of 104, and received the Royal Assent on 13 April.
When it finally came to it—and in contrast to the attempts of
1810, 1821, and 1825—the Catholics had taken almost no
part in the measure. It was an unnegotiated government Bill.
Milner and Poynter were both dead, and their successors made
no co-ordinated or public responses to the government's initiatives. At a meeting in Wolverhampton, which all the Vicars
Apostolic attended, the Oath presented in the new Act was
approved.[131] The Catholic Association welcomed the measure,
so did O'Connell—who regarded it as 'frank, direct, complete'[132] and so did Charles Butler, who wrote to Wiseman in
Rome that 'no business was ever transacted in a more straight-
forward manner, or with kinder views towards the Catholics'.[133] During the debates on the Bill, Pope Leo XII had
died, and his successor, Pius VIII (Cardinal Castiglione) was
reported as being 'perfectly satisfied' with it.[134] The papers
on the bill in the archives of Propaganda make it clear that
Rome had followed its progress closely—and with very full
information.[135] In his circular to the clergy and laity of the
Midland District, announcing the election of the new Pope
—of which a copy survives in the Downside Archives—Bishop
Thomas Walsh expressed sentiments of 'gratitude and attachment' to the Crown for Emancipation, and pointed out to

[128] Ibid. XXXIII, XXXIV.
[129] Ibid. XXXVII.
[130] Charles Butler, *A Memoir*, 43.
[131] Bernard Ward, *Eve*, III. 272.
[132] *Correspondence of Daniel O'Connell*, I. 174.
[133] Ushaw Coll. Archives, Wiseman Papers, 135, Butler to Wiseman, 22 April
1829.   [134] Ibid.
[135] Propaganda, *Scritture* 8 (1823-33), 530-61 (also contains the *Voto* on the
Bill) [in Italian].

the Catholics that they owed 'spiritual obedience, but spiritual obedience only' to the Pope.[136]

Opposition to the Act came from Tory 'ultras': demonstrated by Peel's defeat at the Oxford election, in February, by Sir Robert Inglis. Known originally as 'Orange' Peel, because of his adhesion to the principles of the Protestant Constitution, the Home Secretary was hereafter often referred to as 'turncoat' Peel. Some Catholics opposed the legislation on the grounds that it was no real measure of relief at all—that it was, as William Eusebius Andrews (a Milner supporter who published the *Orthodox Journal*) said, 'the revival of another persecution'.[137] William Langley, objecting to the favourable view of the Act taken by John Birdsall, President of the English Benedictines, denounced the oath not to weaken the Protestant Establishment as the maintenance of heresy; and of the measure in general he wrote: 'It pretends to be a relief Bill, when in fact it is a Bill of pains and penalties.'[138] It was indeed true that the Act left many of the old penal laws still on the statute book, and that they were not repealed in a consolidated measure until 1844 (by 7 & 8 Vict. cap. 102).[139] But the Emancipation Act, as its advocates saw, had rendered them quite inoperable. This was also the view soon to be taken of the clauses against the Religious and Monastic Orders. 'I will stake my existence that I will run a coach-and-six three times told through the Act,' O'Connell declared in reference to the clauses.[140] Butler supposed they were 'a mere dead letter' and believed that if nothing further was said about them they would pass into oblivion.[141] And that proved to be the case. But there was initially great disquiet within the Orders themselves. Some precautions were taken against the ban on the admission of new members due to commence with

[136] Downside Archives, Birt Papers, VIII A, *Letter of Thomas, Vicar Apostolic of the Midland District to the Clergy and Laity*, 21 April 1829.

[137] Ward, *Eve*, III. 260.

[138] Downside Archives, Birt Papers, VIII A, William Langley to John Birdsall, 27 April 1829.

[139] John Hungerford Pollen, 'The Penal Clauses in the Emancipation Bill', in *The Month*, October 1908, 4.

[140] *Correspondence*, I. 174.

[141] Ushaw College Archives, Wiseman Papers, 135, Butler to Wiseman, 22 April 1829.

the passing of the Act: in March 1829, as the Bill was debated
in Parliament, all the boys at Stonyhurst in the higher school
who were candidates for entrance to the Society of Jesus,
were admitted as novitiates *en bloc*.[142] Bishop Thomas Smith
of the Northern District wrote to advise Glover, at Stonyhurst, to seek modifications to the clauses. The contemplation
of the extinction of the orders, he wrote, 'gives me great pain,
as well on account of the esteem and affection I feel for those
Venerable Institutions, as the effect it is calculated to have
upon the interests of our holy Religion in this country'.[143]
The loss of the regular clergy serving the missions would certainly have had a deeply disturbing effect, and the prospect
clearly diminished the antipathy entertained towards the
orders by the secular ecclesiastics. There was talk of the
Benedictines removing themselves to America. Bishop Walsh
wrote to assure the Downside monks of his support in the
crisis—but pointed to the growing doubts as to whether the
clauses would be enforced. The secular clergy, he continued,
would 'adopt any plan' the Benedictines favoured to save
themselves.[144] The President, Birdsall, had anyway produced
two public addresses to Peel in March: the first seeking exemption for the Benedictines from the clauses, and the second dealing with the general threat to monasticism in England.
'This Society', he wrote in the first, 'has no dependence on,
has no interference and no connexion with any Foreign Body
or Society, is under no foreign superior, other than the
supreme head of our Church, a point to which we understand
the attention of His Majesty's Government is more particularly directed.' Most of the monks in England, he further
pointed out, were engaged in ordinary 'pastoral charge, and
the care of congregations.' There was also an appeal to the
recipients' sense of the picturesque and the romantic: 'be it
not forgot that they are descendents of that body of men to
whom the Inhabitants of this Island and all lovers of learning and research are particularly indebted both for valuable

---

[142] Archives of the English Province of the Society of Jesus, Farm Street,
London, *Prov. Angl. S.J. Register*, 118 (entry of 21 Sept. 1829).
[143] Stonyhurst Archives, MS A II, 28 (57), Bishop Thomas Smith to T. Glover,
19 March 1829.
[144] Downside Archives, Birt Papers, VIII A, Walsh to Birdsall, 23 April 1829.

records of lore and the magnificent Buildings which even in ruins yet ornament the land and astonish the beholder.'[145] In letters sent out to the heads of the other regulars in England, Birdsall exhorted them 'to act with common knowledge of what each does or intends to do'.[146] In the event, however, no further action proved necessary, and the clauses were recognized as being a dead letter.

On 4 May 1829, the Earl of Surrey, son of the Duke of Norfolk, was elected for the family pocket borough of Horsham. He was the first Catholic to take his seat in the House of Commons.

[145] Ibid., Birt Papers VIII A, 'Two Printed Letters to Robert Peel by John Birdsall', 16 March 1829.
[146] Ibid., MS Letter of 17 March 1829.

2
Ecclesiastical Administration

The great institutional change of the English Catholic Church came in 1850, with the re-establishment of the hierarchy—a step towards internal self-government; but this was hardly, in the wider context of Christian developments during the century, a particularly unusual phenomenon. For it was a century which saw the first steps to governmental autonomy within the Established Church, with the revivals of Convocation in the 1850s and the evolution of clerical organizations and diocesan conferences—themselves responses to the progressive withdrawal of the state from exclusive protection of the Church of England. In North America, too, the churches were obliged to work out instruments of institutional autonomy as a result of their separation from parent bodies in England and Europe.[1] In 1790 Propaganda had detached the Catholics of the United States from the jurisdiction of the Vicar Apostolic of the London District, and Dr John Carroll, a former Jesuit from an 'Old Catholic' Maryland family, was consecrated as the first Bishop of Baltimore. His see was raised to archiepiscopal status in 1808, and four new dioceses were created: the formal establishment of the American hierarchy.[2] The churches of British North America, also, underwent this transformation, as the grant of Responsible Government indicated that political developments would place Canada and Canadian institutions at a distance from English government. The principle of independent diocesan synods for the Anglicans of Canada was approved at the Quebec Conference of 1851, and in 1853 the first Synod actually met in Toronto.[3] Viewed from the palace of Propaganda in Rome, the development of independent Catholic hierarchies in the expanding world of

---

[1] E. R. Norman, *The Conscience of the State in North America*, Cambridge, 1968, 103 ff.
[2] Ibid. 112.
[3] Ibid. 114.

the nineteenth century was quite familiar. England, it was true, was regarded as something of a special case: but this was not because of any peculiarity in the Catholic condition here —though there were minor problems because of the surviving penal statutes—but because of England's influence in those parts of the world, like Canada, Australia or the Caribbean, where there were considerable Catholic populations. The English bishops were much involved with these overseas churches in the first half of the century.

With ecclesiastical autonomy went an increasing measure of clericalism—though there were other causes of this, too. The growth of priestly over lay control of the churches[4] (seen in Wiseman's policies especially), was evident in the Protestant churches too, both in England, where it was due to the decay of erastianism, and overseas, where it resulted from the central direction required in territorial or missionary expansion. As with Wiseman's 'Romanizing' of the Catholic Church, the transformation wrought in the State Church by the Oxford and High Church movements was sacerdotalist in inspiration and effect.

The last years of government by the Vicars Apostolic in England, therefore, were accompanied by an emphasis on professionalism which was paralleled in society generally and in the other historic churches. That the Catholic Church's institutions of ecclesiastical government had patently been rendered out of date by population growth and shifts in class orientation was also not an unfamiliar phenomenon in the England of the first half of the century: nearly all institutions were creaking with old timbers and awaiting renovation. The clergy of England were governed by Benedict XIV's Bull *Apostolicum Ministerium*, issued in 1753, which assumed the existence of a quasi-hidden Church of the country gentry and their dependants, where the clergy were chaplains to the great houses. The expansion of the urban population, with industrial changes, had left the provisions of the Bull with an extremely anomalous complexion. The Vicars Apostolic had done what they could, with limited finances and limited powers, to develop urban missions, but it was in many places

---

[4] Bossy, *The English Catholic Community, 1570–1850*, 355.

the Religious Orders, the Benedictines or the Jesuits, who moved most effectively into the cities, to found missionary parishes, so laying up problems of jurisdiction between themselves and the bishops. The Vicars Apostolic themselves were appointed directly by Rome, with episcopal rank, and titles *in partibus infidelium*, to govern the four ecclesiastical Districts into which the country was divided: the Northern District, the Midland District, the Western District (which included Wales), and the London District (the Home Counties).[5] Scotland constituted a separate District, and Ireland, of course, had its own, ancient, ecclesiastical hierarchy. As Ullathorne was to argue at the time of the setting up of the new hierarchy in 1850, the recognition of the *Vicars Apostolic* was 'the recognition of a far more extensive Papal power in the country than is the recognition of a hierarchy of titular bishops'. The point was a very acute one. 'For ages the Pope has acted not only as the supreme pastor but also as the immediate Bishop of the English Catholic Church, and has governed through his appointed Vicars,' he continued; 'In establishing the hierarchy, so far from extending his power more over this country, His Holiness has only set it within more canonical limitations.'[6] Each of the bishops in England, therefore, was immediately subject to the Holy See. Their periodic meetings were merely advisory, though their faculties were like those of regularly constituted diocesan bishops. They appointed 'Grand-Vicars' whose functions were precisely those of Vicars-General in a formal arrangement of Church government. An advantage of the system, particularly in a society of social change and mobility like England in the first half of the century, was that the boundaries of Districts and missions could be changed fairly easily—to settle problems arising from proprietary claims of the gentry, or the Religious Orders, rather than from ancient ecclesiastical rights or uses. In view of the sensitive feelings of Protestant Englishmen about papal powers, all Catholics went to some lengths to show that they were *spiritual* only, and that the jurisdiction

[5] There is a map of the English Mission, drawn up in 1829 by Bishop Baines, printed in vol. I of Bernard Ward's *Sequel to Catholic Emancipation*.

[6] Ullathorne Papers, St. Dominic's Convent, Stone. Box X (8) 'Two Draft letters about the Restoration of the Hierarchy' (n.d.).

of the Vicars Apostolic was, accordingly, restricted to their own co-religionists. In March 1821, Bishop Poynter of the London District drew up a paper on the question of the oath to be prescribed in any Relief measure for the guidance of the politicians with whom he was in negotiation. It contained a useful summary of the Pope's delegated authority in England: 'It is chiefly exercised here in appointing Bishops and in giving them powers for the spiritual government of the Catholics in their respective Dioceses or Districts; in superintending the religious conduct of the Catholics; and in granting dispensations from the ecclesiastical impediments of matrimony when necessity requires.'[7]

Under the government of the Vicars Apostolic, England was not subject to the canon law, and it was, indeed, one of the difficulties of reviving a formal hierarchy that the code was in some particulars inapplicable to the conditions in England. Cardinal Acton, in Rome, an opponent of re-establishing the hierarchy, for that and for other reasons, began to construct a new code of canon law, suited to English conditions, in 1843. The pressure of other work led to his abandonment of what was, by any standards, a formidable task. 'The whole body of that legislation', according to Wiseman, writing in 1842, 'has been formed under, and in contemplation of, circumstances totally different from those in which we should have to apply it.' It supposed a background of Roman—rather than common—law; it was intended to operate with the co-operation of the state, in financial as in legal considerations. As Wiseman also pointed out, however, it supposed 'the enforcers and the subjects of the code to be living under a Catholic government, and, alas! such a government as hardly a single Catholic state now presents'.[8] The introduction of canon law to England, therefore, would involve an extremely extensive revision of it—which was why that introduction was in the end delayed until 1918.

Direct Papal authority in England in practice meant government by the Sacred Congregation of Propaganda Fide, under

[7] Westminster Dioc. Archives, Gradwell Papers, Letter Books B3, Poynter to Gradwell, 6 March 1821 (enclosing his paper of 5 March).

[8] 'A Paper on Ecclesiastical Organization', in *Essays on Various Subjects by His Eminence Cardinal Wiseman*, London 1853, I. 346.

whose jurisdiction, as a missionary territory, the country was placed throughout the nineteenth century. Appeals to Propaganda, by bishops against one another, and because of disputes between the regular and the secular clergy, were rather frequent. There are many indications, in the archives of Propaganda, to suggest that the English mission was somewhat more difficult to govern, in this regard, than other areas. This was the result of lack of acquaintance with Roman procedures and protocol, rather than hostility to Roman authority as such, and diminished after the first generations of students trained at the English College in Rome—which reopened in 1818—began to achieve higher ecclesiastical posts in the English Church. Before that, Propaganda had constantly to complain at the irregularities and discourtesies of the English bishops: at their failure to make *ad limina* visits to the Pope, at the loose style of their reports, at the sparse nature of the information they thought fit to send to Rome, and at their promulgation of decrees without the prior authority of the Sacred Congregation. Dr Griffiths, who in 1833 became Bramston's coadjutor in the London District—and who was the first bishop whose education had taken place entirely in England—caused particular offence to Propaganda by writing his *scritture* on a carbon copier.[9] Relations with Rome were not always made more felicitous by the action of the agent employed there by the bishops. His duty was to send information about events at Rome to the Vicars Apostolic, and to present English causes informally to the appropriate Vatican authorities: to ease the way of the many difficult issues sent for decision or adjudication. In practice the holders of the post tended, by inclination or misunderstanding, to get involved in partisan conflicts—this was especially true of Gradwell's opposition to the Jesuits during his period as agent between 1818 and 1828. He had been preceded by Robert Smelt, agent after 1790, and by Paul Macpherson, from 1812. Gradwell was followed by Wiseman, and the agent thereafter was normally Rector of the English College. Wiseman's action in the office was at times controversial, too; in the 1830s some of the Vicars Apostolic declared a wish to avoid his

---

[9] Gwynn, *The Second Spring, 1818–1852*, 161.

involvement, and Propaganda, for its part, asked them to deal directly with itself rather than through the agent.[10] Wiseman was succeeded by Charles Baggs, who in 1843 succeeded Baines as Vicar Apostolic of the Western District. Thomas Grant followed, though only after a prolonged discussion among the Vicars Apostolic about his suitability. He was, in the event, a fair enough agent, but unable to cope with the volume of business attendant upon the final stages of the negotiations for the hierarchy—Ullathorne, as a result, was sent to Rome in 1848 to act on behalf of the English bishops. Grant left Rome in 1851, to become Bishop of Southwark, and Robert Cornthwaite, the new Rector of the Venerabile, became agent. It was during his time at the College that relations with the Jesuits improved, and that proper arrangements were made for the training of the converts for the Catholic priesthood. As agent, however, he gave rise to misgivings, reinforced by the conviction among the English bishops that he was too dependent on Mgr. George Talbot. In 1853 Ullathorne raised the matter directly, and privately, with Wiseman, urging a separation of the agency from the Rectorship. The agent, he argued, should be 'Some person of weight and experience, and of a certain independence of character, in whom the Bishops could have confidence, and whose word would have weight.' There was a 'question', he wrote, as to whether Cornthwaite was 'competent' for such a post.[11] Cornthwaite resigned in 1857, and his successor as Rector, Charles English, proposed that the agency should be separated. Wiseman was opposed to this, fearing the isolation of the Venerabile from the main currents of English Catholic development; so English continued as agent, as did his successor in 1863, Frederick Neve. By then, however, Manning's dependence on Talbot often circumvented the agent anyway. The next agent, Henry O'Callaghan, was put into the Rectorship and agency by the direct intervention of Talbot and Manning in 1868, and continued until 1888; but by then the relations of the bishops with the Roman Congregations had

[10] Michael E. Williams, *The Venerable English College, Rome. A History, 1579–1979*, London 1979, 78.
[11] Westminster Dioc. Archives, Wiseman Papers, Bishops' Letters 130/1, Ullathorne to Wiseman, 20 Dec. 1853.

established themselves to the point at which the agency was scarcely important. The institutional benefits of the re-establishment of the hierarchy in 1850 had by then become evident.

Internal co-ordination of episcopal activity was not impressive, and did not greatly improve after 1850. Bishops' meetings were held in 1804, 1805, and 1810. It was hoped that they could be held annually, but differences of view between the Vicars Apostolic—and particularly between Milner and Poynter over the terms of Catholic Relief legislation—made this inadvisable.[12] 'Cardinal Litta on *many* occasions', Poynter told Gradwell in 1818, 'gave me no other satisfaction that to reproach me with the scandal of uncharitable contentions between Bishops.'[13] They met again in 1825, and the tradition of an annual Low Week meeting thereafter established itself. Their resolutions at these gatherings, however, had no canonical force, and had to be referred to Propaganda. These meetings continued after 1850, and allowed a regular exchange of views without the formal, and by then ecclesiastically regular, consequences of synodical action.

The Missions (or 'parishes', as they were often, though inaccurately called), were entirely dependent upon the rule of the Vicars Apostolic: there were no parochial councils, and in those places where lay committees existed for fund-raising there was an increasing tension with the episcopal authorities as they endeavoured to secure control. It was this direct relationship with the authority of the Vicars Apostolic which exacerbated conflicts with those parishes the regular clergy conducted: friction here exactly paralleled the attrition with the lay finance committees as the authority of the bishops was insisted upon. This shift of influence actually preceded Wiseman and the 'Roman' spirit of advancing Ultramontanism: it was already evident in the conduct of such 'non-Roman' prelates as, in their different ways, Milner and Poynter.

The issue of lay patronage was very serious. It was not, however, unique to England. Known as the problem of

[12] Bernard Ward, *The Eve of Catholic Emancipation*, 183.
[13] Westminster Dioc. Archives, Gradwell papers, Letter Books B3, Poynter to Gradwell, 11 Sept. 1818.

'trusteeism', it plagued the east-coast Catholic dioceses of the United States in the first half of the nineteenth century, too. There, also, prominent and rich laymen had built churches, and groups of lay trustees had been formed to administer ecclesiastical property and incomes.[14] They expected to have a voice, and often a decisive voice, in the appointment of the priests. They had received legal incorporation as the owners of Catholic ecclesiastical property—often the only way in which such property could be secured under the laws of the various states. Competition between Catholics of different national origins, with their different languages and remembered home customs of their origins, compounded the difficulties. The bishops had to put up with 'trusteeism', whilst declining to admit the right of the laity to exercise ecclesiastical patronage.[15] Where the right was insisted upon there were actual schisms: in Philadelphia in 1802 and between 1820 and 1830, and in Baltimore in 1805. In Ireland, too, lay patronage had produced difficulties. There it was a fruit of the penal laws of the eighteenth century, as local lay Catholics, in the more isolated dioceses, finding canonical jurisdiction interrupted, began to appoint their own incumbents. As in America, the voluntary system of religious endowments provided the justification—those who paid the clergy expected a voice in their appointment. Among Galway Catholics, at the start of the nineteenth century, 'the ecclesiastical government partook in some manner of a Presbyterian or rather popular character',[16] with 'vicars' and 'wardens' elected by the congregations, an emulation of the practices of their Protestant dissenting neighbours. Early in the nineteenth century this was ended by the reimposition of proper episcopal authority: a situation not unlike England's existed, with the bishops seeking to bring regularity and ecclesiastical coherence to a Catholic society disrupted by the external forces of state intervention. But in the second half of the eighteenth century

[14] Theodore Maynard, *The Story of American Catholicism*, New York 1960, I. 177.

[15] P. J. Dignan, *A History of the Legal Incorporation of Catholic Church Property in the United States, 1784–1932*, New York 1935, 266.

[16] W. Maziere Brady, *The Episcopal Succession in England, Scotland and Ireland, 1400 to 1875*, Rome 1876, II. 234.

large numbers of parishes in Ireland had suffered disturbances when distant episcopal authorities had appointed or removed priests without confiding in the parishioners or local lay leaders. Catholic gentry sometimes nominated priests to churches on their estates, just like the Protestant lay patrons. The parish priest of Killarney was appointed by Lord Kenmare until the mid-nineteenth century.[17] In England, the practical exercise of lay patronage was the direct legacy of the position the gentry had acquired under the penal laws. The Council of Trent actually allowed the *jus patronatus* to laymen, provided the selected candidate proved fit for office after examination by a bishop,[18] but it was always supposed that it would be exercised within a settled ecclesiastical polity, under a Catholic government, and not, as in England or North America, in conditions of ecclesiastical irregularity. As the law of England stood, at the start of the nineteenth century, neither the Vicars Apostolic, as bishops, nor the Religious Orders, as religious corporations, could hold property, and whatever they did administer was held as the private property of one or more individuals. Every chapel in England was, in consequence, the property either of the layman who built it or of the committee of trustees. In the most restrictive period of the penal laws the Vicars Apostolic were glad of this situation, and willingly left the owners great discretion or absolute right in appointing the priests. It was widely supposed, by the start of the new century, that donations for new religious enterprises would dry up if the rights of the laity over their gifts were curtailed. It was in this atmosphere that the Vicars Apostolic began their campaign to acquire control of ecclesiastical appointments—a necessary condition, from their point of view, for a properly co-ordinated ministry. In 1819 Cardinal Fontana, the Prefect of Propaganda, expressed his opposition to lay patronage in England, declaring that it had indeed 'encroached upon the canonical rights of the bishops'.[19] As an additional cause of suspicion and dissension between the Old Catholic gentry and the centralizing attitudes of the bishops of the nineteenth century, the issue of

---

[17] Norman, *The Conscience of the State in North America*, 120-1.
[18] Section 24, c.18.
[19] Stonyhurst Archives, Glover's *Excerpts* III, 191.

patronage was often the decisive occasion of dispute; for the Religious Orders also, with their stake in their own rights of patronage against the bishops, it was often a crucial matter. Both in the anonymity of their position before the Relief measure of 1791, and in the relative ease of their public service afterwards, the Benedictines of Ampleforth and Downside, and the Jesuits of Stonyhurst, had established and staffed a considerable number of missions. They exercised, and expected to go on exercising, exactly those rights in them that the Catholic gentry enjoyed in the secular missions they had furnished. The Jesuits in particular were insistent on the *jus patronatus*, admitting that 'it militates against the pretensions of the Vicars Apostolic to be absolute masters of every chapel, and of every pious foundation, made by private individuals'.[20] By the 1840s the Vicars Apostolic were beginning to win the contest for control of the missions: in 1844 Bishop Brown of the Lancashire District (which had been created in 1840), published a Pastoral Letter announcing the abolition of all lay committees for the raising and administration of ecclesiastical funds. It is not clear how widely his example was followed by other bishops,[21] but in practice they were, by one means or another, enforcing their will. It was another problem which was already well on the way to being solved before the re-establishment of the hierarchy finally swept lay patronage away for good.[22]

Apart from the problem of contested patronage, it was the difficulties of finance which most complicated the administration of the Church: letters and appeals for cathedral, church, and school building form the largest bulk in all the surviving papers of nineteenth-century bishops. Most of the missions operated on borrowed money. 'It has been my misery ever since I had a mitre to have to deal with enormous debts and deficits,' Ullathorne observed in 1856; adding, however, 'and if it had not been for the good moral state of the clergy of this diocese I know not how I could have gone

[20] Stonyhurst Archives, Glover's *Excerpts* III, 188. See also Bernard Ward, *Eve*, III. 49.

[21] Bossy, 350.

[22] 'Diocesan Organization and Administration', by Morgan V. Sweeney, in *The English Catholics, 1850–1950*, ed. G. A. Beck, London 1950, 121.

through with it.'[23] The raising of large sums by voluntary contributions for church building was not, of course, a problem for the Catholics alone. It characterized the expansion of all English churches in the nineteenth century—even the Established Church, whose receipt of income from Parliament for such purposes ceased in 1824. For the Protestant Dissenters, the voluntary system of endowments became a badge of Christian authenticity, a symbol of religious vitality and freedom from state control. But for the Catholics voluntaryism operated to produce much greater burdens of debt, for they had to appeal to a membership often of the poor Irish of the towns, who were much less able to donate the required sums than the entrepreneurial or landed wealth available to the Dissenters or the State Churchmen. Two particularly grave, and unhappy, controversies illustrated the Catholic difficulties. When, in August 1846, Ullathorne became Vicar Apostolic of the Western District, he inherited the financial liabilities of Prior Park—the college Baines had established in Bath after the failure of his attempt to convert the Benedictine house at Downside into the seminary of the District. The debts were very considerable, and the situation was made more complicated by the curious position of Dr Brindle, the President, who was the legal trustee of the estate, and who had sunk £5,000 of his own money into the College. Asking to examine the financial papers on his arrival in Bath, Ullathorne was told that there were none: all had been destroyed.[24] As Dom Cuthbert Butler put it, 'an unpleasant controversy ensued'.[25] Brindle decided to detach Prior Park from Ullathorne's District altogether, and to conduct it as an independent lay school. Ullathorne appealed to Rome, and in 1847 secured the appointment of an Apostolical Commission to investigate the finances and management of Prior Park and report to Propaganda. The Commissioners—two Vicars Apostolic, and the President of St. Edmund's, Ware—met at Prior Park for a week, and found that liabilities of £60,000 existed. Total assets amounted only to £20,000. But

[23] Cuthbert Butler, *The Life and Times of Bishop Ullathorne, 1806–1889*, I. 167.
[24] *From Cabin-Boy to Archbishop*, 230.
[25] Cuthbert Butler, I. 142.

they made no recommendations, and no action resulted. Ullathorne, against the advice of his friends, sought to close the college down, and was only prevented from taking the appropriate steps by his fortuitous removal to the Central District in 1848. He wrote at length to Propaganda on the sad state of the College's affairs.[26] Among his last official acts in the Western District was to send Wiseman a sad account of the College's hopeless financial plight.[27] In 1856 Prior Park was closed down and sold up by Archbishop Errington.

The other notable case concerned the finances of the diocese of Southwark. When the hierarchy was set up in 1850, the area to the south of the Thames was detached from the London District—now the diocese of Westminster—and became the independent Southwark diocese, with Thomas Grant as Bishop. Grant became, at once, a victim of Wiseman's inattention to detail: the finances of the London District were not adequately divided and the new diocese of Southwark fell into appalling financial straits. Various entreaties made to Wiseman elicited no result. 'Why is a quarrel to be created between yourself and me,' Grant wrote desperately to Wiseman, 'because of a claim that I surely have, to have the books of the London District examined and its property valued in order that it may be known by means of fair and impartial men whether any and what portion of it really belongs to Southwark?' The Cardinal, he insisted, 'will incur all the blame of an unfair division' unless this was arranged.[28] Grant's attempt to raise funds through a 'Southwark Episcopal Fund' ran into the difficulty that potential subscribers held back until they could see exactly what resources would become available once the London funds were unfrozen by Wiseman. 'No business that your Eminence or I can devise is equal in importance to this', Grant implored, in 1853; 'and I beg your Eminence to consider how often I have waited, how little I have troubled you even when letters stating that I was in debt

[26] Propaganda, *Scritture* 12 (1848–51), 109, *Memorial of Ullathorne to the Cardinal Prefect*, 21 June 1848.

[27] Westminster Dioc. Archives, Wiseman Papers, Bishops' Letters, R7913, Ullathorne to Wiseman, 10 Oct. 1848.

[28] Westminster Dioc. Archives, Wiseman Papers, Bishops' Letters, R79/4, Grant to Wiseman, 18 April (n.d.).

were not believed or at all events not answered.' For nearly two years, he contended, Wiseman had been possessed 'of all the papers by which the affair was to be settled'.[29] When the Cardinal did eventually move, it was to instruct Grant, through Mgr. Searle, to settle the debts of St. George's Cathedral in Southwark before there could be any division of 'other funds' belonging to the diocese. 'I have no other resource but to apply to the Holy See', Grant finally told Wiseman; 'it grieves me that time and money shall be spent upon a journey to Rome, and that I should have to appear on the side of my own Diocese against your Eminence.'[30] Wiseman was outraged. 'The very idea of a suffragan of the new Hierarchy, almost within a year, going off to Rome to carry thither a case against his Metropolitan', he expostulated, 'is fraught with scandal.'[31] But it was Grant's view of the matter which was upheld by Propaganda as a result of the inquiry.[32]

It was, in Baines's words, 'the dissatisfaction and disputes which have constantly subsisted'[33] between the bishops and the Religious Orders which, until the mid-century, proved the greatest impediment to the normal conduct of ecclesiastical administration. The conflict of interests over patronage rights in the missions staffed by the regulars was only the visible sign of deeply held mutual suspicions. Many lay Catholics, and some of the bishops, shared the prevalent English distaste for monasticism as such. Indeed, the objections of some of the Cisalpine leaders to the monastic orders went as far as supporting the proposed expulsion of French *émigré* nuns, when Sir H. Mildmay introduced a parliamentary bill for this purpose in 1800: an unusual departure from the normal

[29] Ibid. 130/1, Grant to Wiseman, 9 Jan. 1853.

[30] Westminster Dioc. Archives, Wiseman Papers, Bishops' Letters, 130/2, Grant to Wiseman, 12 Jan. 1853.

[31] Cuthbert Butler, I. 203. Brian Fothergill, *Nicholas Wiseman*, London 1963, 207-8.

[32] Propaganda, *Scritture* 14 (1855-7), 189, Grant to the Cardinal Prefect, 13 Feb. 1854 [in Italian]. For Wiseman's side of the matter, see ibid. 192, *Observations and Proposals*, drawn up by Wiseman, on the division of the finances, 26 March, 1854 [in Italian].

[33] Downside Archives, I.A. MS *Statement of Facts relative to my dispute with the Monks respectfully submitted to the Arbitrators* ('Dr Bains' Defence'), 1835, 1.

hospitality extended in England to the exiled clergy.[34] Bishop Collingridge, Vicar Apostolic of the Western District, was in 1819 quite prepared to accept legislation for Emancipation which, as a condition, would have sacrificed the regular clergy. Though a Franciscan friar himself, he declared he would not accept any new missions founded in his district by regulars.[35] Gradwell in Rome ensured that the dim view entertained by the bishops of the regulars—a view not shared by Milner—was well represented to the Holy See. His 'assiduous insinuations' were turned especially against the Jesuits.[36] He believed 'that the English Jesuits claimed privileges subversive of the authority of the Vicars Apostolic'.[37] Poynter supposed that the Jesuits were 'labouring to raise in our English mission an *imperium in imperio*'.[38] The sores of discord were opened in 1838 when Rome issued two decrees which gave additional privileges to the regular clergy engaged in the mission (in an attempt to foster the 'Roman spirit'), and authorized the regulars to establish new chapels without reference to the bishops. The second decree, in particular, was regarded by the Vicars Apostolic as, in Baines's words, 'a severe reprimand'.[39] The decrees had been issued without prior consultation with the bishops, who were not mollified by Acton's assurance that normally the regulars would operate in co-operation with them. Experience, they contended, had suggested otherwise. In 1840, as an expression of these heightened antipathies, the secular clergy sent a petition to Rome requesting that regulars be no longer elected as bishops in England. In 1841, Dom Thomas Joseph Brown, the Bishop of Newport and Menevia, wearied by the 'long and scandalous dissensions' suggested a procedure for settling disputes between the Vicars Apostolic and the regulars. Aggrieved parties were to submit to arbitrators appointed by Rome: 'let two Ecclesiastics, secular or regular, be chosen by each party, and let them appoint a fifth'. These would then constitute a committee of inquiry, which,

---

[34] Wilfrid Ward, *The Life and Times of Cardinal Wiseman*, I. 203.
[35] Stonyhurst Archives, Glover's *Excerpts* III, 189.
[36] Ibid. III. 241.
[37] Ibid. III. 244.
[38] Westminster Dioc. Archives, Gradwell Papers, Letter Books B3, Poynter to Gradwell, 11 Sept. 1818.
[39] Bernard Ward, *Sequel*, I. 142–3.

he hoped, would in most cases arrive at an amicable and acceptable solution—only if that was not the case should there be a direct appeal to Propaganda.[40] He put his scheme to Fr. Glover, Provincial of the Jesuits, who replied 'that the conclusions of such Arbiters would satisfy no body'.[41]

Suspicions about the Jesuits were the most strongly held: a situation derived partly from international jealousies about the Society's influence, concentrated in Rome itself and carried to the different countries, and partly from the English demonology of anti-Catholicism, in which the Jesuits were depicted in the most disagreeable fashion. The secular clergy and the Old Catholic laity appeared readily to have absorbed these notions. For such, the Society was identifiable with deviousness and intrigue. It was due to the influence of the Vicars Apostolic that the Bull *Sollicitudo Omnium Ecclesiarum* of 1814, which restored the Society of Jesus throughout the world, was ruled by Rome not to apply in England—a position not reversed until early in 1829. In 1826 Poynter wrote to Fr. Charles Brooke, the English Provincial of the Society, refusing to recognize the existence of the Jesuits in the London District precisely because he contended that the dissolution of the Society still applied: 'I am forbidden by the tenor of a letter addressed to my predecessor by the Cardinal Prefect of Propaganda, dated 3 December 1803, to acknowledge the existence of the Society in the London District, or to admit any of its privileges.'[42] Poynter had, anyway, a long record of opposition to the Jesuits because of the 'false accusations' he once claimed they brought at Rome against the English bishops—accusations intended, in pre-emptive strike, 'to protect themselves against any complaints of the Vicars Apostolic against them'.[43] Friction was common. There exists, in the archives of the Jesuits of Stonyhurst, a letter of 1817 by Bishop Gibson, Vicar Apostolic of the Northern District, replying to an accusation that he had refused faculties to a priest on the grounds that he was a member of the

[40] Jesuit Archives, Farm Street, 'Letters of Bishops and Cardinals, 1753–1853', no. 297, Brown to Glover, 26 June 1841.

[41] Ibid., Brown to Glover (reiterating his response), 24 July 1841.

[42] Jesuit Archives, Farm Street, 'Letters of Bishops and Cardinals, 1753–1853', No. 252, Poynter to Brooke, 26 May 1826.

[43] Westminster Dioc. Archives, Gradwell Papers, Letter Books B3, Poynter to Gradwell, 11 Sept. 1818.

Society. The Bishop's explanation was as legalistic as Poynter's: 'I was commanded by the Propaganda and told by them that there were no Jesuits [in England], neither did I know that he was a Jesuit.' He professed friendliness to Stonyhurst, but then went on to complain about the discourtesy of the Society in not informing him who the Provincial of the Society in England was. An enquiry on his part had once elicited the Jesuit response, he claimed, 'that it was their business at Rome to give me information on that head'.[44] The issue resulted in an appeal to Rome.[45] The delation of Fr. Peter Gandolphy's works to Rome for some years focussed anti-Jesuit sentiments. Gandolphy was a Stonyhurst priest who had once aspired to become Rector of the restored Venerabile. His writings on liturgical questions, and especially his views on the sacraments, were objected to by the Vicars Apostolic (with the usual exception of Milner). Always a controversial figure, he was a successful preacher in the Spanish Chapel in London, where he was said to have converted a number of Protestants. It was, in fact, his published sermons which caused offence to Poynter, who believed that as they were delivered in his District he should have been given the chance to authorize their publication. In 1816 Poynter was already addressing objections about Gandolphy to Propaganda; about his attempts to 'humiliate his bishop'; about his 'siding with certain Protestants'.[46] Gandolphy, also writing to Rome, complained about 'the cruel persecutions that are offered to me' by Poynter.[47] Poynter denounced the book to Rome in 1818 for containing heretical doctrine, adding, in a letter to the Roman agent (at a subsequent stage of the proceedings), 'let it be understood that I never meant that the errors which I extracted from Gandolphy's sermons were *all* that might be extracted'.[48] Cardinal Litta, at Propaganda, had

[44] Stonyhurst Archives, C.IV.1 (62), *Bishop Gibson to the Hon. Stephen Tempest*, 6 May 1817.

[45] Ibid. C.IV.1 (63), *Petition of Mr Stephen Tempest to the Pope to be allowed mass in his Chapel at Broughton Hall* [in Italian], 1817.

[46] Propaganda, *Scritture* 6 (1801–17), 746, 23 Nov. 1816 [in Italian]—see also Cardinal Litta's statement about Gandolphy, ibid. 5 Oct. 1816, 798 [in Latin].

[47] Ibid. 762, 26 Dec. 1816 [in Italian].

[48] Westminster Dioc. Archives, Gradwell Papers, Letter Books B3, Poynter to Gradwell, 2 March 1821.

tried to smooth the ruffled waters by bland references to the possibility of error on both sides: a sentiment that had inflamed the situation still more, appearing to Poynter to presage the sort of line Rome might in general take in other questions of dispute concerning 'Bishops and Jesuits'.[49] Assured by the agent that Gandolphy's sermons had been placed on the Index,[50] Poynter suspended him. The Jesuits claimed that the book had not in fact been censured by Rome, but that 'at most some objectionable phrases were ordered to be corrected'.[51] 'Surely the Holy See does not intend to punish me further and unnecessarily!' the poor man wrote to Cardinal Litta in April 1818: 'I have perhaps written inaccurately—but I have copied the inaccuracies of others under the very eye of my own Bishops, and we have not a work in English perhaps that is less inaccurate than mine.'[52] After three appeals to Rome, Gandolphy died, as the Jesuits maintained, 'of a broken heart'; Glover adding, 'and the Bishop is said to have shed tears when he heard of his death'.[53] Glover's defence of the Society against the Vicars Apostolic was in characteristically heightened tones. 'Every engine was at work in Rome, and the vilest and the falsest accusations were employed to effect our ruin,' he recorded of the position in general; 'The imputation of disorderly, violent, rebellious conduct towards the Vicars Apostolic was as false as the gates of Hell . . . they renewed the old pretence that Stonyhurst withdrew young men from their seminaries, and withheld them from their proper districts.'[54] In such an atmosphere of vituperation, it is hardly surprising that relations between the Society and the bishops continued to be difficult. Yet the two sides had a common meeting ground—a ground of conflict, as it often turned out: the missions founded or staffed by members of the Society. Rancorous disputes sometimes occurred, as at

[49] Ibid. B.3, Poynter to Gradwell, 11 Sept. 1818. See Poynter's manifesto on the Gandolphy affair, addressed to Propaganda on 15 Feb. 1820, in Propaganda *Scritture* 7 (1818–22), 450 [in Italian].

[50] Westminster Dioc. Archives, Gradwell Papers, Letter Books B3, Gradwell to Poynter, 22 March 1821.

[51] Stonyhurst Archives, Glover's *Excerpts* III, 247.

[52] Propaganda, *Scritture* 7 (1818–22), 64, 3 April 1818 [in English].

[53] Stonyhurst Archives, Glover's *Excerpts* III, 247.

[54] Ibid. III. 185.

Wigan after 1818, when Bishop Gibson set up a new chapel, run by a secular priest, only a hundred yards distant from the existing Chapel conducted by the Jesuits of Stonyhurst. The *scritture* of Propaganda for 1818 are full of letters about the affair. Feelings, as usual, ran rather high, and in August Charles Plowden was writing from Stonyhurst to Cardinal Litta about the 'falsehoods' in Poynter's account of the Wigan dispute.[55]

The Benedictines of Ampleforth and Downside also had a considerable stake in ordinary mission work, supplying priests to 'parishes' within the Districts of the Vicars Apostolic—especially in the Western District. 'There is hardly any mission in the Western District, to a distance of some twenty miles from our Monastery', the Prior of Downside told Cardinal Capellari in 1829, 'which we have not aided.'[56] Difficulties between themselves and the Vicars Apostolic were less sharp and less frequent than with the Jesuits, but were still not un-common—even in the Western District, where the bishop was normally chosen from among the religious orders. In the second of his reports commissioned by Propaganda in 1847, on the state of the Church in England, Fr. Luigi Gentili claimed that the Benedictines fostered an anti-episcopal spirit, and were always ready to condemn whatever the Vicars Apostolic did.[57] As a member of a different order he might perhaps have exaggerated. But the Benedictines were extremely jeal-ous of their privileges and sought to press ancient territorial claims dating from before the Reformation which, had they succeeded, would have done enormous damage to the bishops' normal conduct of ecclesiastical affairs. Petitioning Gregory XVI against a restoration of the hierarchy, for example, the English Congregation of Benedictines urged an eventual re-turn to them of the same dioceses they had controlled before the Reformation: 'We have ever cherished these peculiar rights of the Benedictine Cathedral Priors and Chapters as the most valuable and glorious privileges of our Benedictine forefathers, and in obedience to your illustrious predecessor, Urban 8th,

---

[55] Propaganda, *Scritture* 7 (1818–22), 53, 9 Aug. 1818 [in English].

[56] See Propaganda, *Scritture* 7 (1818–22), 17: the English Jesuits to the Cardinal Prefect [in Italian].

[57] Leetham, *Luigi Gentili*, 287.

in his "Bulla Plantata", we have carefully kept up the canonical Election of those Cathedral Priors, looking forward to the
ultimate restoration of our ancient Hierarchy, when they
would return to their canonical rights and privileges.'[58] Almost
nothing could have induced greater chill in the hearts of the
Vicars Apostolic than claims like these.

Disputes between the orders themselves also occurred, particularly after the introduction of the new orders in the wake
of Wiseman's 'Romanizing' policy. The new orders did, however, probably have the general effect of easing relations
between the regulars and the seculars because they worked in
ordinary missions with the direct permission of the Vicars
Apostolic—making no claims to patronage or other proprietor-
ial rights as the Jesuits or the Benedictines did. But in some
ways they heightened rivalries between the orders, especially
where there was distrust of the new devotional practices they
did so much to introduce. There is a collection of letters in
the Jesuit archives in Farm Street which interestingly exemp-
lifies this. They are between Fr. Frederick William Faber and
Cardinal Wiseman and relate to objections raised against
Faber's writings by Fr. Waterworth, Superior of the Jesuits.
The correspondence began in August 1856, when Faber appealed formally to Wiseman to inquire into allegations report-
edly made to Mgr. Talbot in Rome, by Waterworth, that
Faber's books—and especially *All For Jesus*—contained heresies. 'How far Fr. Waterworth, from the position he holds, is
simply the mouthpiece and representative of the Society in
England, I do not know', Faber explained, but, as he added,
'my books have had an immense sale, gone through many
editions, and translated into four, some into five, languages.'[59]
Wiseman was appropriately impressed by this last point, and
reported it in his subsequent letter to Waterworth, pointing
out that in consequence 'the charge of heresy in his writings
is a serious one'.[60] He asked merely for a clear explanation.

[58] Downside Archives, VII.A.3.A, Abbots' Papers (File marked 'Hierarchy,
preparatory to'), MS *Address to Gregory XVI from the English Congregation of
Benedictines* (n.d.).
[59] Jesuit Archives, Farm Street, 'Letters of Bishops and Cardinals, 1840–1891'
no. 28, Faber to Wiseman, 'Feast of St. Rose' [23 Aug.], 1856.
[60] Ibid. no. 31, Wiseman to Waterworth, 3 Sept. 1856.

This he got: a lucid denial that he had delated Faber to Talbot. 'I am free, however, to say that in the Confessional these books have caused me much pain, much trouble, and much anxiety,' he added; '*others* felt the books were strange . . . they said they had never been taught what was now propounded.'[61] Faber's baroque spirituality and extravagant emotions were clearly the issues, the underlying cause of antipathy for Catholics of the older styles of English devotional practice. But for Wiseman, at any rate, there was temporary relief: he had defused at least one potential explosion between the contending parties, and wrote hopefully to the English Provincial of the Jesuits announcing that the issue was closed.[62]

In 1881 the Constitution *Romanos Pontifices*, on the position of the regulars engaged in the ordinary parochial work of the English Church, upheld the claims of the bishops by declaring that the missions conducted by the orders were on the same basis as all others. Parish schools run by the orders were also to be subject to episcopal visitation. Furthermore, the missions of the regulars could henceforth be divided by the authority of the bishops and a secular priest appointed to the new mission so created[63]—a crucial change in view of the multiplying problems of the large urban parishes. The number of bishops elevated from among the regulars also declined after 1850: in the hundred years following, all but seven came from the secular clergy.[64] Since around a third of the clergy continued to be members of the religious orders, this in itself testifies to the success of the seculars in gaining control of the Church.

It would be mistaken to dismiss the disputes of the regulars and the seculars as matters of petty jealousy, born of unnecessary rivalries. Some important principles were at issue between the contending parties which, in general, each believed crucial for the furtherance of Catholic truth in England. Motivation was usually inspired by religious principle rather than personal aggrandisement, by the rights of institutions to

---

[61] Ibid. no. 35, Waterworth to Wiseman, 10 Sept. 1856.
[62] Ibid. no. 39, Wiseman to Fr. F. Johnson, 12 Nov. 1856.
[63] Morgan V. Sweeney, in *The English Catholics*, ed. Beck, 140.
[64] Philip Hughes, 'The Bishops of the Century', ibid., 187.

propagate Catholicism in their own tradition. Perhaps the most well-known of these disputes was that between Bishop Baines and the monks of St Gregory's monastery at Downside; and its importance requires a lengthy examination. It illustrates precisely the religious senses involved on both sides, though perceived externally in personal animosities. Peter Augustine Baines was born in Lancashire in 1787, and educated in Hanover and then at Ampleforth—where, in 1804, he was professed in the Benedictine order. In 1817 he was sent to the Bath mission, and it was there, in 1823, that he was consecrated, with the title of Bishop of Siga, as coadjutor to Bishop Collingridge, Vicar Apostolic of the Western District—whom he succeeded in 1829. As a result of his dispute with Downside, and his Pastoral of 1840 which criticized Wiseman's prayers for the conversion of England, Baines acquired an enduring reputation as a difficult man, a controversialist. The Downside monks, not unnaturally, accused him of seeking 'dissensions and party spirit';[65] Ward wrote that 'his episcopate was in fact one continued history of quarrels and disputes.'[66] His sympathy for the Jesuits, which became particularly evident during his visit to Rome in 1826 and 1827, did nothing to endear him to other regulars or to the secular clergy. 'By little and little he became acquainted with all the unfair proceedings which had long been practised in Rome against the English Jesuits,' Glover recorded.[67] Baines in fact was a man of firm principle who was exceedingly anxious about the future conduct of the Church in the Western District. He projected its advance (not in the dramatic style of mass conversions entertained by Wiseman) in careful preparation and gradual consolidation—and, though a Benedictine, envisaged a Church controlled by episcopal authority and integrated fully with the system of Vicariates. Hence the supreme importance he attached to the training of the clergy.

This involved a major problem. There did not exist, in the Western District, a seminary for the clergy, and Baines's first task, on becoming Collingridge's coadjutor, was to try to

---

[65] Downside Archives, VII.A.3.h. Box 1419, 'List of Accusations of Eng. Ben. Cong. against Dr. Baines,' (1832), 2.

[66] Bernard Ward, *Sequel*, I. 12.

[67] Stonyhurst Archives, Glover's *Excerpts* III, 244.

establish one. Since very many of the existing clergy in the missions of the District were regulars, the need had not seemed pressing all the time it was assumed that the future expansion of the missions was to continue as in the past—as an enterprise intended to foster the monopoly of the Benedictines in certain areas. Baines did not believe that this was appropriate to the England of the nineteenth century, with its expanding industrial centres and its powerful Protestant tone. He at once set out to create a proper seminary for the training of secular priests. With the permission of Collingridge, he approached Downside in the hope that the monastery could be converted into a seminary, with himself and his successors as its head.[68] Dr Richard Marsh, the President General of the Benedictines—who 'was looked up to as a man who had done incomparably more for the Order than any other man', as Ullathorne (a monk at Downside himself in these years) recollected[69]—agreed to the plan. So Baines entered into confidential discussion with Prior Barber at Downside in 1823, professing that his proposal was intended 'to benefit the Benedictine body',[70] who would, indeed, receive proper episcopal support and direction for their missionary work. Nor was the plan inconsistent with the Benedictine rule: monasteries had often existed under episcopal superiors even when the bishop was not himself a regular.[71] For the monks of Downside, however, the scheme had quite another complexion. Wounded by what seemed a graceless attitude to their past efforts in the missions, and unable to see why their house should be handed over to Baines, they rejected the plan. They were monks: they could not agree to the withdrawal from the English Benedictine Congregation that Baines's proposals required. 'His restless disposition while within his own monastery at Ampleforth was known to them by repute.'[72] Next, Baines suggested an exchange of property

---

[68] Downside Archives, I. A. MS 'A Statement of Facts relative to my dispute with the Monks, respectfully submitted to the Arbiters ('Dr Baines' Defence'), July 1835, 1. For a general account of the controversy, see J. S. Roche, *A History of Prior Park College and its Founder, Bishop Baines*, London 1931.

[69] *From Cabin-Boy to Archbishop*, 43.

[70] Downside Archives, I.A.3, 'Dr Baines' Defence'.

[71] Bernard Ward, *Sequel*, I. 16.

[72] Ibid. I. 18.

with Ampleforth—who were agreeable both to this and to the original plan—so that the Ampleforth monks, transferred to the Downside buildings, could operate the proposed seminary. Arbitrators were to be approached to arrange the swap. The Downside monks rejected this also. By then the whole Benedictine Congregation in England was divided over the Baines schemes, and Ampleforth, too, was riven by internal dissensions, some of them originating from before the seminary issue. Matters were brought to precipitation in July 1826, when the General Chapter of the Benedictines, which was held every four years, failed to invite Baines to attend, although his predecessors in the Order had always been invited. They simply wanted to discuss the Baines plan—quite apart from routine business—without the inhibiting effect his presence would have had. Baines, not surprisingly, felt he had been badly snubbed. Already the affair had reached the proportions at which personal suspicions were beginning to overshadow the original contentions. Some of the Benedictines, led by Prior Burgess of Ampleforth, presented an address to Baines, regretting his exclusion from the Chapter. The majority proceeded to elect, as their new President-General, one of Baines's most determined opponents. This was John Augustine Birdsall: a person, as Baines himself reflected, 'best suited to wage war with a Bishop'.[73] 'The sternest man I ever knew,' Ullathorne remarked of him; 'so that the younger monks trembled to approach him.' He added, 'I do not think he was aware to what extent his manner and tone were trying to those who had relations of duty with him.'[74] But represented in another fashion, Birdsall's determination to preserve the Benedictine inheritance intact at Downside was exactly what the monks required to match Baines's not dissimilar qualities exercised on behalf of the interests of the District. Birdsall's rigidity, furthermore, sprang from a deep personal commitment to the Benedictine Rule: it was reinforced by the highest motives of religious integrity. The grand issue of the seminary reached stalemate. Reduced to ill-health by the cares of his episcopal duties, Baines departed for

---

[73] Downside Archives, I.A.9, 'Dr Baines' Defence.'
[74] *From Cabin-Boy to Archbishop*, 43.

Rome for what proved to be a lengthy visit—from the autumn of 1826 until the spring of 1829, when, on Collingridge's death, he returned to Bath as Vicar Apostolic.

In Rome, he presented his view of the Downside dispute to Cardinal Capellari, the Prefect of Propaganda, whose initial judgements on the matter he found 'most just and equitable'.[75] The Pope, too, 'loved to converse with him, and listened with attention to every information which the Bishop gave him respecting the English mission in general'.[76] In fact, so favourably did Leo XII come to regard Baines that he was only prevented by death from making him a Cardinal. Capellari seems to have been persuaded of the virtues of Baines's plan for Downside, and agreed to write a conciliatory letter to Prior Barber urging him to give renewed consideration to it. He also appears to have agreed with another of Baines's contentions, derived from research in the Archives of Propaganda undertaken during his sojourn in Rome: that the English Benedictines were irregularly constituted. Though highly formalistic to modern judgement, this sort of case had just the sort of legal authority which most appealed in the Curia at the time: indeed there is some evidence, from both sides in the dispute, that it was Capellari who first suggested to Baines that the case might be made out on such grounds.[77] The contention was quite simply that the Benedictine house at Downside had been re-established in England without the specific permission of the Holy See or the consent of the Vicars Apostolic. If sustained, this would have removed the exemption from episcopal control enjoyed by the monks of Downside and so destroyed the grounds of their resistance to Baines's plans.[78] Baines at first did not question the canonicity of Ampleforth; 'knowing', as the Downside monks argued, that both Benedictine houses had in fact 'been instituted under exactly similar circumstances'.[79] They rushed to scrutinize their ecclesiastical title deeds, instructing Dom Joseph Brown,

[75] Downside Archives, I.A.11, 'Dr Baines' Defence'.
[76] Stonyhurst Archives, Glover's *Excerpts* III, 249.
[77] Downside Archives, I.A.11, 'Dr Baines' Defence'; Allanson Records, I.A.III. 83.
[78] Ibid. VII.A.3.h. Box 1419, 'List of Accusations', 6.
[79] Ibid. 4.

an expert in ecclesiastical law, to report on the matter. After putting questions to senior theologians in Rome he produced a lengthy statement which conceded that the specific permission to reintroduce Benedictine vows to England had *not* been obtained, but arguing that their canonicity had been established by use—that the consent of the bishops had derived from their acceptance of the Benedictine houses, without the need of formal documentary authority.[80] It was a case about as formalistic as Baines's original one. Birdsall had already reinforced it with the claim that a letter sent by Pius VII to Dr Marsh, his predecessor, in 1823, had recognized the transfer of the monks to Downside. All the bishops, he told Propaganda, had before treated the monastery 'with favour and benignly'.[81]

On his return to England in 1829, Baines sent Cardinal Capellari's letter, beseeching the monks to reconsider the seminary plan, on to Downside. Baines, he wrote, had complained of their '*indocilitate*'; and his plans 'seem to me to be very fair, so I urge you, indeed I beg and entreat you, to see that you accede to them with the utmost possible eagerness'.[82] In the next month the Cardinal wrote again, 'Concerning the rights of the parties,' he wrote, 'I do not pronounce in favour of either, but only propose to you an amicable method of avoiding litigation and of pleasant conciliation.'[83] Shortly afterwards, he added (of the possibility of a settlement): 'I do not consider this very difficult.'[84] But he was wrong. Birdsall was unmoved. At the start of October Barber and Brown, representing the Downside monks, called on Baines to state that they would not comply with the Cardinal's advice, but wished to consult with the superiors of the Congregation before deciding upon a reply. 'I had great reason to complain of the behaviour of these gentlemen on this occasion', Baines

[80] Ibid., Allanson Records, I.A.III, 304, Joseph Brown to President Birdsall, on the validity of the vows made in the convents of England, 23 April 1830.

[81] Propaganda, *Scritture* 8 (1823-33), 576, President Birdsall to Cardinal Capellari, 18 June 1829 [in Latin]. For the text of the Rescript, of 13 June 1823 [in Latin] see Allanson Records, ibid. 91.

[82] Downside Archives, Allanson Records, 98, Cardinal Capellari to the Prior and Convent of St. Gregory, 28 July 1829 [in Latin].

[83] Ibid. 96, 8 Aug. 1829 [in Latin].

[84] Ibid. 101, 12 Aug. 1829 [in Latin].

subsequently recalled; 'It was lofty and contemptuous, and on one occasion insolent.'[85] Early in November there was an acrimonious exchange of letters between Baines and Prior Barber—the latter maintaining that Capellari's letter was 'grounded on great misconception of the facts'. He refused to show the grounds on which the monks claimed exemption from episcopal jurisdiction, and announced, instead, that 'the merits of the case are however in process of being submitted to the wisdom of the Holy See'.[86] Stung by the inference that he had fed inaccurate information to the Cardinal, Baines replied: 'Your insinuation that those facts were misconceived would have been better not made.'[87] He proceeded to withdraw 'from every Priest residing in your House whatever Faculties any of you hold from the Vicar Apostolic of this District'.[88] This action, an extremely drastic one, as he later wrote, 'was bringing the question to a fair trial'. For, 'as I had reason to feel quite confident that they were not canonically instituted, I flattered myself that when the Faculties were withdrawn they would not dare to administer the sacraments even within their own House, in which case they would tacitly acknowledge their dependence, and must come to some arrangement'.[89] He was mistaken. The monks continued to administer the sacraments inside the monastery during the period of the Downside interdict; confessions of the servants and lay congregation were received by a priest who came out from Bath and heard them in the brewery 'seated on a tub'.[90] Baines also forbade all Chapel door collections in the missions run by the Benedictines, claiming that they diminished the flow of financial assistance to the District.[91] A dispute ensued about the incumbency of the Benedictine Church in Bath— with yet a further appeal to Propaganda.[92]

[85] Ibid. I.A.13. 'Dr Baines' Defence'.

[86] Ibid. VII.A.3.h. Box 1419, Barber to Baines, 6 Nov. 1829. Also in I.A., Allanson Records, III.145.

[87] Ibid. I.A. Allanson Records, III.146, Baines to Barber, 7 Nov. 1829.

[88] Ibid. 147.

[89] Downside Archives, I.A.17 'Dr Baines' Defence'.

[90] *From Cabin-Boy to Archbishop*, 44.

[91] Downside Archives, VII.A.3.h. Box 1419, 16.

[92] Propaganda, *Scritture* 8 (1823–33), 757, Baines to the Cardinal Prefect, 10 Nov. 1831 [in Italian].

Meanwhile the Downside deputation proceeded to Rome, prepared 'to repudiate the allegations which have sprung up on all sides'.[93] It consisted of Dr Richard Marsh (now the Vice-President and titular Prior of Canterbury Cathedral) and Dom Joseph Brown. Their reception was initially rather less than cordial: their own Order refused to provide them with accommodation. But by January 1830 the degree of their success in persuading Capellari to re-assess his first judgements became clear in the altered tone of his letters to Baines.[94] 'The evil was increased by the system adopted at Propaganda of not allowing the accused party to see the charges brought against him', Baines lamented. 'Under this cover the Benedictine monks grew bold, and poured in a succession of complaints, which, for violence, inaccuracy and hostility, are, I trust, unrivalled.'[95] He was even accused of having dishonestly appropriated £5,000; not to speak of 'abusing the sacred power' entrusted to him as a bishop, and 'countenancing perjury'.[96] 'Of what avail could be the most solemn declarations of a single bishop against the united attestations of a whole General Chapter of Religious men?' he asked.[97] The tables had indeed been turned. The immediate cause of most of the accusations was Baines's implementation of his second plan—for a secular seminary independent of the Downside scheme. This involved (with their agreement) the secularization of four of the Ampleforth monks, including the Prior, and their removal to Bath, together with some thirty boys from their school, to found a school and seminary for the Western District. Baines had spent three months at Ampleforth, just after his return from Rome, setting up the new enterprise. While there, according to the Downside complainants, he endeavoured 'to subvert all the principles of duty and obligation by which Religious houses and Religious are bound together'.[98] The charges of financial malpractice related to a mortgage procured on one of the Ampleforth properties by the departing Prior and to the removal of various articles to Bath; and

[93] Downside Archives, I.A. Allanson Records, III.102, Prior and Convent of St. Gregory to Cardinal Capellari, 27 Oct. 1829 [in Latin].
[94] Ibid. I.A, 19, 'Dr Baines' Defence'.
[95] Downside Archives, I.A.85.
[96] Ibid. 87.
[97] Ibid. 89.
[98] Ibid. VII.A.3.h. Box 1419, 8.

that the pro-Baines party at Ampleforth had 'scratched out and changed various entries in the books of money received and had substituted new ones'.[99] There was even a suggestion that an aged dependant of the monastery, who might have spilled the beans, was abducted.[100] Despite these regrettable allegations, however, Rome sanctioned the removal of the Ampleforth superiors to Bath—to the grandiose mansion which Baines had acquired for his new seminary. Both the purchase of Prior Park and its subsequent maintenance stretched the finances of the Western District rather further than they could bear. The costs of adaptation to ecclesiastical use were also considerable. The existing pagan statues of classical gods and heroes that adorned the façade were 'manipulated with canvas and plaster, and made to represent two rows of saints'. Hercules was crowned with a triple tiara, and a cross placed in his hand (to obscure the club he actually held) and became St. Gregory the Great.[101] It was a bold venture. Unhappily the mansion was extensively damaged by a great fire in 1836, and this effectively ruined its financial viability. Baines's alternative seminary was born to troubles. After the failure of Wiseman to act as intermediary between the bishop and the monks, during his visit to Prior Park in September 1832, Baines managed to get an inquiry by independent arbitrators appointed by Propaganda. Both sides produced lengthy statements of their grievances. Baines was found to be legally correct in most of his claims, especially on the question of canonical regularity, but Rome recognised the *de facto* situation of the Benedictines in England and issued a *sanatio* indemnifying them against past accidental illegalities and guaranteeing their position, independently of episcopal jurisdiction, for the future. Baines died in July 1843. His earthly remains were eventually deposited in the north aisle of Downside Abbey Church; his recumbent effigy represented in gothic vestments—a final sad fate for one whose dislike of the gothic style was maintained with characteristic vigour. He was a very great prelate.

The disputations between the Vicars Apostolic and the

[99] Downside Archives, VII.A.3.h. Box 1419, 10.
[100] Ibid. 11.
[101] *From Cabin-Boy to Archbishop*, 227.

Regulars were among the reasons which eventually converted
the bishops to the need for an English hierarchy—as a way of
consolidating their control over the Church. The movement
for a hierarchy did not originate with them, however, and it
at first had quite different, and rival, purposes. Both the lay
Catholic 'nobility and gentry' who were originally interested
in a proper return to episcopal government, and 'Old Catholic'
clergy, were concerned to secure a more effective voice for the
laity and the lower clergy in the government of the Church.
Their opposition to the continuation of the Vicariates was
precisely because they gave the holders too much summary
authority—the delegated authority of the Pope himself. Hence
the pioneering work of the Catholic Committee for a hierarchy, from 1782. It was concerned with securing lay rights
in the patronage of the missions. Hence, also, the agitation
for a hierarchy of the so-called 'Staffordshire clergy' group—
whom Milner opposed with determination. They looked for a
voice in the election of bishops, for subdivision of the Districts, the election of chapters, and the creation of a normal
parochial system in which the incumbents had rights against
removal by the episcopate. It was the petition of the Northern
Clergy for these 'rights', sent to Propaganda in 1837, that
finally persuaded the Vicars Apostolic of the need to capture
the movement for a hierarchy before it was turned too decisively against their interests. 'Unacquainted as they mostly
were with the principles and practice of ecclesiastical law', as
Ullathorne wrote in his *History of the Restoration of the
Catholic Hierarchy in England*, 'and mainly guided by anal-
ogies drawn from the civil constitution of their country, they
were not unfrequently impressed with the notion that the
Vicars Apostolic were favoured at their expense.'[102] It was a
feeling with which he had some sympathy. He was aware that
many Protestant politicians supposed that an administration
by ordinary Catholic bishops would produce 'a nearer resem-
blance to the character of the British Constitution, and
would set limits to the action of the Pope in English Catholic
affairs'.[103] This was among the reasons—false ones as it turned

[102] Bernard Ullathorne, *History of the Restoration of the Catholic Hierarchy
in England*, London 1871, 4.
[103] Ibid. 15.

out—that persuaded some exponents of the hierarchy that it would prove acceptable to the Protestant temper of the country. Father Mark Tierney, chaplain to the Duke of Norfolk, was a leading clerical advocate of the rights of the clergy, who looked to a hierarchy as the means of securing them; so was Dr Daniel Rock, Chaplain at Alton Towers, seat of the Earl of Shrewsbury. In 1838 Rock joined other priests of the Midland District (and in opposition to Bishop Walsh, the Vicar Apostolic) in agitating for a hierarchy. In 1840 Rock moved to the London District and joined the Adelphi Club—a group of clergy (120 in number by 1843) concerned to promote the idea of hierarchy.[104] In July 1839, in petitioning the Pope in gratitude for the proposal to increase the number of Vicariates, an influential body of the laity—Lord Petre and forty others—took the opportunity to enter a respectful protest about the continued absence of participatory rights. 'More especially,' they told Gregory XVI, 'we find that attempts are being made, with the risk of fomenting dissension among us, to deprive of the expected privilege of voting in the election of chapters and of Vicars Apostolic, those missionaries who belong to religious orders, although when employed on the mission they are as much as the seculars amenable and subject to the legitimate jurisdiction of the Vicars Apostolic.'[105] They urged equal electoral rights for all the lower clergy. It is interesting to notice how readily the laity could combine with the regulars—for whom they at times experienced an 'English' antipathy—when it came to the common defence of patronage rights or other means of limiting the centralizing tendencies of the Vicars Apostolic. For the bishops themselves, the issue of the hierarchy became a crucial one of defending episcopal jurisdiction.

The first episcopal interest in ordinary ecclesiastical government had occurred in the wake of the Relief Act of 1791. In 1815, while in Rome, Poynter had made actual proposals in the form of a draft scheme—never presented because the Pope had left the city for Genoa. The plan included a properly

[104] Kathleen O'Meara, *Thomas Grant*, 52–4.
[105] Downside Archives, VII.A.3.a, Abbots' Papers (File marked 'Hierarchy, Preparatory to'), MS *Petition to Pope Gregory XVI from the Laity*, 26 July 1839.

constituted parochial system.[106] In 1833 a correspondence on the matter took place in the *Catholic Magazine*. But with awareness of the threats to their jurisdiction inherent in the proposals made by the laity and the lower clergy in the later 1830s, episcopal concern to control the movement for a hierarchy increased. At their meeting in January of 1837 the Vicars Apostolic decided to draw up an actual plan. Informed by Wiseman, then still agent in Rome, that the Pope was at least willing to consider increasing the number of bishops in England, Thomas Walsh of the Midland District and Thomas Griffiths of the London District left for Rome, in April. In audience, Gregory XVI told them that he would indeed increase the Vicariates, but was unwilling to contemplate a restoration of the hierarchy[107]—apparently because he feared the British government would try to interfere in the nomination of the new bishops. His supposition was not unreasonably based. The long debates over the Veto at the time of Emancipation had shown how divisive the mere idea of state intervention could be, and in October 1829, in fact (after Emancipation had passed) Wellington, as Prime Minister, had tried to exert pressure at Rome over the selection for the vacant Catholic see of Waterford.[108] The matter continued to give concern. In his reports to Rome in 1847, Gentili stressed the dangers of government intervention in Catholic ecclesiastical jurisdiction,[109] and in their petition to Rome against a hierarchy, the English Benedictines declared their 'serious doubts, when we witness the jealousy and prejudices of our Protestant Fellow Countrymen against our Holy Religion, whether our Civil Rulers might not be forced to interfere on our assumption of the title of Ordinary Bishops, and thus perhaps by new enactments retard the gradual progress of Catholicity amongst us'.[110] In view of the Ecclesiastical Titles Act, in 1851, it was a prophetic statement. Overseas, too, the British government had expected some voice in Catholic episcopal

---

[106] Bernard Ward, *Sequel*, I. 8–9.

[107] Bernard Ward, *Sequel*, I. 127.

[108] Brose, *Church and Parliament*, Stanford 1959, 19.

[109] Leetham, 294.

[110] Downside Archives, VII.A.3.a, Abbots' Papers (File marked 'Hierarchy, Prepartory to'), MS *Address to Gregory XVI from the English Congregation of Benedictines*, n.d.

appointments in those territories where it gave financial assistance to the Church. At the start of the nineteenth century, for example, Sir James Craig, when Governor of Quebec, had demanded the right to nominate Catholic parish priests and had even got the acquiescence of Bishop Denaut; and in 1824 Lord Dalhousie had revived the claim.[111]

Meeting at York in April 1838, the Vicars Apostolic resolved for a division of the existing Districts and the creation of more bishops. They also, in their *Statuta Provisoria*, allowed a voice to the lower clergy in the election of bishops. They were anyway acting in response to an invitation from Cardinal Fransoni at Propaganda, and Rome (in the resulting *Statuta Proposita*) sanctioned the expansion of the Vicariates. In 1840, therefore, the Eastern, Central, Welsh, and Lancastrian Districts were created. External events operated to keep the notion of a proper hierarchy alive: in 1840 a hierarchy for Australia was sanctioned by Rome. The prevailing English voices in Rome were still cautious, however. Cardinal Acton was hostile. Wiseman, while he believed that the existing form of Church government was 'necessarily a temporary and transitory one, preparatory to a settled and normal state', also expressed himself not 'anxious for changes, or desirous of hurrying matters'.[112] Gentili—widely thought to be actively engaged in seeking to persuade Rome against a hierarchy—was indeed opposed, but took no part in the question. But the reports he wrote at the invitation of Cardinal Fransoni, on the condition of the English Church, were certainly little calculated to favour ecclesiastical autonomy—'because the English Clergy are infected with Gallicanism and are dominated by a spirit of ambition and independence'.[113] In his report of June 1847, which deals explicitly with the hierarchy question, Gentili offered the view that if regularized, the bishops would merely change their titles but actually go on exactly as before. He advised Propaganda *not* to tell the English bishops about any schemes for a hierarchy, 'for in

---

[111] Norman, *The Conscience of the State in North America*, 129–30.

[112] Wiseman, *Essays on Various Subjects*, I. 341, 'A Paper on Ecclesiastical Organization' (reprinted from the *Dublin Review* of Aug. 1842).

[113] Claude Leetham, 'Gentili's Reports to Rome', in the *Wiseman Review*, no. 498 (Winter, 1963–4), 398.

England, if anything is planned, it at once gets into the papers
. . . It is one of the weaknesses of this nation that they cannot keep a secret.'[114] No wonder the English mission was the
despair of the Roman officials, for whom secrecy and discretion were the tools of trade.

Wiseman arrived in Rome, accompanied by Bishop James
Sharples, as the representatives of the English Vicars Apostolic, and deputed to present their views on the need for a
hierarchy, in July 1847. The new Pope, Pius IX, was more
sympathetic than his predecessor. After three times offering
mass for light, he decided in favour. The death of Cardinal
Acton assisted matters. In August Walsh died also, and
Wiseman was translated to the London District, a move which
already led some to suppose that Rome was preparing him to
lead the restored hierarchy. In October, Propaganda ordered
the Vicars Apostolic to formulate concrete proposals; they
met in London during November and did so. In Rome, meanwhile, a simple plan for converting the existing eight Vicariates into eight sees had been favoured. On 1 November
Apostolic Letters entitled *Universalis Ecclesiae* were drawn
up, and briefs, nominating bishops to the sees, were dated for
24 November. These were the documents which were shown
to Lord Minto, then in Rome to explore the possibility of
diplomatic relations between the British Crown and the Holy
See. But then began the delays. Doubts were expressed about
the appointment of Wiseman as the first metropolitan archbishop: he was very junior among the existing Vicars Apostolic, and distrust about his style and 'Romanizing', agreeable
though it was to the Curia, had already made him something
of a controversial figure within English Catholicism. There
were also legal problems about the titles of the new sees.
English law, reinforced by the provisions of the Emancipation
Act itself, prohibited the assumption of ecclesiastical titles
already in use by the State Church, yet the Catholics were reluctant to concede the legitimacy of what, to them, appeared
as an alien occupation of ancient sees, with their spiritual and
historical associations with the Catholic past. As the complications stacked up, Grant felt increasingly unable to cope as

[114] Leetham, *Luigi Gentili*, 298.

agent in Rome, and the Vicars Apostolic sent Ullathorne out to conduct matters on their behalf. Grant's role was in consequence slight, but he did draw up some of the subsequent documents[115]—particularly relating to the question of the ancient sees.[116] In Ullathorne's own recollection, he was 'the chief negotiator in bringing the plan to its conclusion';[117] and this is probably correct, at least as far as the English were concerned. The plan was really devised in Rome, however, by the experts at Propaganda, and by the advisory commission of seven cardinals appointed for the purpose by the Pope. Ullathorne arrived in May 1848. For the advice of Barnabò, and to guide the commission of cardinals, he drew up, during the next two months, a number of documents.[118] In correspondence with Wiseman he explained the situation very fully. 'Barnabò told me his object was to establish the Hierarchy and to let the rest develop out of that in due time,' he wrote in July.[119] This was the course favoured by Ullathorne himself: a simple restoration, leaving the subsequent Provincial and diocesan synods to evolve the appropriate detailed provisions of ordinary ecclesiastical jurisdiction. The cardinals desired no further reference to the Vicars Apostolic, since they had Ullathorne as accredited representative, and were happy to expedite matters. Delays continued, however. The cardinals did support the expressed objection of the English bishops 'against lay interference' in the matter.[120] Ullathorne advised against the legal complication of opting for ancient sees. 'The Pope', he told Wiseman, 'is very anxious to see our affairs brought to a conclusion.'[121] Yet the delays continued until, on 17 July, the commission of cardinals finally held their second special meeting and the scheme was approved. Walsh was to be moved to London as the head of the hierarchy, and the titles of the new sees were to be delayed until

[115] O'Meara, *Thomas Grant*, 62.

[116] Gordon Albion, 'The Restoration of the Hierarchy', in *The English Catholics, 1850–1950*, ed. G. A. Beck, 92.

[117] Ullathorne, *History of the Restoration of the Catholic Hierarchy*, iii.

[118] Propaganda, *Scritture* 12 (1848–51), 143–89, 194. The Archives of Propaganda contain 14 documents drawn up by Ullathorne in the period.

[119] Westminster Dioc. Archives, Wiseman Papers, Bishops' Letters R7913, Ullathorne to Wiseman, 14 July 1848.

[120] Ibid. R7913, Ullathorne to Wiseman, 14 July 1844.   [121] Ibid.

their named holders had made suggestions to Rome. Then, while Ullathorne was reporting back to the Vicars Apostolic, assembled for the purpose in Manchester, the revolution broke out in Rome, and with the flight of the Pope to Gaeta, in November 1848, the whole question of the hierarchy, together with most other papal business, lapsed. It was not until after the return of Pius IX to Rome, in April 1850, that the issue was re-activated; and then affairs moved, by Roman standards, swiftly. The brief re-establishing the hierarchy in England was dated 29 September,[122] and on 7 October Wiseman—chosen as the first metropolitan because of the death of Walsh—issued his notorious 'Flaminian Gate' pastoral.[123]

'Catholic England has been restored to its orbit in the ecclesiastical firmament, from which its light had long vanished, and begins anew its course of regularly adjusted action round the centre of unity, the source of jurisdiction, of light and of vigour,' Wiseman wrote in the Pastoral. 'Till such time as the Holy See shall think fit otherwise to provide, we govern and shall continue to govern the counties of Middlesex, Hertford and Essex, as Ordinary thereof, and those of Surrey, Sussex, Kent, Berkshire and Hampshire, with the islands annexed, as Administrator with Ordinary jurisdiction.'[124] Queen Victoria, on hearing it, is said to have asked, 'Am I Queen of England or am I not?'[125] Even Dr Whitty, Wiseman's administrator in London, had doubted the wisdom of publishing the Pastoral, in view of its probable effect upon the Protestant sensibilities of the nation; but, guided by prayer, he had proceeded to execute Wiseman's instructions and published the text just as he had received it.[126] Wiseman meanwhile was making a triumphal tour through Europe, on the way to occupy his new honours, innocently unaware of the effect his florid cadences and extravagant language—more suited to Italian than to English ears—were having. Several

---

[122] Propaganda, *Scritture* 12 (1848–51), 591: *Sanctissimi Domini Nostri PII Divina Providentia* PAPAE IX *Literae Apostolicae quibus Hierarchia Episcopalis in Anglia Restituitur* (signed by Cardinal Lambruschini).

[123] For an account of the subsequent events, as they affected Wiseman, see chapter 3.

[124] For the text of the Pastoral, see Bernard Ward, *Sequel*, II, 283.

[125] Norman, *Anti-Catholicism in Victorian England*, 56.

[126] Wilfrid Ward, *The Life and Times of Cardinal Wiseman*, I. 541.

papers reported the creation of the new hierarchy, but without producing any effect. It was *The Times* which engineered the uproar, so that, as Ullathorne remarked towards the end of October, 'The whole country is in a boil on the subject.'[127] It was the apparent claim to jurisdiction in England—with the insinuation that it partook of a temporal as well as a spiritual character—which *The Times* exploited. 'If the appointment be not intended as a clumsy joke, we confess that we can only regard it as one of the grossest acts of folly and impertinence which the Court of Rome has ventured to commit since the Crown and people of England threw off its yoke,' *The Times* declared: 'The Pope and his advisors have mistaken our complete tolerance for indifference to their designs; they have mistaken the renovated zeal of the Church in this country for a return towards Romish bondage.'[128] Both Wiseman and the Vatican were unprepared for this, recalling —as Wiseman indeed wrote to Lord John Russell on 3 November, just before he was due to arrive in England—that Lord Minto had known of the plans for a hierarchy, and so had the British government, for three years. 'With regard to myself', he wrote, 'I beg to add that I am invested with a purely ecclesiastical dignity.'[129] But the damage was done, and Russell was already publishing a 'Letter to the Bishop of Durham' (4 November) in which he asserted 'There is an assumption of power in all the documents which have come from Rome—a pretension to supremacy over the realm of England, and a claim to sole and individual sway, which is inconsistent with the Queen's supremacy, with the rights of our bishops and clergy, and with the spiritual independence of the nation.' This 'Papal aggression' was, as the Bishop of Durham had originally suggested to Russell, 'insolent and insidious'.[130] ('I don't think the aggression of the Pope was at any rate insidious,' Disraeli later remarked; 'I think it was a frank aggression.'[131]) The Archbishop of Canterbury described the Catholic priesthood as 'subtle, skilful, and insinuating'.

---

[127] *Letters of the Archbishop Ullathorne*, London 1892, 10.
[128] *The Times*, 14 Oct. 1850.
[129] Wilfrid Ward, *Wiseman*, I. 534.
[130] Ibid. I. 547. See also Norman, *Anti-Catholicism*, 57.
[131] Hansard, CXIV, 132 (4 Feb. 1851).

The Archbishop of York said that Rome's 'ever-wakeful ambition is plotting for our captivity and ruin'. The Bishop of London called the priests 'emissaries of darkness'.[132] Still smarting from the effects of the Gorham Judgment, with its candid erastianism, High Church Anglicans were particularly glad of the occasion for a release of emotion against an agreed adversary. Pulpits of all branches of Protestantism hammered away at the Pope and his English followers throughout the last two months of the year.[133] Demonstrations were got up all over the country, and even among English-speaking Protestants overseas (like the citizens of towns in Ontario). The Pope and Wiseman were burned in effigy. Clerics were pelted in the streets; 'small boys forsook the delights of marbles and tops to join in the service, and scrawled the magic words *No Popery!* on the flag-stones'.[134] For some years public ostracism of Catholics was common: Catholic domestic servants found it difficult to get employment.[135] Some Old Catholics shared the Protestant outrage. Lord Beaumont thought the hierarchy would jeopardize the civil liberties of Catholics, and the Duke of Norfolk supposed that the Ultramontane opinions he thought lurked behind the scheme were incompatible with allegiance to the Crown.[136] 'Ill-advised things have been done by us to provoke much of it,' the Earl of Shrewsbury wrote to Ambrose Phillipps de Lisle in February 1851, citing 'the pompous Pastoral from outside the Flaminian Gate'.[137] 'So you English imagine I meant to insult Queen Victoria and violate the laws of your country,' Pius IX said in Rome, 'You are a very strange people. You seem to me to understand nothing thoroughly but commerce.'[138]

Wiseman did what he could to repair the damage. He had

---

[132] Wilfrid Ward, *Wiseman*, I. 549.

[133] For an example of these sermons, see Norman, op. cit. 167 (Document 10, 'A Sermon on Papal Aggression', by the Rev. William Bennett, entitled *Popery as set forth in Scripture: Its Guilt and Its Doom* [1850]).

[134] O'Meara, 76.

[135] Wilfrid Ward, *Wiseman*, II. 43.

[136] S. W. Jackman, *Nicholas Wiseman. A Victorian Prelate and his Writings*, Dublin 1977, 35.

[137] E. S. Purcell, *Life and Letters of Ambrose Phillips de Lisle*, London 1900, I. 321.

[138] O'Meara, 74.

seen, in a few short weeks, the final disintegration of the illusion that the mass conversion of England was imminent. He wrote *An Appeal to the Reason and Good Feeling of the English People* immediately upon his arrival in London, and, in December, delivered a course of lectures at St. George's Cathedral in Southwark on the subject of the hierarchy, seeking to dispel mistaken impressions.[139] The Government responded, in February of the next year, with the Ecclesiastical Titles Act. On the bright side, from the Catholics' point of view, there was at least the conversion of Manning—prompted when he was obliged to convene an anti-Catholic meeting of the clergy of Sussex in November 1850 (he was Archdeacon of Chichester), and effected in April 1851. The converts, in fact, were delighted by the hierarchy, and by the style in which Wiseman had chosen to introduce it. Their triumphalism, however, was not shared by many of the Catholic laity and clergy whose claims to a proper parochial system, and rights to a voice in the election of bishops, had been ignored. A few petitions, over the following years, continued to be addressed to Rome on the question, but with no satisfactory outcome.[140]

In institutional terms, the effects of the hierarchy were not dramatic. The London District was divided into the dioceses of Westminster and Southwark. The Northern District became the diocese of Hexham and the Yorkshire District the diocese of Beverley. The Lancashire District ceded Cheshire to the diocese of Shrewsbury, which also got North Wales and Shropshire. The remainder of the old Lancashire District was divided into the dioceses of Liverpool and Salford. The Central District was reapportioned into the dioceses of Birmingham and Nottingham. Most of the Eastern District became the diocese of Northampton. The Western District was divided between Plymouth, Clifton, and Newport—which included South Wales.[141] At the top of the English hierarchy was the Westminster Metropolitan, but the suffragans (diocesans of

---

[139] See chapter 3 following.
[140] Holmes, *More Roman than Rome*, 86–7.
[141] For the arrangement of diocesan affairs, see R. J. Schieffen, 'The Organization and Administration of Roman Catholic Dioceses in England and Wales in the mid-nineteenth century' (London University Ph.D. thesis, 1970).

the Provinces) were only in a very limited sense subject to his authority: a point Wiseman never quite understood. The Metropolitan could convoke provincial synods, had appellate jurisdiction, and enjoyed certain rights of precedence. But he was not the national representative of the English Catholic Church, and was not treated as such by the other bishops or by Rome—even though he often was by the press and by public opinion.[142] Each Bishop held his authority from Rome. The 'rights' of the lower clergy were no more conciliated than under the preceding arrangements, and rumbles of discontent continued throughout the rest of the century. Though never amounting to a serious questioning of authority, the bishops were aware of it. 'The reported discontent on the part of the Clergy, respecting the absolute want of canonical judicial proceeding in this country, was spoken of' at the Low Week Meeting of the Bishops in April 1869. 'But it was thought premature to consider it.'[143] Thomas Grant, still in Rome before assuming the duties of Bishop of Southwark, began to write a paper, in January 1851, about the practical effects of the hierarchy, 'so as to give the clergy the satisfaction of knowing that they would get some of the favours and advantages of the *Jus Commune*'.[144] He abandoned the project because he believed that Wiseman's lectures at St. George's would meet the need, but his notes still exist, in the Westminster Diocesan Archives, and they offer an interesting reflection on the way the officials in Rome, with whose views he was familiar, expected things to go in England. 'What will be the working effect of the re-establishment of the Hierarchy?' he asked. 'The *jus commune* of the Church has been restored among us,' he continued, even though the full force of canon law had not. The Pope, he wrote, was anxious to allow local conditions to be accommodated, 'to leave us to work out the provisions of the canon law with reference to our local circumstances and wants'. The synods, and especially the Provincial Synods, when they met, would formulate the

---

[142] Morgan V. Sweeney, in *The English Catholics, 1850–1950*, 124.

[143] Westminster Dioc. Archives, ACTA, *Meeting of the Bishops in Low Week, 1869*, 27.

[144] Westminster Dioc. Archives, Wiseman Papers, Bishops' Letters, 137/1/24, Grant to Wiseman, 14 Jan. 1851.

appropriate directives suited to English conditions. He advised
the bishops to emulate the rules established by St. Charles
Borromeo for the Church of Milan in the sixteenth century,
and the legislation of the Synod of Baltimore at the start of
the nineteenth—the latter especially because it provided
ecclesiastical instruments for an English-speaking Catholic
Church operating in not too dissimilar circumstances from
the Church in England. 'It will be said that we look to the
synods for every thing', he wrote.[145] And so they did. The
First Provincial Synod, at Oscott in July 1852, confirmed
the defeat of the laity and the lower clergy over the questions
of parochial rights. The bishops ruled that the missions were
not yet ready to be arranged into ordinary canonical parishes.[146] Some slight concessions were later made. Certain
missions in each diocese were allocated to the administration
of 'Missionary Rectors', who were removable not by the
bishop's *dictat*, but by a special procedure involving committees of inquiry. This followed instructions of August 1853,
sent by Propaganda. It was not a very substantial change, and
for all practical purposes 'parochial rights' were not conceded. Nor were parish councils set up. But Rural Deans
provided a link between the missions and episcopal authority
which eased some of the misunderstandings common before
the hierarchy. The absence of canonical parishes was not the
only sign that the restoration of the hierarchy had still left
England without complete autonomy. Cathedral canons were
appointed in an unusual manner, with no common life
and with less independence of the bishops than their counterparts enjoyed in fully regular schemes of ecclesiastical government.

Diocesan synods began to be held after 1853, and thereafter met every five or six years, but the legislation passed
showed great deference to the decrees of Provincial Synods,
and generally merely reiterated their provisions. The early
Synods also show how closely the bishops still regarded
themselves as being subject to Propaganda. The archives
of Propaganda contain papers from each diocese in turn,

[145] Ibid. 137, 25a–d, 'Notes on the practical consequences of the restoration
of the Hierarchy' (Feb. 1851).
[146] Decrees XIII and XIV.

enclosing, as in the case of Westminster,[147] copies of decrees passed, and, as in the cases, for example, of Clifton[148] and of Southwark,[149] detailed explanations of the procedures adopted. The effective use of synods in creating a consolidated diocesan administration was well illustrated by the work of Bishop Alexander Goss in Liverpool. Goss had entered Ushaw in 1827 at the age of twelve, and had completed his studies in Rome. But he was never 'Roman' in spirit— merely employing the centralized authority of Rome for tactical advantage in his attempts to preserve a measure of independence from Westminster. He had become Coadjutor in Liverpool at the age of thirty-nine, in 1853, and his model for diocesan administration was indeed that of St. Charles Borromeo: he was authoritarian and inflexible in his determination to secure clerical obedience and institutional coherence.[150] The diocesan synods were held regularly, as were deanery conferences. Annual retreats for the clergy were begun, and Goss himself conducted triennial visitations, and initiated searching and extensive statistical enquiries into the work and needs of the parishes. He died in 1872. It was only after the Fourth Provincial Synod that diocesan legislation, especially in matters touching stipends and clergy discipline, began to show confidence and independence.[151] But the most obvious sign that England's position was still irregular was the continued supervision of the Church by Propaganda. That continued until Pius X's *Sapienti Consilio* in 1908. It was not until the *Codex Juris Canonici* in 1918 that canon law applied fully in England, and ordinary parishes, in consequence, came into existence.

[147] Propaganda, *Scritture* 13 (1852-4), 842 [in English].

[148] Ibid. 894, Bishop Thomas Burgess to the Cardinal Prefect, 1 Jan. 1854 [in Latin].

[149] Ibid. 902, Bishop Thomas Grant to the Cardinal Prefect, 14 Jan. 1854 [in Italian].

[150] See P. H. Doyle, 'Bishop Goss of Liverpool and the importance of being English', in Stuart Mews (ed.), *Religion and National Identity. Studies in Church History*, 18 (1982), 433-49.

[151] Sweeney, op. cit., 130.

3

Cardinal Wiseman: Catholic Consolidation

'His life's work, and even his name,' according to Denis
Gwynn, 'was little more than a memory when his successor
Cardinal Manning died in 1892.'[1] Wiseman divided English
Catholic opinion in his own day, and subsequent commentary
upon his life has continued to reflect those divisions.[2] The
general drift of interpretation, however, has been towards
the diminution of his reputation, as writers of diminishing
degrees of Ultramontanism have surveyed what he did to
English Catholicism. Wiseman's great contribution was to
bring the English Catholics into a disciplined acquaintance
with the spirituality and ecclesiastical style of the Papal Catholicism of the decades which succeeded the restoration of the
Church after the French Revolution. His work paralleled that
of Cardinal Paul Cullen in Ireland—whom he had known as a
young man, when they were both students in Rome.[3] Cullen
returned to Ireland as Archbishop of Armagh in 1850, and in
1852 he was translated to the Archbishopric of Dublin with
the specific mandate, as Legate, to unify the Irish Catholics
and to impose regular ecclesiastical discipline on a Church
which had, as an inheritance of the Penal Days of the preceding century, developed both national and local sympathies
and practices inimical to the Ultramontanism of the Roman
order demanded by Propaganda.[4] He encountered considerable Irish opposition. Wiseman, similarly, sought to bring centralized discipline to a Church which had survived for a couple
of centuries with little experience of Rome. He, too, encountered opposition, and from those who were able to point to

[1] Denis Gwynn, *Cardinal Wiseman*, London 1929, ix.
[2] Dr. Richard Schiefen has a forthcoming study of Wiseman which will doubtless—in view of the previous scholarly contributions of this author—become a
standard and important work.
[3] Wilfrid Ward, *The Life and Times of Cardinal Wiseman*, I. 72.
[4] On Cullen's mandate, see E. R. Norman, *The Catholic Church and Ireland
in the Age of Rebellion, 1859–1873*, London 1965, 17-20.

his seemingly slight qualifications for the task he undertook. Both men were favourites of the Roman court; both had resided for most of their lives outside their respective countries and could be represented as more 'Italian' than national in their outlook—as lacking real knowledge about the Churches and the societies to whom they were sent. It is arguable that Wiseman's version of Catholicism reflected only an ephemeral moment of Italian Catholicism: it has been noticed that the Rome described in his book of reminiscences, *Recollections of the Last Four Popes and of Rome in their Times* (published in 1858) 'was indeed the last age of Papal Rome. He was witnessing a peculiar form of Roman Catholicism that was shortly to disappear.'[5] It is also arguable that the English and Irish Catholic Churches would have been assimilated to the practices of Roman centralism without either Wiseman or Cullen—that these two men were entrusted with a work which the general movement of things would anyway have accomplished.

The idiosyncrasies of Wiseman's personality, of which much has been made by recent writers not altogether in sympathy with his ideals, cannot have added to his effectiveness; yet it was not these, but his apparent insensitivity to English Catholic traditions, which inspired opposition. He had a following of isolated devotees, but had no party within the Church. He came from the splendours without and never fully understood the emotional investments which those who had always been within had made in their threadbare tabernacle. At least one distinguished modern historian has characterized his personal power in English Catholicism as 'a breach in continuity'.[6] The breach, however, was set to happen anyway. Wiseman was only the particular agent of the most dynamic force within nineteenth-century Catholicism: Ultramontanist sympathies were inevitably to affect the English, as all other Churches in the Catholic world. As the agent, Wiseman was also credited with Catholic advances which were already on the way—the revival of spirituality and the growth of numbers which were a feature of the century, but which affected

[5] Williams, *The Venerable English College, Rome*, 95–6.
[6] Bossy, *The English Catholic Community, 1570–1850*, 360.

all other denominations and were inseparable from the general
phenomenon of the Victorian boom in Christianity. Wiseman
certainly encouraged the converts, at a time when others did
not, and that in itself was enough to authenticate some of the
claims of his contemporaries that he should be 'recognized as
the true architect of the Catholic revival'.[7] He also helped to
lay 'the foundations of regular ecclesiastical life'.[8] The belief
of one of his most recent biographers that he 'brought the
English Roman Catholic community out of the wilderness'[9]
can also be given some substance—though it rather under-
values changes already in progress before he arrived upon the
scene. Unlike most English Catholic prelates in the nineteenth
century, Wiseman had a European reputation, and in that
wider theatre he was usually credited with having wrought a
revolution within the English Church—as Wiseman was himself aware. When Father Hermann, Prior of the Discalced
Carmelites in London, told the Malines Congress in 1863 'that
the advantages gained for the Catholic cause are in great part
the work of the Cardinal himself',[10] he uttered more than
a conventional piety: it was a general impression outside
England. From that viewpoint—though not, of course, from
within the walls of Propaganda—the English Catholic advance
was uncomplicated by the internal strife which accompanied
so many of Wiseman's actions. 'We may date, then,' Father
Hermann continued, 'the happy change we have signalled,
from the time when His Eminence began to guide the Catholic
movement.'[11]

Despite his rather imperfect acquaintance with English conditions, at least until he moved to Oscott in 1840, Wiseman
was robustly English in sympathy. His love for English qualities forms a constant theme in his writings and sermons. He
had, indeed, all that self-consciousness of nationality which

[7] Brian Fothergill, 'Wiseman: The Man and his Mission', in the *Wiseman Review*, 493, Autumn 1962, 236.

[8] Gordon Wheeler, 'The Archdiocese of Westminster', in *The English Catholics, 1850–1950*, ed. Beck, 153.

[9] Jackman, *Nicholas Cardinal Wiseman. A Victorian Prelate and his Writings*, 46.

[10] *Catholicism in England, An Address delivered 3rd September, AD 1863, at the Catholic Congress at Malines, by Father Hermann*, London 1864, 4.

[11] Ibid. 7.

those achieve who are not by immediate background integrated with the national values they esteem. He was born in Spain, of Irish parentage. Yet he referred to the English College in Rome as 'home'; 'it was English ground, a part of the fatherland'.[12] The College did in fact echo the style of some English institutions: Macaulay, on a visit in 1838, remarked that it was 'much like the halls of the small colleges at Cambridge in my time—that of Peterhouse, for example'.[13] The national note was happily sounded by Pius VII when he received Wiseman, together with the other new students who had arrived in 1818 to reopen the College after its closure during the French occupation. 'I hope you will do honour both to Rome and to your own country', the Pope said—words which Wiseman regarded as a lifelong guide.[14] He was impressed by a sense of England's achievements, and of the possibilities and duties they implied for Catholics as members of the national community. 'There is no doubt, my brethren', he told a Salford congregation in July 1850, preparatory to reminding them of the need for moral and social regeneration, 'that never in the history of nations, was any people advanced beyond ours, at the present time, in all that constitutes social and intellectual greatness.'[15] He called for more gratitude to God as the bestower of such riches, and contrasted the material progress with moral corruptions of society. This sense of great achievement allied with lost moral qualities recurred in Wiseman's judgement of the English Protestants' attitude to Catholics. This was true even at the time of the 'Papal Aggression' uproar in 1850. The whole of his famous *Appeal* was directed to the reasonableness of the English public; and there is a letter in the Ushaw College archives, addressed at the very height of the clamour to the Revd. Thomas Slater, a Co. Durham priest, in which he declared: 'depend upon it, justice will be done to us, by the good sense

[12] Wilfrid Ward, *Wiseman*, I. 15.
[13] Ibid. I. 272.
[14] *Recollections of the Last Four Popes and of Rome in their times, by H. E. Cardinal Wiseman*, 14.
[15] *The Social and Intellectual State of England, Compared with its Moral Condition. A Sermon delivered in St. John's Catholic Church, Salford, on Sunday, July 28th 1850, by the Right Rev. N. Wiseman D.D.*, London 1850, 5.

of our fellow-countrymen.'[16] In 1863, in his address to the Malines Congress, Wiseman paraded his belief in the essential fairness of Englishmen. 'We know that individuals may have their minds thoroughly penetrated with prejudices from early education, and later influences, particularly from the press', he said, 'But experience has proved that at the bottom, buried beneath this confused heap of false, and even absurd convictions, there is a powerful sense of justice, which, if properly evoked, will make its way through these erroneous teachings, and, standing above them, will tread them under foot.'[17] It was his co-religionists in England of whom Wiseman seems sometimes almost to have despaired; his belief in the basic fairness of the Protestant culture of the English nation—as opposed to his knowledge of Anglican theological controversy —was 'very much of a closed book to him', as one of his biographers has noticed.[18]

These sorts of contrast—between material and moral progress, and between English prejudice and English sense of justice—are frequently encountered in Wiseman's thought. They are very much a feature of his dramatic cast of mind: a characteristic which made him such an effective polemicist. As a student in Rome he had been lastingly impressed by Pius VII's rearrangement of the memorials and statues in the long corridor leading to the Vatican library, with Christian monuments on one side and pagan ones on the other. 'You may walk along an avenue, one side adorned by the stately and mature or even decaying memorials of heathen dominion, the other by the young and growing and vigorous monuments of early Christian culture,' he later recalled, 'There they stand face to face, as if in hostile array, about to begin a battle long since fought and won.'[19] In the circumstances of later European religious conflict the contrasts were seen to reappear. The Reformation, he told Protestants in 1838, should

[16] Ushaw College Archives, Wiseman Papers, 966, Wiseman to Slater, 16 Nov. 1850.

[17] *The Religious and Social Position of Catholics in England. An Address Delivered to the Catholic Congress at Malines, August 21, 1863, by H. E. Cardinal Wiseman*, 52.

[18] Fothergill, *Nicholas Wiseman*, 22.

[19] *Recollections of the Last Four Popes*, 107. See also Wilfrid Ward, *Wiseman*, I. 38.

be understood as a series of contrasts. 'Ours was a *conserva- tive reform*; we pruned away the decayed part; we placed the vessel in the furnace, and, the dross being melted off, we drew it out bright and pure.' (It was not a description of counter- Reformation Catholicism that English Protestants were likely to recognize). 'Yours', Wiseman continued, 'was *radical* to the extreme; you tore up entire plants by the roots, because you said there was a blight on some one branch; you threw the whole vessel into the fire, and made merry at its blaze.' He also said, 'we could run through some hundred such com- parisons, to show the opposite characters of our two re- forms.'[20] It is not surprising that he got on so well with Pugin —whose *Contrasts* was published during Wiseman's tour of England in 1836.[21]

Wiseman was, or became, a writer on religious controversy rather than a theologian or historian in any conventional scholarly sense. He had an excellent and very clear mind, which went at once to the essentials of a question under scrutiny. But after his early research in the Vatican library, which resulted in the publication of the *Horae Syriacae* in 1827, he undertook very little new scholarly activity, deriving most of his subsequent knowledge from a reading of period- ical literature and the public prints. His linguistic capabilities were extraordinary. He could speak some half a dozen languages perfectly. Yet these talents were not employed academically even in his later years in Rome—before the ecclesiastical duties of his English life would anyway have compelled a limit to scholarship. His mind was anyway rather unoriginal;[22] his interests rather eclectic. In this last charac- teristic, as in other things, he showed himself to have a taste for the 'useful knowledge' (that some admired, and others regretted) enthusiasm of the spirit of the age. The twelve lectures on science and religion which he delivered in Rome in 1836 gave early indication of the range of topics on which he was willing to offer published opinions. One is on the comparative study of languages; another on natural history;

[20] *Essays on Various Subjects*, II. 58.

[21] Gwynn, *The Second Spring, 1818–1852*, 66. Bernard Ward, *The Sequel to Catholic Emancipation*, I. 87. Wilfrid Ward, *Wiseman*, I. 354.

[22] Jackman, *Nicholas Cardinal Wiseman*, 47, 64.

others on the natural sciences, early history, archaeology, and oriental literature. He was a great gatherer of factual information. In 1851 he followed the Arctic Expedition closely; he drew up a memorandum for Rowland on the Post Office.[23] The publication of his collected *Essays on Various Subjects*, in 1853, in three enormous volumes, was a further testimony to his breadth of knowledge: the third contains an assortment of diverse titles—'Remarks on Lady Morgan's statement regarding St. Peter's Chair', 'Spanish and English National Art', 'Italian Gesticulation', and so forth. On the Irish tour of 1858, he took time off in Dublin to deliver a public lecture on 'The Ornamental Glass found in the Catacombs'.[24] But this astonishing range was achieved at the expense both of depth and of development.[25] When compiling the essays for publication in 1853, he observed 'I have not formed an opinion or a feeling that I have ceased to entertain.'[26] In addition to his academic interests, Wiseman was also musical. He played the organ in the chapel of the English College at service times. There survives, in the Westminster Diocesan Archives, a copy of his certificate from the Roman Academy of Music. His most successful literary venture was the novel *Fabiola*, written mostly at Monte Porzio and completed on holiday at Filey in 1854. Published early in the following year, the book had an immediate and lasting success. It went through numerous editions and there were translations into a number of languages (including Esperanto in 1911 and Irish in 1939). In 1949 it was made into a motion picture in Italy. But *Fabiola*, which is a moralistic story about the sufferings and victories of the early Christians in the catacombs of Rome, can scarcely be valued for its literary merits. As Professor Jackman has observed in his analysis of the novel, 'all the Christians tend to speak in an unnatural fashion, best described as clerical'.[27] It was a religious work, intended to cultivate religious sensibilities, and it certainly achieved that.

[23] Wilfrid Ward, *Wiseman*, II. 154.

[24] *The Sermons, Lectures and Speeches delivered by His Eminence, Cardinal Wiseman, Archbishop of Westminster, during his Tour in Ireland in August and September, 1858*, Boston 1859, 147.

[25] Fothergill lists a selection of Wiseman's writings to display this range; see *Nicholas Wiseman*, 285.

[26] *Essays on Various Subjects*, I. xi.

[27] Jackman, 103.

Recent historical opinion has tended to refer frankly to aspects of Wiseman's personality as the cause of his friction with the English bishops, and it is doubtless necessary to do so. But it must also be remembered that in the twenty-two years of his residence in Rome, where his character was set, he was known for the ease of his personal relationships and his social charm. His tact and judgement, in fact, as displayed to the Roman officials, led to his advancement. Gladstone, entertained by him during a visit to Rome in 1838, was struck by his reasonableness and his breadth of vision. The implication is that—however much, once arrived in England, he over-emphasized his Roman pre-eminences and prerogatives— the bishops must bear some of the burden of the subsequent personal difficulties. They were themselves not the easiest of men. Wiseman, certainly, 'sometimes allowed his emotional feelings to get the better of his intellectual judgement'.[28] Dr Whitty, his Vicar-General at Westminster, recalling conversations in the summer of 1850, as Wiseman prepared to go to Rome for the red hat, remarked 'In many respects he remained a child all his life.' And of the journey to Rome: 'it struck me as being very like a boy's anticipation of his journey home in vacation'.[29] He had a taste for reading children's books. He relaxed only in the company of the young— at Rome, in his later years as Rector of the English College, he took the students on 'outings', sometimes to Fiumicino, at the mouth of the Tiber, for a bathe in the sea. His love of the College is perhaps to be seen in this context; a place where the young could discover the beauties of Rome and the pleasures of the Italian countryside.[30] His early years as President of Oscott perpetuated something of this feeling. Again, he was among the young in the security of institutional life. 'There was the playfulness of the child, and the wisdom of the sage most admirably combined in him', as one who was a boy at Oscott during Wiseman's time there recalled after the Cardinal's death. 'The short excursion, the salubrious drive, the goodly share of sweetmeats or Spanish toys, and an occasional game at hand-ball'—these were Wiseman's manner

[28] Fothergill, in *Wiseman Review*, 493 (1962), 240.
[29] Wilfrid Ward, *Wiseman*, I. 523.
[30] *Recollections of the Last Four Popes*, 183–5.

of appreciating the company of the young. By those years, too, he had become rather fat—'a ruddy, strapping divine', as Macaulay called him.[31] He ate well and hugely enjoyed convivial company; but this is not to suggest that he was worldly. The spiritual life, and his devotional exercises, were the most important elements of the daily routine. Throughout his life he was ill. Sometimes he went to Rome to help recover health, as well as to attend to the business of the Church; in 1856 he went to Vichy for the water, and in 1863 to Broadstairs for the sea air. In London, as illness came on, he retired more and more frequently to his country residence, Etloe House in Walthamstow. He had also, in classic nineteenth-century style, experienced fits of religious scepticism— especially in Rome in 1827, during the dispute over the chair of Oriental Languages, when he was also seized with a conviction that he was about to go insane.[32] Doubts returned again in 1840, just as he was to be made a bishop.

Those who have found Wiseman's character unattractive have also noted his love of show—a quality easily indulged by a prince of the church, for whom ceremonial and dressing-up are inseparable from the practice of vocation. Wiseman did, it is true, take particular pleasure in this aspect of his duties. Father Faber once remarked that 'when in full tog he looked like some Japanese God'.[33] (Wiseman said of Faber that his 'letters to me are insulting to insanity'.[34]) Cardinal Antonelli, the Papal Secretary of State, advised Wiseman to eschew unnecessary public display in order to avoid offending English Protestant sensibilities,[35] but Wiseman regarded open manifestations of Catholicism as an effective means of witnessing to truth. Financial restraints set a limit to it. 'The state and splendour of a Cardinal is scarcely attainable with your limited means in London,' Grant wrote to him from Rome early in 1851; 'and even if attainable, is scarcely desirable, whereas a Cardinal who lives as much as possible for the poor and

[31] Wilfrid Ward, *Wiseman*, I. 272.

[32] Ibid. I. 64.

[33] Jackman, 20.

[34] Cardinal Gasquet, 'Unpublished Letters of Cardinal Wiseman to Dr Manning', in *Dublin Review*, Oct.–Dec. 1921, 180, (Letter of 22 March 1862).

[35] Holmes, *More Roman than Rome*, 87.

amongst them is sure to have his weight and consideration even amongst the most unfavourable of our censors.' He recommended that Wiseman should model himself upon the lives of St. Charles Borromeo and St. Francis de Sales.[36] Wiseman did not get on with Grant. His sense of the external show of spiritual authority was popular with the poor in the slums he visited as part of his duties as Archbishop of Westminster. The crowds pressed forward to touch his robes, seeking some tangible link with the mystery of religion.[37] At the height of his dispute with the Westminster Chapter, in 1859, when Manning was dispatched to Rome to represent the cardinals' case, Wiseman wrote urging him to bring back some '*fiocchetti*, little frizzled gold knots, to put at the end of alb or rochet strings etc.'.[38] It was entirely characteristic of him. It was around this time—actually in the summer of 1858—that Wiseman went on a tour of Ireland, and there he got just the public acclaim for Catholic magnificence, in a series of grand occasions, that his English Catholic followers failed to provide. The visit was ostensibly to open a new church at Ballinasloe, but 'his visit became a triumphant progress through the country'.[39] As in Italy, or Spain (which he visited for the first time since his childhood in 1844), Wiseman was at his most responsive and most relaxed among a Catholic people of peasant spirituality and unreserved enthusiasm.

Wiseman's capacity to inspire opposition in others, as has been noticed, was largely a phenomenon of his English years. Some English Catholics had always been wary of his influence in Rome. But it was when he left Oscott, to become Vicar Apostolic of the London District, in 1849, that the suspicions he inspired in others passed into a more critical phase. Wiseman was himself changed to some extent by the experience. To depart from Oscott was to live, for the first time in his life, outside an institution. In the less companionable world to which he now departed he was both lonely and

---

[36] Westminster Dioc. Archives, Wiseman Papers, Bishops' Letters, 137/1/24, Grant to Wiseman, 14 Jan. 1851.

[37] Sheridan Gilley, 'Vulgar Piety and the Brompton Oratory, 1850-1860', in *Durham University Journal*, XLIII (Dec. 1981), 20.

[38] Wilfrid Ward, *Wiseman*, II. 330.

[39] Patrick K. Egan, *The Parish of Ballinasloe. Its History from the Earliest Times to the Present Day*, Dublin 1960, 249.

without personal bearings. His sufferings, in consequence, grew more acute with each year, and lasted until his death. In such an atmosphere, his suspicions of the Catholic bishops matched theirs of him. The difficulty was a mutual one. There were, of course, overt causes of conflict. As Lesourd has written, 'la personne de Wiseman n'était pas unanimement appréciée parmi les catholiques anglais: on lui reprochait d'être trop "Romain", trop favorable aux converts, trop soumis aux vœux du gouvernement anglais'.[40] These matters, however, were enormously exaggerated by suspicions of Wiseman himself—who was, as Bishop Patterson remarked, 'not sufficiently alive to the effect upon others of his manner'.[41] Further opposition was caused by his failure to help those who looked to him. Newman, who was most notably let down by him on a number of occasions, rather kindly described his impulses as 'evanescent'.[42] Others were less restrained. By the later 1840s, Wiseman was speaking of 'my *total isolation* as regards support and counsel, as well as sympathy and concurrence in views and plans'.[43] Things got even worse, as he was to discover, in the next decade. 'God grant us peace,' he wrote to Manning in 1862, 'for I shall not much longer stand this pelting from all sides.'[44]

The division of Wiseman's life into Roman and English dimensions—made for obvious purposes of chronological analysis—was something of which he was himself actively aware. In the first part of his life, in Rome, he came gradually to a restless desire for work in England; in the second part, in England, he yearned for the past happiness and the religious grandeur of Rome. Nicholas Wiseman was born at Seville in 1802, son of a merchant whose father had migrated to Spain for business reasons. The family came from Waterford in Ireland. His mother, Xaviera, took the child and laid him on the altar of Seville cathedral, and dedicated him to the service of the Church. Wiseman's early childhood thereafter seems to

---

[40] Jean Alain Lesourd, *Les Catholiques dans la société anglaise, 1765–1865*, II. 681.

[41] Wilfrid Ward, *Wiseman*, II. 78.

[42] Ibid. II. 43.

[43] Ibid. I. 447.

[44] Gasquet, 'Unpublished Letters . . .', 180.

have been conventional enough: it is interesting to notice, however, that the family knew Blanco White in Seville—indeed he acted as spiritual director to them.[45] When, over twenty years later, Daniel Rock wrote to Wiseman asking him 'to collect every possible information' about Blanco White, 'from the most authentic sources', Wiseman must have been well-placed to comply.[46] After his father's death, Xaviera moved to Ireland with her two sons, Nicholas and James (the elder child), and for two years Wiseman went to a local boarding school in Waterford. 'When I first came to Ireland as a child I did not know a single word of the English language', he told an Irish audience half a century later.[47] In 1810 Wiseman was removed to Ushaw College, where he fell under the influence of Lingard and first met, as a contemporary schoolboy, George Errington. He was happy at Ushaw and always recalled his time there with pleasure. These details of Wiseman's early life may seem unnecessary: but they indicate the extent to which he stood, by background, outside the Old Catholic English world to which he was later called.

Sheltering one day in a cottage to avoid a storm which had blown up during a walk from Ushaw, he recognized a vocation to the priesthood.[48] In 1818, in consequence, and at the age of sixteen, he was chosen to be one of the first group of seminarists to travel to Rome and inaugurate the studies of the English College, reopened under the patronage of Cardinal Consalvi. He was to live there for twenty-two years; and since his mother had now moved again, to Paris, he had, during all those years, almost no family links with England. In a letter of commendation the Vice-President of Ushaw declared of the young Wiseman: 'His talents are unrivalled in Ushaw College . . . his character as a Christian scholar quite without fault.'[49] He was, in fact, however, a very average student. But at the English College he began to disclose some considerable intellectual talents, as well as becoming absorbed in the

[45] Gwynn, *The Second Spring*, 46.
[46] Ushaw College Archives, Wiseman Papers, 40A, Rock to Wiseman, 4 Feb. 1827.
[47] *Tour in Ireland*, 45.
[48] Wilfrid Ward, *Wiseman*, I. 9.
[49] Milburn, *A History of Ushaw College*, 144.

history of Papal Rome and acquiring a delight in classical antiquities. In 1824 he received the Doctorate of Divinity after the usual august public examination,[50] and in the following year was ordained to the priesthood. Only two years later, in 1827, he was made Vice-Rector of the College, and the year after that became Rector. It was a brilliant start to his career, and he was already winning golden opinions from the officials of the Curia. As Rector, he also became the agent of the English bishops in Rome, and it was the work this involved which attracted him increasingly over the years that followed to English affairs. His academic reputation was confirmed in 1822 with the publication of the research he had undertaken under Cardinal Mai's guidance. This book, the *Horae Syriacae*, resulted in the expectation that he would be appointed to the Chair of Oriental Languages in the Roman University, and when he was not, he appealed successfully to Leo XII. In 1827, when the Pope decided there should be a course of sermons in the English language to enable foreign visitors to Rome to become acquainted with the truths of the faith, it was Wiseman who was appointed to give them—in the Church of Gesù e Maria. They were his first real exercise in public speaking, and from their institution dates Wiseman's impressive career as a lecturer. The sermons were regarded, as Cardinal Acton wrote to assure Wiseman, as a 'great success':[51] with every step his career advanced to greater achievements. The new Pope (Pius VIII) was happy with the provisions of the Catholic Emancipation Act in 1829, and it fell to Wiseman not only to communicate details of the passage of the legislation to the Pontiff, but also to announce the final victory. The celebrations at the English College were, as Wiseman wrote, 'unintelligible to the multitude', however; 'the words "Emancipazione Catholica", which were emblazoned in lamps along the front, were read by the people with difficulty, and interpreted by conjecture'.[52] It was the series of *Lectures on the Connexion between Science and Revealed Religion*, given in Cardinal Weld's apartments during

[50] Of which he gave a description in *Recollections*, 190.
[51] Ushaw College Archives, Wiseman Papers, 757, Charles Acton to Wiseman 15 April 1818.
[52] *Recollections of the Last Four Popes*, 249.

Lent 1835, which further heightened Wiseman's reputation for learning, and which became the *vorspiel* for his more celebrated lectures in England during the Advent of the same year. These, which were first delivered in the Sardinian Embassy Chapel, and repeated, in virtue of their great success, at Moorfields Church in Lent 1836, were the first public presentation of Catholic doctrines in England, intended for non-Catholic audiences, and achieved much attention. They were a sign of Wiseman's ability to converse successfully with Protestants, and assisted the way of some who were later to become converts. Lord Brougham, who attended regularly, was not among them. The lectures confirmed what the Roman experiences had already indicated—that the style of public address was to be Wiseman's 'most regular means of influencing public opinion'.[53]

It was the idea of founding a Catholic University in England, first conceived in 1834, (perhaps because of Bishop Baines's undertakings), which in part lay behind Wiseman's tour of England in 1835-6. He went, on arrival, almost at once to Prior Park. But his stay there was not happy. Whereas Wiseman envisaged a university as the centre of a national cultivation of Catholic learning and research, Baines had a narrower vision, a scheme which despite his early hope of admitting laymen, went little further than the provision of a seminary training for the clergy of the Western District. The difference of view was that which was later to recur between Newman and Cardinal Cullen over the Irish University venture. The notion that Wiseman might become Baines's coadjutor passed away, and after Baines's suggestion that Wiseman was on a probationary period only at Prior Park,[54] the university scheme disappeared from his mind. The tour proceeded elsewhere. 'I intend to quarter myself', Wiseman wrote humorously to Monckton Milnes, 'upon such of the nobility or gentry of these realms as can sufficiently appreciate such an honour.'[55] Returning eventually to London, where he acted as temporary chaplain to the Sardinian Chapel, he threw himself into the foundation of the *Dublin Review*.

[53] Wilfrid Ward, *Wiseman*, II. 47.
[54] Gwynn, *Father Luigi Gentili and his Mission (1801-1848)*, 98.
[55] Wilfrid Ward, *Wiseman*, I. 215.

It was, indeed, the huge number of articles he wrote for the journal in the years which followed—some seventy altogether, and most of them before 1850—which established his reputation with the English Catholics. The idea of a new Catholic magazine was, by Wiseman's own account, first entertained by Michael J. Quin, in 1836—who then approached both Wiseman and O'Connell to join him. 'I was in England only for a short time, and saw the difficulty of connecting myself with an enterprise so far removed from my permanent residence in Rome,' Wiseman wrote. But the importance of the new journal for 'Catholic principles and sentiments' was too pressing for him to allow the opportunity to lapse.[56] He wrote two articles before his own departure; the first number of the *Dublin* appeared in May 1836. As a serious vehicle of Catholic thought, the journal performed an enormous service to English Catholicism: in 1961, in his honour, its name was changed to the *Wiseman Review*.

In 1840 Wiseman returned permanently to England, and the second phase of his career began. He became coadjutor to Walsh in the Central District of the rearranged Vicariates. At his consecration to the episcopate in the English College Chapel, by Cardinal Fransoni, he took the title of Bishop of Melipotamus. His chief work, in England, was to preside at Oscott College—where he was duly received, amidst just the sort of ceremonial formality he most liked, in September 1840. His time as President was reasonably happy, gathering the circle of Anglican converts to himself and entertaining, just as he had done in Rome, distinguished visitors. It was during this period that Pugin became a close friend. There is some reason to suppose that the professors of the College were at times out of sympathy with Wiseman's rather large interests, absorbed, as they were, in their teaching activities,[57] and declining to regard the College as the centre of a Catholic revival. These external interests of Wiseman led to his departure to Rome in July 1847, with Bishop James Sharples (coadjutor to Bishop George Brown of the Lancashire District), as representative of the English Bishops. They were to consult

---

[56] *Essays on Various Subjects*, I. v. (Preface, which contains a brief history of the foundation of the *Review*.)
[57] Wilfrid Ward, *Wiseman*, I. 346.

with the Holy See about a hierarchy for England. The death of Cardinal Acton at Naples, about which they heard during their journey, enhanced the prospects for a successful mission, since Acton had always advised the Papacy against an English hierarchy. Wiseman was also helped by having the confidence of Mgr. Barnabò, new Secretary of Propaganda. It was in the course of this visit to Rome that Wiseman was entrusted by the Pope with the task of seeking to interest the British Government in diplomatic relations. Clearly Wiseman's importance in the Vatican's English strategy was increasing, and on his return to England he became temporary Vicar Apostolic of the London District—an appointment made permanent on Walsh's death in 1849. In May of the following year he was informed by Cardinal Antonelli that he was to become a cardinal, but it was with some misgiving that he left for Rome in August, believing that his work in England was at an end. To his evident surprise, on arrival in Rome, he learned from Pius IX that the hierarchy was to be restored to England and that he was to be its head. The Papal Brief setting up the hierarchy was dated 29 September 1850: a sequence of events, perhaps the most well known in the English Catholic history of the nineteenth century, were set in motion. Wiseman was to become a national figure, but a figure of notoriety.

'Wherever a Bishop appears', Wiseman said in 1863, 'a true religious oasis is immediately formed around him.'[58] It is hardly surprising that he was unprepared for the hostile clamour with which Protestant England greeted the bishops of 1850. On his journey back to England, bearing his new honours, his thoughts turned mostly to the financial difficulties of maintaining his position.[59] The shock he sustained on reading *The Times'* attack, and the fortitude with which he faced both that and the subsequent threats made to his person by extremists, were real enough. 'I received letters announcing that the moment I entered the pulpit a pistol would put an end to my course,' he later disclosed.[60] There was at least one compensation: the collections (or 'take' as Wiseman called them) made in churches during the uproar,

---

[58] *The Religious and Social Position of Catholics in England*, 25.
[59] Wilfrid Ward, *Wiseman*, I. 531.
[60] *Tour in Ireland*, 305.

when people were packed in to see the new Cardinal, went up appreciably.[61] He was also able to play a heroic role—'I have borne the entire brunt of the excitement; the other bishops have escaped unnoticed.'[62] He wrote at the start of his *Appeal to the Reason and Good Feeling of the English People* about the agitation, 'perhaps unparalleled in our times', that 'its violence has been that of a whirlwind, during which it would have been almost folly to claim a hearing'.[63] The *Appeal*, which he began to write the very day he arrived back in London, and which Ullathorne described as 'inaccurate, as regards the order of facts as well as the persons to whom he ascribed them,'[64] enjoyed an enormous circulation (30,000 copies were sold in the first week) and the full text appeared in all five leading London newspapers.[65]

The Pope, he contended in the *Appeal*, was not to blame for the hierarchy: the restoration had resulted from a petition of the English Vicars Apostolic, to which the Papacy had responded.[66] (Eight years later, at a banquet in Waterford, he was to declare 'I must disclaim any merit in the great measure itself. It was the spontaneous act of the present Pontiff'.)[67] The hierarchy, he wrote, was a simple matter of ecclesiastical jurisdiction and administration, not looked upon by the bishops 'as a matter of triumph'[68]—a straightforward attempt to offset the impression of quasi-temporal grandeur left by his Flaminian Gate Pastoral announcing the new arrangement. It was a matter of governing England through regular ecclesiastical structures.[69] No attack upon the Royal Supremacy or the Established Church was intended: the hierarchy did not and could not alter either.[70] He was also able to point out that Catholic hierarchies existed in Ireland and in the Colonies

[61] Cardinal Gasquet, 'Letters of Cardinal Wiseman', in *Dublin Review*, Jan.–March, 1919, 9 (Wiseman to Talbot, 9 Dec. 1850).

[62] Ibid. 11.

[63] *An Appeal to the Reason and Good Feeling of the English People on the Subject of the Catholic Hierarchy*, 7.

[64] Ullathorne, *History of the Restoration of the Catholic Hierarchy in England*, VI. The first draft of the book is in the Archives of St. Dominic's Convent at Stone, Box VII.

[65] On Nov. 20 1850.

[66] *Appeal*, 20.

[67] *Tour in Ireland*, 304.

[68] *Appeal*, 2.   [69] Ibid. 4.   [70] Ibid. 10, 17.

without hazard to Protestant interests.[71] The *Appeal* was, as it was intended to be, reasonable and full of sound points; and to some extent it helped to quieten the agitation. In December he reinforced the message by delivering three lectures at St. George's Cathedral in Southwark. They were an elaboration of the points he had already made, and he took the opportunity to emphasize again how the English agitation had ignored the general practice of Rome. He cited the recent creation of Archiepiscopal provinces in the United States, remarking, inaccurately as it happened, that 'not a voice has been raised against this act of Supremacy'.[72] But his broad perspectives were right, so was his belief that 'Time will disperse the mist, and show the transaction in its true light.'[73] Caught up in the success of the first lecture, however, he wrongly calculated that 'there is now no apprehension of any Government or Parliamentary measures against us'.[74] The Ecclesiastical Titles Act was introduced to the House of Commons on 7 February 1851—Wiseman himself being present in the gallery—and passed its second reading by 433 to 95 votes.[75]

The real nature of Wiseman's success over the restoration of the hierarchy lay not in his part in eventually allaying the Protestant fears he had anyway helped to provoke, nor in his preceding representations at Rome, but in his ability to turn a scheme of local ecclesiastical government (originally promoted by those seeking less centralized control) into an instrument for the diffusion of Ultramontanism. To some extent he overplayed his hand. The history of the succeeding decade may easily be interpreted as a decade of internal conflicts, with Wiseman emerging as an isolated and less and less effective figure. The bishops believed he was autocratic, and the cardinal, for his part, certainly supposed that they were

---

[71] Ibid. 24.

[72] *Three Lectures on the Catholic Hierarchy by Cardinal Wiseman*, London 1850, Lecture I. 10. See Norman, *The Conscience of the State in North America*, 99–101; Sydney E. Ahlstrom, *A Religious History of the American People*, Yale 1972, 564–5.

[73] *Appeal*, 6.

[74] Gasquet, *Dublin Review*, (1919) 10 (Wiseman to Talbot, 9 Dec. 1850).

[75] Wilfrid Ward, *Wiseman*, II. 24, 29. For a general account of the 'Papal Aggression' agitation, see Norman, *Anti-Catholicism in Victorian England*, iii. 52–80.

insufficiently loyal to the Roman authority which he represented, as he believed, in his person. Part of the trouble lay
with the very events of 1850. Public opinion treated Wiseman
as the leader of English Catholicism and he began to act according to this image. The bishops were correct in contending
that their jurisdiction and powers derived directly from Rome,
and that Wiseman's powers were largely limited to his own
archdiocese.[76]

In the administration of Westminster, as the years passed,
he became more and more dependent upon others—his secretary, Searle, his coadjutor Errington, and above all, Manning.
In the English Church generally, the First Provincial Synod
of 1852 was his only real success[77] (at least in the sense that
whatever differences of view or incompatibilities of personal
temperament lurked below, nothing broke the surface of the
accord which was then manifested). It was his 'masterpiece'—
the word used by Ullathorne, who recalled 'The unity and
harmony that pervaded that Chapter is one of the most
delightful reminiscences of my episcopal life.'[78] It was at the
opening of the second session of this Synod that Newman
preached his 'Second Spring' sermon. Wiseman and many of
the bishops wept. But after the Synod there was, as Dom
Cuthbert Butler put it, 'a certain reaction against Wiseman'.[79]
Some have seen the disputes between Wiseman and the
bishops in the years between 1853 and 1862 as 'the inevitable
growing pains of the new ecclesiastical order'.[80] But they
were not really that: they were the consequence of the manner in which Wiseman sought to impose Roman discipline
and the fact that it was being imposed at all. In these last
years of his English work, Wiseman was often ill. Yet still he
managed to travel—to Rome for the definition of the Immaculate Conception in 1854, for his presentation of the case
against his chapter in 1859, and for the canonization of the
Japanese Martyrs in 1862; to Ireland in 1858, to Malines in

[76] E. E. Reynolds, *Three Cardinals*, London 1958, 119.
[77] See Richard Schiefen, 'The First Provincial Synod of Westminster (1852)',
in *Annuarium Historiae Conciliorum* (1972), 188-213.
[78] *From Cabin-Boy to Archbishop*, 299.
[79] Cuthbert Butler, *The Life and Times of Bishop Ullathorne, 1806-1889*,
I. 199.
[80] Fothergill, in the *Wiseman Review*, 493 (1962), 243.

1863. His last years, in Manning's lovely words, were 'like the hours of a still afternoon, when the work of the day begins to linger, and the silence of evening is near'.[81] Exhausted, lonely, and subject to occasional depressions of spirit, he died in February 1865.[82]

It is not easy to evaluate the work of this extraordinary and great prelate. Yet the disputations of his later years have remained the freshest feature of the collective memory, and their causes do require careful explanation. They actually began quite early—in the later 1830s—when a number of the English bishops began to feel that Wiseman was too independent in his management of their dealings with Rome, when acting as their agent. It was certainly true that Wiseman progressively behaved as if he was the agent of the Holy See, revealing Papal directives and attitudes to the English bishops, rather than acting as the Roman letter-box they considered as constituting his proper function. There was, at that time, apparently, a general feeling among the Vicars Apostolic that Wiseman should be found a post in England, but also a general reluctance to accept him as a coadjutor.[83] There were particular suspicions that he favoured the religious orders too much, and the two Edicts of 1838, which circumscribed episcopal authority over the Regulars and allowed new missions to be opened by them autonomously, were regarded as not only offensive in themselves but as indicating Wiseman's influence. In 1838, therefore, the Vicars Apostolic resolved that in future their agent should not be the President of the English College: a direct rejection of Wiseman. Wiseman's own knowledge of English affairs was a little too dependent on the opinion of such as Phillipps de Lisle, Spencer, and Rock: all of whom he cited as authorities in an account of the English mission he made for Propaganda in 1839.[84] His seeming partiality to the religious orders, of course, accounts for much of the later difficulty over the Oblates of St. Charles. To some

---

[81] Wilfrid Ward, *Wiseman*, II. 453.

[82] The account of Wiseman's funeral, in *The Times* (24 Feb. 1865), describes the remarkable public sympathy it elicited: 'Not since the state funeral of the late Duke of Wellington has the same interest been evinced.'

[83] Holmes, *More Roman than Rome*, 63.

[84] Propaganda, *Scritture* 9 (1834–41) 525, *Cenni sullo stato religioso dell' Inghilterra tratti da particolari lettere scritte di recente*, 12 Jan. 1839.

of the London clergy, when he was Vicar Apostolic in 1849, it was this feature of the 'Romanizing' that was the hardest to stomach—for practical reasons as well as ideological. For the rules of the orders did not envisage their undertaking the ordinary parochial work of the English missions, and their styles of ministry were, as a result, often quite out of sympathy with existing practices. Bishop Griffiths had been opposed to the establishment of the Jesuits at Farm Street. Wiseman ignored such feelings. He regarded the orders, and especially the new Italian ones, as vital spearheads of the missionary advance in England. He set up Fr. Dominic Barberi and the Passionists at Highgate.[85] He supported Fr. Faber against the opposition of the London clergy when the Oratory of St. Philip Neri was settled in London in 1849.[86] He also helped the Redemptorists and the Marists to establish themselves in London. During his years at Westminster, in fact, fifteen communities of men and twenty-three of women were founded.[87] It was an impressive achievement, but it was bought at some cost to domestic peace. A number of the bishops were as suspicious as many of the secular clergy. Dislike of Wiseman's 'Romanizing', and his lack of respect for the independence of the episcopate, underlay the difficulties of the 1850s, whose overt disputes were rationalized by both sides into disputes about principles. The first sign of trouble came in 1853, when the bishops decided to deal with the government directly, over the question of Catholic chaplains for the armed forces. There were fears partly about Wiseman's sense of his own authority, but also about his efficiency in such matters. In Rome, during the autumn of that year, Wiseman tried to explain the party divisions of the English Church to Propaganda—an indication of their sharpened dimensions.

Wiseman's dispute with the Chapter of Westminster, which lasted over a period of ten years, was the most notorious of these occasions of disharmony. The questions in dispute were focussed particularly clearly. 'The fundamental issue', as Dr Schiefen wrote in his illuminating examination of the episode,

---

[85] Bernard Ward, *Sequel to Catholic Emancipation*, II. 178.
[86] Chapman, *Father Faber*, 230, 232.
[87] *The English Catholics, 1850–1950*, ed. Beck, 154.

'involved the right of the Chapter to interfere in matters which, as they appeared to Wiseman, were clearly within the sole jurisdiction of the bishop.'[88] In his own diocese, that is to say, Wiseman was defending episcopal independence against the Chapter in much the same way as in the larger context of the English Church in general he defended the senior Archbishop's superiority over the other bishops. Issue was first joined over the question of Catholic Colleges. Wiseman had always believed that the English clergy needed reforming, and that an infusion of 'Roman' spirit in the seminaries would go a long way to preparing them for the ideal of priesthood which he imagined to reside in Italian practice. In 1851 he managed to dismiss the President of St. Edmund's College, Edward Cox. At that time, also, he appointed the convert, W. G. Ward, as lecturer—and later professor—of Dogmatic Theology. In 1858 another appointment was made which seemed to suggest a defined plan by Wiseman to mould the College to his own image: that of the young Herbert Vaughan as Vice-President. In letters to Talbot during these years, Wiseman was explicit about his intentions. With Cox's removal, he wrote in 1851, the College was 'cleared of its terrible obstruction'. He continued, 'The whole system will be reformed, and a sound, high-toned ecclesiastical spirit will be introduced.'[89] The widespread suspicions about Wiseman's intentions crystallized in the mind of his coadjutor (after 1855) George Errington, titular Archbishop of Trebizond. Though a contemporary of Wiseman's at Ushaw and at the Venerabile, and his Prefect of Studies at Oscott—where he was a close confidant of Wiseman's—Errington was a very different kind of man. Efficient and disciplined in business, more 'English' than 'Roman' in outlook, and unmovable on points of principle, Errington was once described by Mother Margaret Hallahan as 'hewn out of a rock'.[90] Through his blue-tinted spectacles he viewed the accumulating evidence of Wiseman's baneful attempt, as he judged it, to take over

[88] R. J. Schiefen, 'Some Aspects of the Controversy between Cardinal Wiseman and the Westminster Chapter', in *Journal of Ecclesiastical History*, XXI. 2, April 1970, 125.

[89] Gasquet, *Dublin Review* (1919), 22 (Wiseman to Talbot, 3 Aug. 1851).

[90] Wilfrid Ward, *Wiseman*, II. 259.

St. Edmund's College as a microcosm of the fate of the entire English Church. In 1855 he imposed restrictions on Ward's teaching—which was, clearly, Ultramontanist in tone. Ward resigned. Wiseman reinstated him. Errington suggested his own resignation as coadjutor in a letter to Talbot: 'The Ward affair was in reality, as the public I find has considered it, a trial of strength between my influence and one opposed to it.'[91] Instead of resignation, however, he retired temporarily to the diocese of Clifton, returning to London, at Wiseman's request, after Ward's resignation from St. Edmund's in 1856. Ward then withdrew his resignation.

Manning entered the story in 1857 with the establishment in Bayswater of the Oblates of St. Charles. In the same year Dr Whitty joined the Society of Jesus and Manning, a convert of six years, who at that time was scarcely known to the clergy was, through Wiseman's influence, appointed by Rome as Provost of Westminster—in which capacity he presided over the Chapter. When three members of the St. Edmund's staff, including Vaughan, joined the Oblates, it appeared to Errington, as to others, that Wiseman's circle was seeking to hand the College over to the Order. Errington devoted much time to a critical examination of the rules of the Oblates to determine if there were departures from the original rules of St. Charles Borromeo which might incapacitate the English Oblates from undertaking the duties of St. Edmund's. Successfully discovering a few discrepancies, Errington got a modification of the rules in May 1858 which subjected members of the order engaged in mission work to the jurisdiction of the bishop. But he remained unsatisfied. Even Mgr. Searle, Wiseman's secretary, shared his deepening suspicions. In July 1858, the Chapter of Westminster took the question into its consideration formally, with Errington behind the successful resolution to institute an inquiry into the status of St. Edmund's College.[92] The issue between Wiseman and his critics now rearranged itself around an interpretation of the decrees of the Council of Trent. By their provision, each diocese was to set up a seminary, which was to be under the

[91] Ibid. II. 261.
[92] Schiefen, 'Some Aspects of the Controversy . . .', 128.

control of the bishop: Wiseman, apparently acting under this understanding, had originally entrusted to some of the canons in the Chapter certain powers in relation to the affairs of St. Edmund's. In 1858 the Chapter produced these as evidence against the possibility of linking the seminary with an order, and drew up a petition seeking the Oblates' exclusion. Wiseman denied this by arguing that the Tridentine decree did not apply: St. Edmund's was not a seminary in the ordinary sense, but a mixed college for the education of lay boys and priests.

The principles having now surfaced upon the sea of suspicions and ideological incompatibilities, the details of the subsequent dispute between Wiseman and the Chapter were of less significance. An absurd row about the authenticity of the Chapter Book Wiseman had demanded to see[93] indicated the depth of the fissures that had opened up. 'The fermentation of spirits in the Diocese is extreme,' the Bishop of Emmaus (Patterson) reported to Talbot in March 1859; 'reports from the Chapter of the most exaggerated description are circulated, and the old cry is raised that the Cardinal is acting tyrannically and arbitrarily.'[94] In December 1858, Wiseman annulled the proceedings of the Chapter, and both sides appealed to Rome. 'It is then of great moment to me to know', as Wiseman wrote to Errington at this juncture, 'whether you have assisted by your advice my Chapter (through any of its members) in the course that body has lately been pursuing in my regard.' He asked especially about the preparation of the documents being sent to Rome.[95] First Patterson, and then Manning, were dispatched by Wiseman to represent his case to the Holy See. Canon John Maguire wrote to Talbot to say 'that the step taken by the Chapter is no act of defiance or hostile feeling or prejudice, no result of faction or collusion'. He expressed pain at 'estrangement' from Wiseman—who 'it has been my pride and my endeavours to serve faithfully and assiduously'.[96]

[93] Ibid. 129.
[94] English Coll. Archives, Talbot Papers, 565, Patterson to Talbot, 18 March 1859.
[95] Errington Papers, Bristol Record Office, 35721, 9, Wiseman to Errington, 9 Dec. 1858.
[96] English Coll. Archives, Talbot Papers, 472, Maguire to Talbot, 28 Dec. 1858.

In Rome, Propaganda decided to refer the matter back to the English Church—to the Third Provincial Synod. When this met, at Oscott in July 1859, the bishops anticipated frightful disagreements. Ullathorne believed that the points at issue should be treated, first, according to canon law, and, secondly, as 'equity and expediency require'. Such calculation did not match the emotions of the others. Ullathorne, indeed, was, as he wrote at the time, not 'involved personally in the controversy'—'happily for myself', he added. 'I think I see some of the signs of danger.'[97] Wiseman visited him four months before the Synod was due to meet, but Ullathorne's attempts 'to modify some of his views'[98] were not successful. At the Synod, Errington spoke out against Wiseman's case, despite Wiseman's preparatory reminder to him that he would expect his support—since he was his coadjutor. Some of the bishops wanted to pass formal Decrees about the Colleges; others thought it more politic simply to address a letter to Propaganda giving their conclusions in a less formal manner. A majority, including Ullathorne—who regretted it—voted for the formal procedure.[99] Decree XV was passed against Wiseman's opposition—it was actually framed by Errington and Grant. It provided for a Board of bishops to manage the colleges, although the right of canons to become involved in the management of colleges was denied, so upholding Wiseman's contention that existing institutions were not within the Tridentine provisions. 'The Synod', Manning wrote to Wiseman just after the end of the meetings, 'was the last conflict in a year's campaign.' He added: 'it seems to me to have been a complete justification of all you have done, and I hope you will now dismiss all thought and anxiety'. As for the Chapter of Westminster—'they are more likely to return to a right mind if they are left awhile to themselves'.[100] But the going was not easy. By 1862 relations had become so bad

[97] Westminster Dioc. Archives, Wiseman Papers, Bishops' Letters, 130/1, Ullathorne to an unnamed bishop, 15 April 1859.

[98] Ibid.

[99] Birmingham Dioc. Archives, B.3915 'Draft Letter to the Cardinal [Prefect of Propaganda] about the Decrees of the Third Synod of Westminster, concerning the government of the English Colleges' (n.d., but 1859).

[100] Westminster Dioc. Archives, Wiseman Papers, Bishops' Letters WB/40, Manning to Wiseman, 28 July 1859.

that most of the bishops found excuses from attendance at the annual Low Week meeting. In Rome, there were delays, the matter remaining *sub judice*, as Propaganda wrote to remind the Chapter in January 1861. All must wait until 'the deliberations of the Provincial Synod and the deliberations of the Holy See shall have been adjusted'.[101] Wiseman, meanwhile, became increasingly restive—particularly with Grant. 'We differ on every point—he has never manifested the least anxiety on the state or wants of our clerical education,' he complained to Talbot, in August 1863, from Broadstairs. 'What can I do but let things go on as they have done in times past, till a greater-hearted spirit and feeling prevail and my successor in future times will be allowed to work for the Church in confidence that he will be trusted in what he does.'[102] In September 1863, Propaganda approved the Decrees.

Contemporaneously with the St. Edmund's question, Wiseman was also involved with the five northern bishops, in a parallel dispute about the government of Ushaw. In 1850 he had been appointed 'Apostolic Visitor' of St. Cuthbert's College and in 1854, at the Low Week meeting of the hierarchy, had defended the President, Dr Newsham, in his claim that the College was independent of the northern bishops—on the grounds that it was not a seminary in the Tridentine sense. It was this dispute which, at the Synod in 1859, made the northern bishops determined to side with the opposition to Wiseman on the Colleges issue.[103]

As a result of these sorry events, Wiseman was determined to dispose of his coadjutor. Errington, incensed by the cardinal's dealings with him, and particularly offended by the charge (made explicitly by Wiseman) that he was 'anti-Roman',[104] refused to resign. Talbot, from Rome, tried to persuade him to accept the archbishopric of Trinidad, in April 1859. By then, Errington, sensing he had the sympathy and support of a majority of the clergy in England—which may

[101] English Coll. Archives, Talbot Papers, 552, Frederick Oakley to Talbot, 24 Jan. 1861.
[102] Ibid. 1109, Wiseman to Talbot, 23 Aug. 1863.
[103] Milburn, *A History of Ushaw College*, 203, 208, 242, 244, 272.
[104] Wilfrid Ward, *Wiseman*, II. 331.

well have been the case—regarded himself as standing up for
traditional English Catholics. That was, indeed, precisely
what Talbot had imagined he was doing. 'I firmly believe that
the animus of the whole movement against the Cardinal is the
Anglo-Gallican retrograde spirit which still reigns in the old
clergy of London', he wrote to Searle in January 1859; 'Dr
Errington sympathised in their views, and Dr Errington has
found that they sympathise with him.'[105] This opinion
reached Errington's notice and he wrote at once to Talbot.
Talbot hastened to reply soothingly to him, expressing 'sorrow' if he had, in what was, after all, as he pointed out, a
private letter to Searle, hurt his feelings. 'I do not believe that
you are anti-Roman in theory or principle', he declared, but
'you will never get on with Cardinal Wiseman', and so was
'not suited for London'.[106] Errington was not mollified. 'I had
written to complain to yourself of your having made very
serious and false charges and insinuations against me', he
wrote to Talbot, 'and you write back as if I had been merely
writing about some matter in which you had unintentionally
said something painful to my feelings.'[107] Talbot, later in the
year, objected to Errington's public 'speaking against me',
and added; 'I have always acted with the most ingenuous charity in your regard.'[108] In December 1859, both men were in
Rome to make their respective representations: Cardinal
Barnabò plainly sided with Wiseman, whose four months
spent compiling a *scrittura* for Propaganda on the affair were
therefore not in vain. In February 1860, Manning arrived to
put the case to the Pope as well. On 8 March, Errington was
summoned to Pius IX's presence and urged to accept the
archbishopric of Trinidad. He refused. Those waiting in the
antechamber were astonished to hear raised voices. Within,
Errington produced a pocket-book and began to take down
the Holy Father's words. His notes on the interview survive
—in the Clifton Diocesan Archives. He was, he recorded,

[105] Errington Papers, Bristol Record Office, 35721, 12, Talbot to Searle,
13 Jan. 1859.
[106] Ibid. 16, Talbot to Errington, 15 March 1859.
[107] Errington Papers, Bristol Record Office, 35721, 17, Errington to Talbot,
30 March 1859.
[108] Ibid. 28, Talbot to Errington, 22 Dec. 1859.

'Kindly received but kept standing.' The Pope stated that the reason for requiring his resignation was the 'incompatibility' of himself and Wiseman. 'Would you like to see him die?', the Pope asked heatedly. 'I said I had my own honour, and that my friends would not allow me to sign my own condemnation,' Errington replied. His Holiness denied that Talbot had been responsible for giving him prejudicial information—he had not spoken with him on the matter for two months. 'The Pope grew severe and energetic', Errington recorded, 'and asked me how he could allow me to be at Westminster after the Cardinal's time, with this obstinate character, and how could he count upon my doing what he asked if I would not do so now?' Errington then again refused to resign unless commanded. The Pope was outraged. 'He then rose and with great animation told me that I was most obstinate; that to refuse a favour to the Vicar of Christ was great and bad obstinacy, that it was the mark of a bad disposition, and showed me to be unfit for the position; and he would always consider me as of a bad disposition, with a bad heart.' The Pope's words should be borne in mind: they account for his wrath with the Chapter of Westminster in 1865, when they sent Errington's name to Rome as Wiseman's successor. The interview came summarily to a conclusion: 'He rang his bell and I knelt down to kiss his foot, which he extended.'[109]

Pius IX, despite his outrage at such an unprecedented affront, agreed to Errington's plea for a formal inquiry—'thus providing' as Errington wrote to Clifford, 'for some of the ordinary safeguards of an accused person'[110]—and three cardinals were appointed to examine the conflicting evidence of the events in England. In July 1860, on the basis of their findings, Errington was removed from the coadjutorship—but without the stipulation of any offence. The Decree referred simply to incompatibilities with the Cardinal. He retired to Prior Park in the diocese of his friend, Dr Clifford, the Bishop of Clifton; and there he quietly taught theology until his death in 1886,

[109] Errington Papers, Bristol Record Office, 35721, 36, 'Minutes of audience on 8 March, 1860'.
[110] Clifford Papers, Bristol Record Office, 35721, Errington to Clifford, 6 June 1860.

a quarter of a century later.[111] There is a letter of 1863 in the Talbot papers (at the English College in Rome) from Canon John Morris of the Westminster Chapter, speculating about the 'great scandal' and 'embarrassment to the Holy See' which would arise should Errington press his claims to succeed Wiseman. He added—in a summary of the differences between the style of the two men—'that Dr. Errington's appointment would be a very serious injury to the spirit that the Cardinal has been so successful in introducing'.[112] The Roman spirit, however, continued its success.

With the evidence of such dramatic episodes as these, it is hardly surprising that Wiseman's period as leader of the English Church has been regarded as an especially acrimonious one. To what extent was Wiseman himself to blame? Clearly his manner and his 'Roman' policy were bound to provoke difficulties. But Wiseman was, it must be remembered, a man noted in Rome for his diplomatic skills. In 1832 he acted as intermediary in the dispute between Bishop Baines and the Downside Benedictines.[113] This was not successful; but then the nature of that controversy was such that no conciliation could really have been expected to succeed. In 1847 he was entrusted by the Holy See with the task of persuading Lord Palmerston to support the Papacy against the threat of the Austrian army, then occupying Ferrara. The Whigs had just formed their administration in England, and were sympathetic to Pius IX because of his known liberal opinions. Yet diplomatic approaches to the British government were difficult because no formal relations existed—business had to be arranged through the Hanoverian ambassador—so Wiseman's achievement here was considerable. Lord Minto, who was about to visit Italy, was instructed by Palmerston to go to Rome as well. Wiseman's further suggestion, the institution of formal diplomatic relations, was also given a friendly reception by the British government, and after Minto's three

---

[111] For a full account of the Errington case, see Wilfrid Ward's *Wiseman*, II. 257. It is largely based on Errington's own narrative, written in 1860 for submission to the Pope.

[112] English College Archives, Talbot Papers, 510, Morris to Talbot, 26 June 1863.

[113] Bernard Ward, *Sequel*, I. 41.

months in Rome (where he resorted to the salons of prominent liberal politicians, to the increasing embarrassment of the Pope), legislation was introduced in 1848. It was opposed in Ireland, where it was seen as a crafty device of the English to govern the Irish through the good offices of Rome, and in England by some ultra-Protestants and some Old Catholics.[114] Wiseman wrote a public reply to a 'Memorial of the Catholics of London', in which he sternly told them 'the Pope is a temporal sovereign, as well as our spiritual Head: and in *that* capacity has a right to hold relations as he judges best'.[115] Wiseman showed his knowledge of Papal diplomacy in 1855, when he gave a course of public lectures in London on concordats, explaining their nature and effects to a public whose anti-Austrian sensibilities had been offended by the concordat made in that year between the Papacy and the Habsburg court. In 1862 he was sent by the Pope to see Napoleon III, and sought to influence him against Piedmontese policy in Italy. The Emperor was unmoved. But as further testimony to Wiseman's abilities as a diplomatist the episode ought to be remembered—the more so since it took place immediately after the worst phase of the English troubles.

Over Wiseman's administrative capabilities, however, there need be little doubt. Due to what Archbishop Mathew called his 'insecure command of detail' in ecclesiastical business,[116] Wiseman was always at his least effective in the daily conduct of affairs. Enormous amounts of time were absorbed by nineteenth-century clerics in worrying about the financing of their institutions: Wiseman, who probably founded more than anyone else, declined to bother. In small things, too, his dislike for money matters was evident, and extended even to paying cab bills—'It seemed', recalled Bernard Smith, 'out of keeping with his rather grandiose habits that he should do so himself.'[117] Similar characteristics tended to appear in his dealings with government departments. He had a natural respect for

[114] Bernard Ward, *Sequel*, II. 191–203.

[115] *Words of Peace and Justice addressed to the Catholic Clergy and Laity of the London District on the Subject of Diplomatic Relations with the Holy See,* by the Rt. Rev. Nicholas Wiseman, D.D., Bishop of Melipotamus, London 1848, 11.

[116] David Mathew, *Catholicism in England, 1535–1935*, 194.

[117] Wilfrid Ward, *Wiseman*, I. 350.

authority, but believed his position was such that he could rely upon more influence than he possessed. There is, for example, a manuscript letter in the Westminster Diocesan Archives which formed the basis of a consultation with the bishops about Catholic co-operation with the Royal Commission on popular education, set up in 1858 (the Newcastle Commission, which reported in 1861), in which Wiseman suggested that they should make the appointment of a Catholic Commissioner 'a necessary condition of our co-operation'.[118] Most dealings with government departments were made by individual bishops after 1853, and Grant, in particular, looked after the important contacts necessary for securing concessions over military and institutional chaplaincies.

It was Wiseman's economy of business sense which involved him in some of his more well-known difficulties with others. There was his failure to get the facts right in relation to Newman's chimerical bishopric; his loss of documents landed Newman on another occasion with the disagreeable loss of the lawsuit brought against him by Achilli in 1851; and it was Newman, yet again, who suffered when Wiseman inexplicably abandoned a project, on which Newman had already commenced work in 1857, for a new translation of the Bible. Incredibly, their friendship survived. In 1854 Wiseman was taken to court by one of his own clergy—Fr. Boyle, assistant priest at Islington. The issue was really about opposition to Wiseman's attempt to introduce the new devotions to the diocese, but Boyle raised legal points about the cardinal's right to dispossess him, and it was, once more, Wiseman's inattention to accuracy and detail which led him to the three libel actions that followed. The archives of Propaganda for 1851 contain numerous papers on the Boyle affair.[119] These instances were dramatic indications of his daily practice of inefficiency. Hence the need for an assistant. Ill-health, too, made it imperative by the mid 1850s. Talbot, with wisdom which later developments amply confirmed, suggested an auxiliary bishop, who would be easily removable; Wiseman insisted on a coadjutor, with rights of succession. This led

[118] Westminster Dioc. Archives, Wiseman papers, R79/6 (1 Oct. 1858).
[119] Propaganda, *Scritture* 12 (1848–51), 669 ff.

to the appointment of Errington in 1855. It proved the most unhappy of Wiseman's miscalculations in his judgement of people, but the ease of their relations at Oscott presumably suggested that he and Errington could work well together.[120] The choice was not unreasonable, from that perspective. Wiseman came increasingly to depend on others. It was from Mgr. George Talbot, the convert son of Lord Talbot of Malahide, that he derived more and more of his information about Rome; and from Sir George Bowyer (a Member of Parliament between 1852 and 1868, and also a political consultant of Cardinal Cullen's) that he took his political knowledge. The correspondence from Bowyer, in the Westminster Archives, though not extensive, shows the degree of Wiseman's dependence on him. At Rome, too, as Odo Russell remarked in his despatch to the Foreign Office, Bowyer was 'very active' and 'constantly with the Pope and Antonelli'.[121] There were, it is true, shadows upon this relationship, especially as both Manning and Talbot came to distrust Bowyer. Bowyer, in turn, 'was loud-mouthed in his denunciations of Manning; and carried his abuse even into the smoking-room of the Reform Club'.[122] It was, of course, to Manning that Wiseman finally, and decisively turned, and on whom his dependence became most marked. It was, as Cardinal Gasquet remarked, to Manning that Wiseman 'poured forth his woes',[123] and whose complete loyalty he secured. But the influence was two-way. Manning hardened the cardinal's attitudes, leading to his withdrawal of support for Newman's scheme of an Oxford oratory, to his acquiescence in the censure of Phillipps de Lisle's attitudes to Christian Reunion, and to his approval for the prohibition of Catholic students at Oxford and Cambridge colleges. The bishops' dislike of Manning's influence considerably intensified their opposition to Wiseman's policies and conduct in the later 1850s. Pressed by Talbot to consider the appointment of a new coadjutor, however, Wiseman

[120] For a full account of Errington's period as coadjutor, see Cuthbert Butler, *Life and Times of Bishop Ullathorne*, I. 278-306.

[121] *The Roman Question. Extracts from the despatches of Odo Russell from Rome, 1858-1870*, ed. Noel Blakiston, London, 1962, 80. This refers to 1860.

[122] Purcell, *Life of Cardinal Manning, Archbishop of Westminster*, II. 404.

[123] Gasquet in *Dublin Review* (1921), op. cit., 161.

was reluctant: in June 1863, he wrote of his 'greatest objections' to the idea. 'In my present relations with many of the bishops, this is a grave matter,' he added, for to name a man as his intimate at this state would be divisive—and hazardous, for there was no guarantee of full support in Rome for any candidate he might name. 'You know that Cardinal Barnabò has been always inclined to take the side of the Suffragans, and count up the numbers of those against me, and complain that I did not make enough of their numbers etc.' He concluded: 'I want peace above all things.'[124]

There were, then, clear deficiencies in Wiseman's administrative capacity and in the manner of his exercise of authority. It was his great misfortune, however, that in the matter to which above all else he gave both personal and public priority—the spiritual life—there was also controversy and division. Wiseman's greatest endeavour was to stimulate the introduction of the new devotions to England, and to see their spread throughout the Church. Later generations of Catholics have sometimes chosen to abandon the new styles, or to regret their 'Italianate' triumphalism: but there can be little doubt about the spiritual importance of the emphasis given to the devotional life in England by their introduction. The quality of the prayers and spiritual disciplines themselves are quite independent of this—it was Wiseman's highest task, as he saw it, to revivify English devotional life, and that he did. The revival was centred in his own personal devotion to the Virgin and to the Counter-Reformation saints. The Forty Hours' Devotion was introduced, and the Rosary—'the devotion so little understood, nay, often so much slighted, even by good people in our country'[125]—was encouraged by the foundation of rosary confraternities. Wiseman himself wrote two books of popular devotions for the laity, in furtherance of his conviction that existing Catholic prayers needed to be replaced because they were tainted with Protestantism. 'Now it has seemed to us as though some of the leaven which, while it fermented, soured the sweet bread of old devotion among

---

[124] English Coll. Archives, Talbot Papers, 1107, Wiseman to Talbot, 26 June 1863.

[125] *Essays on Various Subjects*, I. 496: 'Essay on the Minor Rites and Offices of the Church', Part I (1843).

our neighbours, had unfortunately slipped in among ourselves,' he wrote in 1842: 'It appears to us as though most
of our modern English prayers came too much from the
head.'[126] It was devotions of the heart that had so impressed
themselves upon Wiseman when he recognized their effect in
the religion of the ordinary people in Italy and Spain. Particularly during the summer visits to the English College's
villa at Monte Porzio, during his Roman years, he had seen
the power of popular spirituality among the poor. His hope,
in England, was to create a peoples' spirituality—something
evidently lacking in the State Church. In his polemical writings he set out to defend the folk devotions of Catholicism
overseas from the normal English assumption, shared by
Protestants and Catholics alike, that they were a mere compil-
ation of superstition. In reply to Newman's belief—expressed
while still a Protestant—that these practices went far beyond
the Tridentine spirit, in their supposed excesses and their
simple credulity, Wiseman declared that in popular Catholicism 'devotional feelings are taken as tests of their convictions
and faith'. He added, 'interrogate those who have manifested
those powerful feelings about their faith, and you will soon
find that it is *Tridentine* and sound'.[127] He was aware that
contemporary English culture assumed all Catholicism overseas to be superstitious and empty. In reality, he argued, it
was different: 'Travellers go forth with a standard formed in
their mind upon models at home.' But it was 'the religion of
England' which was 'the religion of one day in the week'.[128]
The Catholicism of Spain, he said in another place, was assumed to have resulted in the 'abject degradation to which
a people could be brought by not reading the Bible, and
allowing themselves to be blindly led by designing priests'. It
was supposed that Spanish religious life 'consisted in outward show, that the poor were beguiled by magnificent cer-
emonials', and that the country exhibited 'a melancholy
picture of spiritual abandonment and abjection'.[129] Nor were

[126] Ibid. I. 383, 'On Prayer and Prayer-Books' (1842).
[127] N. Wiseman, *A Letter Respectfully Addressed to the Rev. J. H. Newman*,
London, 3rd edn. 1841, 25.
[128] *Essays*, III. 516, 'Religion in Italy' (1836).
[129] Ibid. III. 4–5, 'Papers on History, Antiquities, and Art' (1845).

these ideas caricatures of Wiseman's own devising: he was correct in supposing that his new devotions would encounter the charge that they were an attempt to subject Englishmen to the superstitious level of European peasants. At the same time, he encouraged Biblical study, including what he thought of as 'critical study', and regretted that 'it was not more cultivated among us'—provided that it avoided 'extreme views'.[130] In this, however, as in his spiritual exercises, there was a great emphasis on the miraculous. That was not a feature which particularly separated his vision from that of most contemporaneous Christianity; but the extremes of his adherence to the ecclesiastical and folk miracles of the post-Reformation Church were sometimes at variance with the conventional Catholicism, not to speak of the Protestantism, of the England to which he came in the mid-century. He had a special devotion to the miracles of St. Philomena (now no longer included within the calendar of the saints) and rejoiced in 1848 when Gladstone's sister—'a most superior and most interesting convert', as he wrote to the Earl of Shrewsbury[131]—was cured from sickness through the application of one of the relics of the saint. Such occurrences, he claimed, indicated that English Catholics should do more to cultivate '*full* reverence to the Saints, and interest concerning them'.[132] For Ushaw, he procured a collection of relics, which included 20 of Christ, 3 of the Virgin, and 860 of the saints, and which Talbot 'declared to be equal to that in any Roman basilica'.[133] At the time of the college's Jubilee, in 1858, Wiseman managed to get the canonesses of St. Augustine in Paris to part with the ring of St. Cuthbert (though it was never claimed that the saint had worn it while alive: it had adorned his finger after one of the medieval reopenings of his tomb).[134] This he presented as an addition to the relic collection. For the new Lady Chapel at St. Edmund's, in 1860, he got the left leg of St. Edmund from the Archbishop of Sens.[135] It was not at all

---

[130] Ibid. I. 167–8, 'The Miracles of the New Testament' (1849).
[131] Ushaw College Archives, Wiseman Papers, 464, Wiseman to the Earl of Shrewsbury, 3 Jan. (n.d.).
[132] Wilfrid Ward, *Wiseman*, I. 507.
[133] Ibid. II. 167.
[134] Milburn, *A History of Ushaw College*, 227.
[135] Bernard Ward, *History of St. Edmund's College, Old Hall*, 277.

the spiritual style to which the English Catholics were accustomed.

The atmosphere of exultation and triumphalism, inherent in Wiseman's conception of the spiritual life, extended to every part of his understanding of the institutional Church. He was the great English apostle of Ultramontanism. National Churches were, by his definition, simply not Catholic. 'According to our view', he wrote in reply to Anglican claims, in 1842, 'the Catholic Church is one and indivisible, one spirit animating one body, giving to it all one life, discernible not merely by similarity of outward and visible operations, but by intercommunion of inward principles, the assent to one doctrine, based upon one authority, guaranteed by one infallibility, secured by one bond of love, strengthened by one hope.'[136] Nor were the truths of Christianity separable from the institutional structure of holiness. 'The government of the Church'—a feature which most English Protestants regarded as the most corrupt feature of Catholicism—'is so essential a part of her very being, that if a sense of her value be lost, we must fear that with it much else that is practically important will be gone.'[137] At the centre of this structure was the temporal dominion of the Papacy, whose 'independence must be real and not imaginary, to guarantee liberty and security of action', and which was assigned by 'Providence'.[138] In his view of the Church it was the clergy who directed and the laity who followed—a very decisive reversal of the roles which the Catholic gentry had imposed upon English Catholicism, howbeit of necessity, in the eighteenth century. 'We will call you forth when the Church of God wants your aid,' Wiseman told 'the nobility and laity' in 1848; 'we will always gladly see you working with us, but we cannot permit you to lead, where religious interests are concerned.'[139] He saw, indeed 'the influx into ecclesiastical and spiritual affairs of principles belonging to temporal and social interests' as being

---

[136] *Essays*, II. 310, 'The Anglican System' (1842).

[137] Ibid. III. 16, 'Papers on History, Antiquities, and Art' (1845).

[138] *Pastoral Letter of His Eminence the Cardinal Archbishop of Westminster enjoining a collection throughout the diocese for His Holiness the Pope*, London 1860, 24–5. (In response to this appeal, the Westminster clergy raised £6,340.)

[139] *Words of Peace and Justice*, 16.

'one of the great dangers of our time'.[140] The clergy, linked by their superiors to the spiritual refeshment of Rome, and guided by Roman discipline, were to cultivate a Church free from the laicization of the encompassing erastian religiosity of England. The devotional life of the Roman Church was to be the central driving force. Those who opposed Wiseman's vision here were correct in regarding it as the directional principle of his life.

English Catholicism, if regarded from this standpoint, had certain deficiencies. In Wiseman's diagnosis, it simply was not spiritual enough: people seemed to require too many worldly props. 'Our Catholicity is as cold as our politics are hot,' he remarked in a letter to Shrewsbury, about the possibility of remoulding *The Tablet* into an exclusively spiritual journal; 'consequently it will be difficult to draw forth any sympathy from our public for anything purely religious, without some exciting ingredient.'[141] In the summer of 1840, before leaving Rome for his work at Oscott, Wiseman drew up a list of his priorities for the Church he was to serve. The devotional life came first: more honour of the Virgin, the introduction of retreats, missions, the Forty Hours and the rosary. Then came the reform of the clergy: better (i.e. 'Roman') clerical training, the adoption of proper clerical dress, the conducting of regular episcopal visitations and diocesan synods. It was a fair enough summary of his attitude to the reforms that he believed necessary. 'What I am most anxious to accomplish', he had written to Dr Newsham two years previously, 'is to establish a small community of missioners, who, living at a common home, should go *bini* [in twos] from place to place giving lectures, retreats, etc., in different dioceses.'[142] Such a scheme, which was eventually fulfilled by the Italian orders Wiseman helped to introduce to England, was almost perfectly calculated to arouse the suspicions of the bishops and of local Catholic sentiment. Wiseman could not understand them. To be near to the spirit of Roman practice seemed, to him, an approximation to an infallible model of the Christian life.

---

[140] Ibid. 15.

[141] Ushaw College Archives, Wiseman Papers, 464, Wiseman to the Earl of Shrewsbury, 3 Jan. n.d. [1840s].

[142] Wilfrid Ward, *Wiseman*, I. 266.

Yet, unlike most of his Catholic contemporaries, Wiseman was sympathetic to the difficulties of Anglicans—he took the Oxford movement seriously, and used his critique of its leading assumptions as the occasion, once more, to project an enormous contrast with authentic Catholic principles and practices. The true Church thus laid out for Anglican inspection, however, was an Ultramontane assemblage which many of his own co-religionists found less than satisfactory. It was that which accounted for the sad paradox, from Wiseman's point of view, that his very success in addressing Protestant Englishmen involved the generation of suspicions within his own communion. Wiseman's criticism of the Church of England derived from his essential position on the nature of Catholicism: that since the Church was single and universal it could have no 'branches' as Anglicans supposed. 'A branch is a part of something else, of a plant', he argued; 'of what is the Anglican Church a branch?'[143] The evidences of his view, he pointed out in 1850 (in his second public lecture on the hierarchy) were plainly present in conventional Protestant attitudes to Catholicism. 'To say that one Church which calls another a teacher of doctrines "repugnant to God's word, of blasphemous fables and dangerous deceits," considers that and itself to be only two branches of one tree, would be contrary to every good feeling as much as to reason.'[144] At different times he pointed out that both the question of the Jerusalem bishopric scheme of 1841, when the Church of England had put itself into 'active communion' with German Protestantism,[145] and the Gorham Judgment in 1850, which had underlined the subordination of Anglican doctrine to the State—Anglicans having 'cut themselves so completely off from that authority, and that tribunal, to which alone an appeal in matters of faith would lie'[146]—showed how far removed English Protestantism was from the universal Church. As late as 1864 he was still hammering the message home, this time in the circumstances of the publication of *Essays and Reviews*: the Protestant Church had been revealed as 'a

[143] *Essays*, II. 306, 'The Anglican System' (1842).
[144] *Three Lectures on the Catholic Hierarchy*, Lecture II, 14.
[145] *Essays*, II. 368, 'Protestantism of the Anglican Church' (1842).
[146] Wiseman, quoted in Wilfrid Ward, I. 520.

canker of rationalism': 'learned men, in high dignity, have lifted up, if they have not thrown off, the cloak, which wrapped up in decent concealment the hideous sore'.[147] Wiseman regarded the foundation of the *Dublin Review* in 1836 as a splendid opportunity to present a reasoned case in support of Catholic views of the Church and so to help re-direct the course of the Oxford movement: 'To watch its progress, to observe its phases, to influence, if possible, its direction, to move it gently towards complete attainment of its unconscious aims.'[148] It was in the *Review*, of course, that he made his famous comparison between the Anglicans and the Donatists, which, according to Newman, upon whom it operated to produce one of the decisive steps on the road to conversion, 'absolutely pulverized' the Anglican theory of the *via media*.[149] The voice of antiquity was clear. St. Augustine's judgement of the Donatists was exactly the sort of authority to which Wiseman always appealed as the basis of his view of an indivisible Church: *Qua propter securus judicat orbis terrarum, bonos non esse qui se dividunt ab orbe terrarum, in quacumque parte orbis terrarum.*[150] 'Here then', Wiseman added, 'is a general rule applicable not merely to the Donatist case, but to all future possible divisions of the Church.'[151] It was a position he had always maintained, insisting, when he entertained Newman and Froude during their visit to Rome in 1833, that the whole teaching of the Council of Trent must be accepted entire, for it was the voice of the Universal Church.[152] But the seriousness of his two visitors convinced Wiseman that 'a new era had commenced in England'.[153] In his polemical writing on Anglican claims, thereafter, he sought to show that by their own appeals to antiquity and to true Catholic principles, the High Church divines were revealing that it was 'beyond human power' to repair 'the worn-out constitution of the poor old English Church'.[154] He referred

---

[147] *Pastoral Letter of H. E. Cardinal Wiseman enjoining the Collection for the building of Churches and Schools in the Archdiocese*, London 1864, 12-13.

[148] *Essays*, I. viii.

[149] J. H. Newman, *Apologia Pro Vita Sua*, New York, 1956 edn., 219.

[150] *Dublin Review*, Aug. 1834; reprinted in *Essays*, II. 224.

[151] Ibid. II. 225.   [152] Reynolds, 40.

[153] Wilfrid Ward, *Wiseman*, I. 119.

[154] *Essays*, II. 29, 'Tracts for the Times', Part I (1838).

to the *Charges* of the Anglican bishops, of 1841, to show the detestation in which the official leaders of the state church held the views expounded from Oxford.[155] His condemnation of Protestantism was the more severe because of the contrast with true religion; his loathing of 'that terrible event in English history, the horrors of which have been gilded by the name of Reformation,'[156] was the more intense because it deprived the English nation of its real inheritance. To such extremes the Old Catholics, with their quiet existence and their familiarity with the prevailing Protestant culture, were unused. Their suspicions of Wiseman were heightened, not diminished, by his Catholic exclusivity.

Yet it must still be concluded that, despite the difficulties with his own co-religionists, it was a considerable achievement of Wiseman's to have reawakened popular spirituality, with his 'Italian' devotions, and to have introduced Ultramontane discipline to the English Church, while at the same time managing to conduct a reasoned dialogue with the High Church Protestants. The Oxford movement, for its part, convinced him of the possibility of the conversion of England. Encouraged in Rome by Father Ignatius Spencer's accounts of the floods of converts to come (though he never fully shared Spencer's rather unrestrained optimism), and impressed by contacts with such as Lamennais, Montalembert, Lacordaire, and Döllinger, that a general European Catholic revival was likely to have an English dimension if the right stimulants were applied, Wiseman developed extremely high hopes of the prospects. The Oxford movement appeared to show that Protestantism was about to disintegrate. The early years of the 1840s seemed pregnant with new life. 'Experience has shown', Wiseman declared, 'that the country population are ready to receive without murmuring, indeed with pleasure, the Catholic views propounded from Oxford.'[157] The great temperance movement of Fr. Mathew in Ireland, with its rivivalistic fervour, and the Disruption of the Presbyterian Establishment in Scotland, added to the impression that some

---

[155] *Essays*, II. 347. For a full statement of these, see W. S. Bricknell, *The Judgment of the Bishops upon Tractarian Theology*, Oxford 1845.
[156] *Essays*, I. 360, 'The Fate of Sacrilege' (1846).
[157] Bernard Ward, *Sequel*, II. 100.

great new departure in religion was imminent. Wiseman, as usual, caught the spirit of the times. In his enthusiasm he was even ready 'to fall into the shade and take up our position in the background'; to hand over the leadership of Catholicism to the Oxford converts.[158] It was, indeed, another of Wiseman's achievements to have been among the first Catholic leaders in England to have ventured forth to attract converts and to have succeeded. Characteristically, he placed prayer above action (or even above journalism) as the means by which the conversions were to be encouraged: he wrote to the European bishops soliciting intercessions for the conversion of England, and issued a prayer for use within the Church at home. His old teacher, Lingard, and many others, warned him against treating the Oxford men too seriously. He ignored them and was right to do so. The cost, however, was levied within the Church, in jealousies between the Old Catholics and the converts—which Wiseman hoped would be overcome by joint submission to 'Roman' influence—and by a general resentment, among those who had borne the heat and burden of the day, that he was, as an Old Catholic lady put it, 'cockering up the converts'.[159] The favour shown to Ward, Manning, and Talbot was especially held to be unfortunate. Sometimes Wiseman's enthusiasm was embarrassingly punctured by events. Richard Waldo Sibthorp, Fellow of Magdalen College, Oxford, converted on a visit to Oscott in 1841, returned to the Church of England again in 1843. Wiseman had to spend a day in bed recovering from the shock of Sibthorp's defection. He was in bed again, but alas in the throes of death, when his last hours were lightened by news of Sibthorp's reconversion to Catholicism, after an interlude of twenty years.

It is important to realize, in evaluating Wiseman as a public figure, that part of his accomplishment in speaking successfully—despite the fracas of 1850—to a Protestant society hitherto given to extreme phobia about cardinals and Spaniards, lay in his own personal indebtedness to some of the liberal values of the 'Steam Age mentality'. Despite his adhesion to an exclusive view of the Church, there was

---

[158] Purcell, *Life and Letters of Ambrose Phillipps de Lisle*, I. 290.
[159] Reynolds, 143 (Mrs Barbara Charlton).

nothing of 'medievalism' (—the word used by Gladstone of the Catholic Church as late as 1874—) in his social and political outlook. At the end of 1850, as he stood back from the 'Papal Aggression' episode in order to assess its real significance, he saw that no real harm had befallen the Catholics. 'We have not been dragged before tribunals', he observed, and attributed this good fortune 'to the spirit of the age'.[160] In his earlier *Appeal* he had pointed to the Catholics' ability, in modern society, to act 'on an acknowledged right of liberty of conscience'.[161] Now spirits of the age and liberties of conscience were items which, as the *Syllabus of Errors* was to make clear in 1864, were not exactly nearest to the heart of Ultramontane Catholicism; but Wiseman was a stalwart adherent of nineteenth-century liberalism—at least in its English version. In his defence of the Temporal Power of the Papacy, of course, the Italian liberals were cast in a very different light. But then he also seems to have regarded the States of the Church as being administered according to liberal precepts. 'Without entering into any general considerations on the subject of government, or discussing its best forms', he recalled in 1858, 'one may say unhesitatingly that the government of Pius VII, through his minister Consalvi, was just, liberal, and enlightened.'[162] What was true of Pius VII can hardly have been less true of Pius IX, the acknowledged, if chastened, liberal.

Unlike the paternalistic Tories of his day, who lamented the passing of the old order and loathed the new England of commerce and 'useful knowledge', Wiseman felt at home in the nineteenth-century arrangements of things. At Salford, he once declared, 'I believe that the truest and surest type of a great and prosperous nation will be the union of the two symbols which are here: on the one side those vast and darkened piles of building, which fill your city, with their full columns above which the banner of industry ever streams in the wind; and, on the other, the vast magnificent church of God, with its spire bearing the symbol of peace and

---

[160] *Three Lectures on the Catholic Hierarchy*, Lecture III (22 Dec. 1850), 13.
[161] *An Appeal to the Reason and Good Feeling of the English People* (1850), 4.
[162] *Recollections of the Last Four Popes*, 82.

salvation.'[163] Factory and Church—to decode Wiseman's overflowing style: the union which the age needed. Very many bishops, both Anglican and Catholic, would have found such an image difficult to project—to them the world of the factories disclosed an alien atmosphere, an unwelcome intrusion in the small cities and rural heartlands of traditional English Christianity. Wiseman's rhetoric was full of allusions to the Victorian culture of achievement, expansion, and technical expertise. In 1849, for example, when writing in the *Dublin Review* about aspects of Biblical criticism, he produced a startlingly contemporary, if rather laboured, reference to Telford's Menai Straits bridge: 'Yet as surely as did the steam-engine and the hydraulic press, and the pontoons, and the many capstans with their many crews, lately bring the Britannia tube-bridges into their right position, and firmly plant them there; because, though to a mere bystander they appeared pulling in various and conflicting ways, yet they were all under the direction of a master-mind; even so do the many strange powers, to all appearance discordantly at work for ages upon the texts of Old and New Testaments, appear to the devout scholar, overruled and made subservient, by a wise and unseen control, to the placing and preserving in its high and noble position in the Church, that holy and venerated record of God's mercies.'[164] The compatibility of modern science and revealed truth: it was a constant theme in Wiseman's thought.

He believed the Church should also build upon what most seemed truthful and beneficial in the accomplishments and culture of each age. From the first public lectures he gave, in Cardinal Weld's apartments in Rome, in 1835, it is possible to discern the extent of his indebtedness to this concept. Those lectures were themselves a defence of science. It was, however, science as understood by Wiseman and as developed by the time he spoke; and it was a science whose interpretation was to be guided by revealed truth. Yet his attempt, he said, was 'to bring theology somehow into the circle of other sciences, by showing how beautifully it is illustrated, supported,

[163] *The Social and Intellectual State of England*, 19.
[164] *Essays*, I. 178, 'The Miracles of the New Testament' (from the *Dublin Review*, Dec. 1849).

and adorned by them all'.[165] His purpose was 'to show the correspondence between the progress of science, and the development of the Christian evidences';[166] and his conclusion was 'that the Christian religion can have no interest in repressing the cultivation of science and literature, nor any reason to dread their general diffusion, so long as this is accompanied by due attention to sound moral principles and correctness of faith'.[167] In detail, of course, he sometimes took issue with scientific speculation. He denied Lamarckian theories in order to contend that geological discoveries—of which he approved—nevertheless supported Biblical accounts of the Creation, and 'the truth and certainty of the primitive records of man'.[168] By his later years, he had come to see more hazards in modern knowledge than had hitherto occurred to him. The 'conflict between religion and reason', he still believed, was because of unnecessarily large claims made by the latter. 'We cannot shut our eyes to the aim or tendency of modern science; which is, to demand not equality but supremacy, not a fair balance but a loaded scale,' he observed.[169] The Wilberforce—Huxley controversy, and the publication of *Essays and Reviews*, had clearly left their mark on his fears. But 'eternal truth will still prevail, when temporal science shall have revised its wisdom, and brought it into harmony with the moral evidences which surround and support revelation'.[170] He never rejected his early belief in science, or his fascination for scientific discovery. His later caution derived from a pressing sense that some interpreters of science were promoting an unnecessarily secular scheme of values by imposing false claims in areas of experience and learning. He once told the students at Oscott that forty years hence 'the professors of this place will be endeavouring to prove, not transubstantiation, but the existence of God'.[171]

---

[165] *Twelve Lectures on the Connexion between Science and Revealed Religion delivered in Rome by Nicholas Wiseman D.D.*, London 1836, I. 4.

[166] Ibid. I. 6.

[167] Ibid. II. 296.

[168] *Pastoral Letter of H. E. Cardinal Wiseman enjoining the Collection for the building of Churches and Schools in the Archdiocese*, 9.

[169] Ibid. 6.

[170] Ibid. 10.

[171] Wilfrid Ward, *Wiseman*, I. 360.

In politics, Wiseman was a liberal. This, too, was in contrast to the prevailing political conservatism within the higher clergy of the English Catholic Church. His favourite orator, indeed, was Lord John Russell. He always regarded English Catholicism as deeply indebted to the liberal political ideals which had secured both Emancipation and the various subsequent concessions in relation to oaths, institutional chaplaincies, and so forth. But he was not 'political'; he urged, indeed, that politics should be kept out of religious enterprises. The most famous evidence of this was the *Dublin Review* itself. At the foundation of the journal, in 1836, it was agreed between the associating partnership of himself, Quin, and O'Connell 'that no extreme political views should be introduced into the *Review*'. In 1853 he was able to remark that 'this condition has, in most trying times, been faithfully observed'.[172] Despite O'Connell's English reputation for political radicalism (—though he was regarded as a moderate in Ireland—) Wiseman was a consistent friend and supporter. When O'Connell made a public visit to Oscott during the time of Wiseman's presidency, both men were seen 'arm in arm, telling good stories to each other and laughing heartily'.[173] Wiseman, who had a great sense of occasion, had (—as he wrote to the Earl of Shrewsbury, who presided at the dinner in O'Connell's honour—) beforehand kept the visit a secret from the students 'as it would cause great excitement'.[174] Wiseman's liberal sympathies were also disclosed in a liking for Napoleon III, and in 1855 he had a *Te Deum* sung to celebrate the birth of the Prince Imperial. Many English Catholics, sympathetic to the monarchists in France, were upset. But the issue of the Temporal Power of the Papacy eventually induced Wiseman to change his political allegiance. In 1858 the Derby administration represented legitimacy in the Italian question, and the Liberals, especially after Gladstone's attack on the States of the Church and Russell's speeches in support of the *Risorgimento*, represented opposition to the States of the Church. In the 1859 elections he urged the Italian

---

[172] *Essays*, I. vi.

[173] Wilfrid Ward, *Wiseman*, I. 350.

[174] Ushaw College Archives, Wiseman Papers, 465, Wiseman to the Earl of Shrewsbury, n.d.

question as an issue at the polls, and intervened dramatically, in the Conservative interest, at the Waterford contest in Ireland.[175] For the Conservatives it was a dubious assistance: the *Rambler* suggesting that Wiseman's involvement 'doubtless had its effect in adding to their unpopularity'.[176] Cardinal Cullen, who himself supported the Liberals during the campaign, told Propaganda that 'the row which Cardinal Wiseman made during the election in Ireland had caused much damage'.[177] It was Wiseman's only attempt at overt political activity, apart, perhaps, from his condemnation of Garibaldi during his visit to England in 1864—as 'one who today advocates and perpetuates the destruction of thrones, and gives public rewards for the attempted assassination of kings, and tomorrow exhorts his fellow-subjects to reject the constitutional government of his country, and centre all authority in a despotic dictatorship'.[178] But then Wiseman regarded the question of the States of the Church as religious rather than political.

There is a golden passage in Wiseman's *Appeal*, about the slums of London, which is some clue to his attitudes to social issues. He was defending the choice of Westminster for the title of his archiepiscopal see against the Protestant Dean and Chapter of Westminster Abbey, who had been among the first to object to its use. 'Close under the Abbey of Westminster', he wrote, 'there lie concealed labyrinths of lanes and courts, and alleys and slums, nests of ignorance, vice, depravity, and crime, as well as of squalor, wretchedness, and disease; whose atmosphere is typhus, whose ventilation is cholera; in which swarms a huge and almost countless population, in great measure, nominally at least, Catholic; haunts of filth, which no sewage committee can reach—dark corners, which no lighting-board can brighten.' He continued: 'This is the part of Westminster which alone I covet.'[179] Nor were these phrases mere florid rhetoric. Wiseman had a real feeling for the poor.

---

[175] Norman, *The Catholic Church and Ireland in the Age of Rebellion*, 35.
[176] *Rambler*, new series, I. 253 (July 1859).
[177] Propaganda Archives, *Scritture riferite nei congressi, Irlanda*, 33. f.888 (3 June, 1859).
[178] *Pastoral Letter of H. E. Cardinal Wiseman*, London 1864, 17.
[179] *Appeal*, 30.

'Who thinks of them?' he asked his people in 1850; 'They are considered as a class beneath you.'[180] And again: 'Society wishes to overlook them and, as in our proud metropolis we seek to drive them from the thoroughfares and streets through which fashion passes, and so pack them still closer together in hidden corners, where the corruption will fester more sorely.'[181] He linked environment and criminality, perceiving the impossibility of moral life in those whose conditions of work and dwelling gave no opportunity to cultivate it. In 1851 he reviewed Henry Mayhew's *London Labour and London Poor*, and its revelations confirmed his views. In 1853 he gave a series of lectures on *Home Education of the Poor*. Like most sections of educated opinion in the first half of the nineteenth century, he accepted the leading doctrine of the Political Economists, and entertained no intimation of the sort of collectivist solutions to social evils which reformers in the second half of the century promoted. Manning reflected the attitudes of this developing critique of *laissez-faire* practice. Wiseman still regarded private and organized charitable enterprise as the means by which the sufferings of the poor were to be alleviated and their moral capacities enhanced. There were exceptions in his strict adhesion to Political Economy—as there were quite commonly with others of philanthropic instinct in his day. He was critical of the new Poor Law of 1834, contrasting its provisions with the charitable institutions of Catholic countries. The poor in England, he wrote, regarded the workhouse 'as something little better than a gaol'. The overseers of the Poor Law Unions were 'not much disposed to look upon their inmates as their children or friends'. In Spain, in another of his contrasts, 'the feeling of kindness to the poor and sick is the genuine fruit of charity'.[182] In a sermon on the *Difficulty of Salvation of the Rich* he pointed to the responsibilities attached to the possession of money—moral hazards were 'infinitely more numerous than the poor have to encounter'.[183] He recommended the

---

[180] *The Social and Intellectual State of England*, 15.
[181] Ibid. 16.
[182] *Essays*, III. 146–7, 'Papers on History, Antiquity, and Art' (1845).
[183] *Sermons on Moral Subjects by His Eminence Cardinal Wiseman*, Dublin 1864, 40.

exercise of charity, 'the queen of virtues'.[184] Such sentiments placed Wiseman pretty centrally within the English liberal paternalism of his class and time. His promotion of work to help the poor was, however, not a fringe concern: it lay near to the centre of his view of Christian responsibility. Hence his zeal for Christian education, and the enormous encouragement he gave to the clergy to found Catholic schools—whose purposes included the moral enlightenment of the poor as much as counteracting the secularizing and proselytizing 'spirit of irreligion' fostered, as he believed, in the Protestant schools.[185] Wiseman, who was particularly careful about his dress, even employed tailors who were members of the Working Men's Associations—the Christian socialist enterprise got up by Maurice, Ludlow, and Neale—in order to express his sympathy for working-class self-help movements.[186] For a man only too often remembered by posterity for his grand manner and his capacity to inspire distrust in others, his was a life of quite remarkable service to the cause of his Church and to the ordinary Catholic people whose lives he sought to touch with some intimation of spiritual dignity.

[184] Ibid. 53.
[185] *Pastoral Letter of H. E. Cardinal Wiseman*, London 1864, 19.
[186] John Ludlow, *The Autobiography of a Christian Socialist*, ed. A. D. Murray, London 1981, 170.

4

Catholics, Government, and Society

Throughout the nineteenth century, Catholics in England were drawn more and more frequently into contact with government and the agencies of government. This was caused, first, by the expansion of Catholic institutions—the schools, orphanages, reformatories, and refuges, service and other public chaplaincies, and the multiplication of endowments and funds requiring the protection of the law. It was also caused by the expansion of the activities of the State: the piecemeal but inexorable growth of collectivism in the nineteenth century, as the government assumed increasing powers of intervention in social and economic relationships, meant that areas once the exclusive responsibility of the Churches—like education or health care—became the centres where religious and public bodies met and had to re-define their relationships. The Catholics, with their spreading network of institutions, no less than the Protestants, were impelled into the political sphere through this. The Church was also drawn into public life through the rising expectations of the Catholic bourgeoisie: at all levels Catholics were beginning to break out of their customary social pockets and to require their own religious leaders to adjust Catholic conditions to the realities of a competitive professional world. They did not seek to re-draw the map of professional life but to occupy a share of the existing one; this meant the entry of the Church into middle-class secondary education and the provision of some sort of university education. It was, indeed, in the world of education that the Church and the government of the country came most frequently into contact—and sometimes into collision.

The nineteenth-century state, in the broadest perspective, may be seen to have encountered two major difficulties in its educational policies. That it had policies at all, in education, was itself new: when the century began it was still supposed by everyone (apart from a very small group of philosophical radicals) that education was the responsibility of the Protestant Established Church. The first difficulty lay in the expansion of the population and the increasing complexity of economic life; for both simultaneously outstripped the resources of the State Church to act as the national educational agency. The second difficulty was the rise of religious diversity, for the number of those whose resistance to the claims of the national church was liable to attain a degree of militancy was rapidly increasing, mostly among the Protestant Dissenters, but also among some Catholics. At first the response of Parliament was limited and still informed by traditionalist presuppositions. In 1833 a sum of £20,000 a year was voted for education, to be distributed to the schools of the State Church, to those conducted by the National Society, and to those of the British and Foreign Society—a body which, though achieving the support of many liberal churchmen, was undenominational and employed (like the Irish State primary schools set up by the government in 1831) a 'common Christianity' formula of agreed Biblical instruction. As Manning once explained to Wiseman, 'it is altogether a mistake to think that the British and Foreign school system is one of *Indifference*'. It was, on the contrary, established on the principle 'that all education must be based upon the Bible'. He added that its attempt to exclude doctrine was 'an example of the intellectual inconsequence of Protestantism'.[1] In 1839 the parliamentary grant was increased by £10,000 and the Committee of the Privy Council for Education created to provide for the administration of the awards and the inspection of the schools making application.[2] By the 1860s, and as the Newcastle Commissioners' report made clear in 1861, a more collectivist response was appropriate, and in Forster's Act of 1870 the State itself entered education with the setting up of a 'dual system' of Voluntary Schools (the denominational, largely Anglican and Catholic schools eligible for parliamentary maintenance grants) and

---

[1] Westminster Dioc. Archives, Wiseman Papers, Bishops' Letters WB/40, Manning to Wiseman, 28 March 1856.

[2] E. R. Norman, *Church and Society in England, 1770–1970*, Oxford 1976, 113.

and Board Schools (paid for by a local education rate and responsible to government). The Board Schools adopted the non-denominational formula of 'common Christianity', and were therefore offensive to the consciences both of Catholics and of many Anglicans. The last quarter of the century saw a conflict of these two Churches with the government in an attempt, not to change the system, but to win parity within its financial arrangements for the Voluntary Schools. Their objectives were vehemently opposed by the Liberal Party, but proved sympathetic to the Conservatives: education became, therefore, a highly political matter after 1870. Under a Conservative administration, in Balfour's Act of 1902, the Voluntary Schools achieved most of their claims to parity.

The Catholic Hierarchy did not immediately apply for the grants made available by the committee of Privy Council in 1839. It was not clear that their schools were eligible; and there was, anyway, a division of opinion among the bishops as to whether they should be accepted. Some believed that state inspection, the condition of the grants, was potentially hazardous to the independence of the schools. In the circumstances of England's national Protestant culture, these fears were entirely reasonable. Some entertained them, however, in an extreme form. Thus Mother Margaret Hallahan, a great influence for Catholic education, expressed the deepest suspicions. 'I can hardly put into words my very great dislike of having anything to do with the government or committees, or anything where there are a great many opinions and a multiplicity of voices and speeches,' she wrote to one of her religious in the 1860s. The government, she continued, about the grants, 'could never mean any good to the Catholic Church, but merely holds this plan out as a bribe to try and destroy our Holy Church, and to sap it at its very foundation by endeavouring to make its little ones unfaithful.' It was, she believed, 'a deep-laid scheme of the devil'.[3] It was left to Ullathorne, who actually shared her suspicions though in a less exacting fashion, to bring the schools she founded into

[3] St. Dominic's Convent, Stone, Mother Margaret Hallhan Papers, T.977/1, Letter to one of her Sisters (n.d. but ? 1864). For a similar version of these sentiments, see F. R. Drane, *Life of Mother Margaret Mary Hallahan*, London, 2nd edn. 1929, 208.

association with the government grant scheme shortly after her death in 1868.

Ullathorne's importance in the Catholics' attitudes to the educational policies of the State is such that some lengthy account must be given of this great prelate. He was, anyway, 'for forty years the standard reference for the Catholic tradition in England'—an opinion which was not an exaggeration.[4] He was always thought to embody the robust, simple Catholicism of Yorkshire recusancy, yet to have occupied a middle ground between the values of the Old Catholics and the influence of the Roman outlook and the converts. He transmitted something of the atmosphere of the old Church into the vitality of the new: when Bishop Brown of Newport died in 1880, Ullathorne was the last of the Vicars Apostolic from the era before the re-establishment of the Hierarchy— 'the sole surviving link with the Catholic past'.[5]

William Bernard Ullathorne's autobiography, entitled *From Cabin-Boy to Archbishop*—not, perhaps, a very radical transition—contains the record of a dedicated and effective Christian life. He wrote it in 1868, and spent the last years of his life, in the later 1880s, revising it for publication. When he died, in 1889, in the dignity of titular Archbishop of Cabasa, he was rightly recognized, as Edward Ilsley (the new Bishop of Birmingham) reported to Rome, as 'virum optimum et fortem et jurium Ecclesiae propagandorum'.[6] As he lay dying, indeed, he had interrupted the prayers to say 'the devil's an ass'.[7] He was very English. The family was descended from St. Thomas More, and was proudly conscious of its Catholic inheritance. His father ran a small draper's business in Pocklington, Yorkshire, and it was there that Ullathorne was born in 1806. His education, at the village school in nearby Burnby, was fairly rudimentary, though he later supplemented it by study at Downside and by a lifelong attention to the reading of the Fathers; so although it may be true, as Bernard Ward concluded, that he 'had never fully overcome

---

[4] Mathew, *Catholicism in England, 1535–1935*, 194.
[5] Cuthbert Butler, *The Life and Times of Bishop Ullathorne, 1806–1889*, II. 265.
[6] Propaganda, *Scritture* 28 (1888–90), 293 (27 March 1889).
[7] Mathew, 196.

the want in his early education',[8] he was certainly not, by the time of his elevation to the priesthood, an uneducated man. He did, however retain a regional accent which, to London ears, always sounded rather unsophisticated. At the age of twelve he joined his father's business, which had by then been moved to Scarborough; but, inspired by reading *Robinson Crusoe*, he left it after a year to go to sea. He became cabin-boy on the brig *Leghorn*, and sailed to the Mediterranean. It was during the course of a voyage to the Baltic on his second vessel, the *Anne's Resolution*, that he went ashore at Memel with the ship's mate—a man called Craythorne, who had been to Stonyhurst—to attend mass, and underwent some sort of religious reawakening: 'I saw the claims of God upon me, and felt a deep reproach within my soul.'[9] He began to read religious books, left the ship to return to the draper's business in Scarborough, and then, in 1823, feeling his vocational impulsions ever more urgently, entered the school at Downside. He was still only sixteen years old. In 1824 he became a Benedictine postulant and was professed in the following year. It was while teaching at Ampleforth in 1831 that he was ordained priest, at Ushaw, and then returned to Downside as a teacher.

The next phase of his life began in Australia. The suggestion of a mission to the convicts in Australia—many of whom, being Irish, were Catholic—first came from Dr Polding, the novice-master at Downside. There were other events which drew Ullathorne's thoughts overseas. In 1831 Bishop Slater of Mauritius, an Ampleforth Benedictine, had died and was succeeded by a member of the Downside community, Bishop William Placid Morris. Ullathorne volunteered to go out too. In the end he went to Australia: as Vicar-General, with a government grant for his passage and a letter of introduction from the Colonial Office to the Governor of New South Wales—an interesting indication of the preparedness of the British government to assist the work of the Catholic Church in the colonies. He arrived in New South Wales in February 1833, aged twenty-six, and began his work among the convicts.

---

[8] Bernard Ward, *The Sequel to Catholic Emancipation*, II. 161.
[9] *From Cabin-Boy to Archbishop*, 21.

The colonial administration duly rendered much assistance, both financial and practical. After seeing the condition of the convicts on Norfolk Island he became, and remained all his life, a penal reformer. On a visit to England in 1838 he gave evidence to Sir William Molesworth's Parliamentary Committee on Transportation.[10] He wrote *The Horrors of Transportation Briefly Unfolded to the People*. In his subsequent book, *Management of Criminals*, he gave an account of the unpopularity his liberal opinions on the convict question involved him in on his return to Australia. This climate of hostile opinion, and the sense that the work in England was also urgent, led to his permanent return in 1840. He was still young. Indeed, on a visit to Rome in 1837 he had called on Cardinal Fransoni, the Prefect of Propaganda, who had, in Ullathorne's own account, 'looked at me coldly for an instant, and then said: "what a youth"'. His reception by Gregory XVI was no more reassuring. When the Holy Father saw him he said 'Quel giovane.'[11]

So there began, on arrival in England, six years of work in Coventry, a Benedictine mission since 1803. He had the enormous advantage of the presence, first as his housekeeper, of Sister Margaret Hallahan. She was also head of the primary school for girls and sacristan of the Church. She introduced Rosary evenings to Coventry.[12] It was her influence which modified Ullathorne's own original dislike of the new devotional outlook. He looked more than merely askance at some of Father Faber's practices—a matter that came before him as Bishop of Birmingham since that was where Faber lived, in the Oratory—and believed the *Lives of Modern Saints* were unsuited to the English religious atmosphere, as being too luxuriant in Latin folk spirituality. But under the influence of Sister Margaret Hallahan he gave a limited encouragement to the new devotions in Coventry. It was also her influence, perhaps, which prompted Ullathorne to take up the idea of missions—which brought Gentili to Coventry in 1845. The mission was also designed as a Catholic response to the

---

[10] St. Dominic's Convent, Stone; Ullathorne Papers. Box VII (5) is a copy of his evidence to the Molesworth Committee (8 Feb. 1838).

[11] *From Cabin-boy to Archbishop*, 127.

[12] Drane, *Life of Mother Margaret Mary Hallahan*, 73.

annual Lady Godiva procession, 'which in those days was openly indecent'.[13] Sister Margaret had an image of the Blessed Virgin fixed in a cart, and then had it pulled around the Church in a rival procession. When, in 1846, Ullathorne became Vicar Apostolic of the Western District, and moved first to Bath and then to Bristol, Mother Margaret's Dominican sisters—now regularly constituted—moved with him, too, and set up in a large house next to the cathedral which Ullathorne built in Clifton. The two years in the Western District were not happy ones. Shocked by the financial mess left by Baines and Baggs, and unable to overcome the intransigence of many of the clergy, Ullathorne's attempts, in the Prior Park inquiry of 1847, to bring some sort of coherence to the troubled affairs of the District met further opposition. In 1848 he was in Rome, acting for the English bishops in the negotiations preceding the re-establishment of the Hierarchy, but when he returned to England it was to Birmingham, where, in the new ecclesiastical system finally set up in 1850, he became Bishop—a post he held for the next thirty-seven years. Mother Margaret Hallahan's nuns moved with him to the Midlands in 1853, establishing the Dominican convent at Stone in Staffordshire, where Ullathorne lies buried. He was a very successful bishop, quietly providing for the expanding needs of the Catholic population, with schools and new missions; and establishing a friendship with Newman, who also lived in Birmingham, which was extremely close—and survived even the difficulties over the *Rambler* episode in 1859.[14]

Ullathorne was very much a Benedictine, yet he spent only eight years of his long life in the cloister. In 1862 he would have resigned his see and returned to Downside but for the public objection of the Pope—who ended a mass in St. Peter's basilica by rejecting Ullathorne's application. The call of the cell remained. In 1853, indeed, it was involuntarily answered. He was imprisoned in Warwick Gaol, together with Dr Moore the President of Oscott, for liability as a shareholder (on behalf of the Church) in the bankruptcy of the Monmouthshire and Glamorgan Banking Company. 'We are not worse accommodated than a Carthusian monk,' he wrote

[13] Cuthbert Butler, *Ullathorne*, I. 132.   [14] See chapter 7.

to the Abbess of Stanbrook, 'our cells are quite as good as those of a convent.'[15] But they had their meals sent in from a hotel. Ullathorne was also addicted to snuff.

In politics he was a paternalist Tory, who loathed the rise of Gladstonian Liberal politics (—in sharp contrast to Manning—) and, on being sent some literature by the Anglican Guild of St. Matthew, in 1887, observed: 'It takes me back to the time of Richard II and John Ball.'[16] He disliked democracy as the rule of ignorance. Yet he had some insight into the new industrial world of the Birmingham in which he ministered: he perceived the future of an urban Catholicism, adapted to a society whose styles and expectations were quite without precedent. To that world he brought the *stabilitas* of the Benedictine mind. 'A bishop ought to see through Our Lord's eyes, and should be free from the spirit of the age in which he lives, which is but the passing fashion of the passing world', he wrote.[17]

In 1850 Ullathorne published *Remarks on the Proposed Education Bill*, an attempt to pre-empt the coming debate about the position of religion in the schools by upholding parental rights to denominational instruction for their children. It was a tract against the secularization of primary education. In 1857 came his much more important work, *Notes on the Education Question*—a lengthy and balanced account of government policy which was ultimately critical of the terms upon which Catholic schools accepted maintenance grants from the state. The chief danger he saw was of government interference. 'After ages of exclusion, as Catholics, from the funds at the command of the State, we are beginning to receive its aid towards educating the poor of our Church', he wrote; 'And in return for that aid, as a matter of course, we are giving up something of that absolute freedom and independence of action, which, whatever else we have suffered, has been our greatest earthly blessing.'[18] He did acknowledge that government inspection had 'stimulated

---

[15] *Letters of Archbishop Ullathorne*, 35.
[16] Ibid. 492.
[17] Ibid. 46.
[18] *Notes on the Education Question by the Right Rev. Bishop Ullathorne*, London 1857, 7.

and braced up the tone of our schools'.[19] The danger lay in 'those hidden springs within the machinery over which the Government holds the direct, the exclusive and perpetual control'.[20] He concluded: 'Government inspection is one thing, but Government control would be another; and that we can never accept.'[21] His motives, like those of some others who were sceptical of the grants, were compounded of suspicion of the government because of the traditional anti-Catholic prejudices of English government, and suspicion of the rise of the power of the state as such. These difficulties were not so apparent to Wiseman. At the annual Low Week Meeting of the Hierarchy in 1857 Wiseman and Ullathorne differed over the continued acceptance of grants and Ullathorne's *Notes* were disapproved. When, afterwards, Wiseman published a letter in *The Tablet* declaring that the grants were safe, it was taken as a public rebuke to Ullathorne—who had, by then, become recognized as the leader of that large party within the Church who adhered to independence in educational questions. In 1870 Ullathorne was opposed to the Education Act, whereas Manning accepted it: the split within the Hierarchy continued. At a great meeting in the Birmingham Town Hall, in November 1869, Ullathorne had spoken of the evil effects of separating religious and secular instruction: the very principle of the education movement of Jesse Collings and Joseph Chamberlain, originating also in Birmingham. Ullathorne, on his return to England from the Vatican Council, worked to keep the Catholic schools out of the new dual system. 'Understand it plainly, my brethren,' he warned in a Pastoral letter of October 1870, 'that it now depends on our own exertions, whether our Catholic children shall be taught by Catholic teachers, or shall be put under a system of education which will not only deprive them of Catholic influence, but will be directly injurious to their Catholic sense and faith.'[22] The warning was not heeded, and large numbers of

[19] Ibid. 60.
[20] Ibid. 61.
[21] Ibid. 67.
[22] Birmingham Diocesan Archives, B.4854, *A Pastoral Letter to the Faithful of the Diocese of Birmingham, by William Bernard Ullathorne* (27 Oct. 1870), 4.

Catholic primary schools continued to receive both grants and inspection under the terms of the new legislation.

Grants had first been applied for, and received, by the Catholics in 1847. One of the immediate consequences was the creation of the Catholic Poor School Committee—a body to treat with government over the education question, to monitor the grants, and to co-ordinate action between the bishops and the schools. Later in the century its name was changed, in recognition of circumstances, to the Catholic School Committee, and later still, in 1905, to the Catholic Education Council. The immediate predecessor to the Catholic Poor School Committee was the Catholic Institute of 1838, a body of laymen organized by the Hon. Charles Langdale, MP for Knaresborough. He was to become, as President of the Poor School Committee, the most important Catholic educationalist of the century. Assisted by Thomas William Allies, the secretary from 1853 to 1890, he may be credited with the creation of an effective and successful agency to publicize Catholic educational endeavour. In 1845 the Catholic Institute made a special educational appeal, declaring that although there were 30,000 Catholic children being educated in England, there were also 35,000 who were not. Langdale became chairman of the standing educational committee set up by the Institute, and in that capacity, in 1846, began correspondence with the Committee of Privy Council for Education about the possibility of Catholic schools receiving maintenance grants. In February 1847, there was a test case: a Catholic school at Blackburn applied for a grant—the result of Lord Lansdowne's suggestion that the Catholics should test the rules. The bishops were able to show that the school was not limited to Catholics and that Protestant children could be exempted from the religious instruction. After some temporizing, the principle of the grants was conceded. In June 1847, Frederick Lucas got up a more vigorous agitation—the 'Association of St. Thomas of Canterbury for the vindication of Catholic Rights'. More democratic in style than the Institute, and with a greater appeal to the Catholic middle class, it urged *political* action—that candidates at election should be asked to support Catholic education claims. Its example was successful overseas—very far overseas: a branch was founded by the Catholic clergy of Chile early in the 1850s.[23] The success of the Association in England led to the demise of the Catholic Institute; but the bishops were wary of the political tactics and militancy of Lucas's organization and sought the creation of a body under their own immediate supervision to deal with educational questions. The Catholic Poor School Committee of 1847 was the result. As Bishop Thomas Griffiths wrote to Wiseman: 'I think the time has arisen when, for the sake of peace, the Bishops should proceed at once to appoint those Priests and Laymen whom they judge best qualified.' This would make it clear, he continued, that 'those who wish to form a "Catholic Association" to watch over elections etc.' would 'do so without being under the patronage of the Bishops'.[24] In a letter to the Poor School Committee, in 1848, the Hierarchy defined the relationship of the Committee and the bishops: 'We recognize your committee as the organ sanctioned by us of communication with the Government; and we have every confidence that your committee, in your communications and negotiations with Government for any Government Grants will be fully aware of our determination not to yield to the Ministers of the day any portion, however small, either of our ecclesiastical liberty, or of our episcopal control over the religious education of the children of the poorer members of our flock.'[25] The Committee was also responsible for the distribution of the voluntary sums donated for Catholic education.

The Poor School Committee secured an immediate concession from the Committee of Privy Council—that the salaried inspectors of Catholic schools would themselves be Catholics. The Committee also framed a model trust deed for Catholic schools to use when applying for grants, known as the 'Kemerton Trust'. In 1869 the bishops agreed to set up a Council for Education in each diocese—in some they already

[23] Jaime Eyzaguirre, *Historia de las instituciones políticas y sociales de Chile*, Santiago 1967, 118.

[24] Ushaw College Archives, Wiseman Papers, 422, Griffiths to Wiseman (n.d., but 1847).

[25] Westminster Dioc. Archives, ACTA, Meeting of the Bishops in Low Week, 1869 (9 April), 25 (which reproduces the text of the 1848 Letter).

existed—which would, apart from generally supervising and stimulating educational efforts, collect educational statistics to be forwarded to the Poor School Committee. In 1888 the bishops modified the constitution of the Committee and broadened its function. The Bishop of Salford, Herbert Vaughan, who had been charged with assessing possible courses, reported in favour of the Committee appointing 'a standing sub-committee, to meet from time to time during the course of the year to discuss matters affecting Public Elementary Education', with 'a similar standing sub-committee' appointed by the bishops 'for the same purpose'.[26] In 1897 Vaughan—by then Archbishop of Westminster—recommended that the Catholic School Committee (as it had itself suggested) should become 'a bond of union between the various Catholic Associations, so that the Catholic community shall present a united front before the country and the government in matters affecting public elementary education'.[27] Indeed, relations between the Committee and the bishops were throughout extremely harmonious, due, largely, to the close control the Hierarchy actually exercised over its actions—deputations of the Committee, led by the chairman, attended the Low Week meetings of the bishops each year—and due to the administrative wisdom of Langdale and Allies. Even in 1870, with severe internal dissensions among the English Catholics about the wisdom of accepting Forster's Act, the Committee, which met in nine special sessions, retained a balanced and united front. Even Ullathorne, the opponent of the central purpose of the Committee's existence, the acceptance of state grants, paid tribute to its fairness and success: 'It is only by our organization that, in this question of education, we can stand in our freedom', he wrote of the Committee in his *Notes*.[28]

The injection of financial aid was an enormous benefit to the schools. In the first fifteen years of the grants, sums totalling £239,757 were received for primary education, and

---

[26] Westminster Dioc. Archives, ACTA, Meeting of the Bishops in Low Week, 1888 (10 April), I. 8.

[27] Westminster Dioc. Archives, Vaughan Papers, 54a, Draft Circular letter to the Bishops (1 July 1897), 3 (a).

[28] Ullathorne, *Notes on the Education Question*, 71.

£21,543 for normal (teacher training) schools.[29] Despite Ullathorne's misgivings, the inspection of the schools receiving grants did not in itself lead to significant government encroachment on their Catholic character. In 1852 the bishops set up their own inspectors of religious instruction, on a diocesan basis, to guarantee standards both in those schools in receipt of aid and in those which were not. Bishops were occasionally upset by unfavourable reports. In 1854, in fact, Wiseman himself was moved to considerable displeasure when the Revd. T. W. Marshall, the first Catholic Inspector, reported to the Privy Council Committee on the slow rate of educational improvement among the Catholics of London— a conclusion Wiseman regarded as 'most unjust, and I am tempted to use a stronger term, towards the zealous clergy and laity of my Diocese'. He proceed to generalize: 'I observe a growing jealousy of Government interference in our education, a tendency to make Government master of our teachers, through the advantage it offers to mere secular education, and so leading to great power of interference in our religious matters.' Ullathorne could not have put it more forcefully. 'Now there appears to me to exist a new, and unexpected and dangerous exercise of power.'[30] These sentiments, directed to Charles Langdale at the Poor School Committee, elicited a reassuring response, and an assertion that no new encroachment by the state was intended.[31] Wiseman was similarly disturbed in 1858, when the inspection of education in the Reformatories was transferred from the Privy Council to the Home Office, and came thereafter into the control of the Inspectorate of Prisons. The officer responsible was a Protestant clergyman. Although he declared his intention of exercising his powers through a Catholic priest, acting in his presence, Wiseman objected and threatened to withdraw the Catholic Reformatories from the receipt of state aid altogether—'at the cost of all or part of the principles which have hitherto formed the basis of our relation

[29] Wiseman, *The Religious and Social Position of Catholics in England*, 30.
[30] Westminster Dioc. Archives, Wiseman Papers, W3/31/52a, Wiseman to Langdale, 4 Feb. 1854.
[31] Ibid. W3/3159a, Langdale to Wiseman, 24 Feb. 1854.

with the Government on the subject of Education'.[32] William Clifford, the Bishop of Clifton, who had himself been appointed to the Prison Inspectorate in 1857, explained to the Protestant clergyman at the centre of the difficulty (the Revd. P. Turner) the nature of the Catholics' objections. 'Such differences might perhaps be avoided through the moderation of individual inspectors, but Government would still claim the *right* thus to interfere in religious questions even if the Inspector refrained from *using* it,' he wrote of possible friction between the inspector and the examining priest; 'This is what Catholics object to.'[33] The Church had come a long way from the penal days.

When the Newcastle Commission was set up by Parliament in 1858 to inquire into the whole question of popular education in England, Wiseman circularized the bishops advising them to co-operate. The Commission had applied to the Poor School Committee seeking their help in gaining access to the Catholic schools. Wiseman had consulted with Errington, Clifford, Grant, and Langdale, and examined the questionnaires sent out by the Commission. Apart from an item about school endowments, which they thought it might be hazardous to answer because of the state of the law on Catholic bequests, they recommended that the Commissioners' work should be assisted. They also agreed 'that the questions should be transmitted to the respective schools through the bishops, and the answers returned to them, to be forwarded by them to the Secretary of the Poor School Committee for the Commission,'[34] thus retaining episcopal oversight of the entire matter. The Newcastle Commission Report of 1861 was the prelude to the Forster Act of 1870. There was, in 1869, legislation intended to rationalize the trusts of the endowed schools—a matter mostly affecting the Church of England, but the Catholic bishops were worried about their own colleges, and got them exempted from the new law on the grounds that they were also places for the training of the clergy.[35]

---

[32] Ibid. R79/6, Wiseman to Bishop James Gillis, 1 Oct. 1858.

[33] Ibid. 130/1, Clifford to Turner, 6 Dec. 1858.

[34] Westminster Dioc. Archives, Wiseman Papers, R79/6, Wiseman to Gillis, 1 Oct. 1858.

[35] Ibid. ACTA, Meeting of the Bishops in Low Week, 1869 (6 April), 4.

Sensing the threat to denominational education in the Dissenters', Liberals' and secularists' campaigns for radical legislation upon the basis of the Newcastle Commission findings, the bishops also agreed, in 1869, to issue a Pastoral Letter, on the Feast of the Sacred Heart, on the dangers facing the Catholic schools.[36] When Forster's Bill for the creation of the 'dual system' of primary education was introduced to Parliament in 1870, the bishops were in Rome for the Vatican Council. Opinions among them were divided; a majority were sceptical about the wisdom of continuing to accept state grants for their schools within the new system. That was Ullathorne's view. But Manning had already—as he explained to a meeting of the bishops in Rome during February, called to consider the Bill—agreed to the principle of the legislation with the government before he left London.[37] By standing aloof from the new School Boards, as he explained to Ullathorne, 'we should be exposed to the danger of their hostility'.[38] With the Hierarchy in Rome, the Poor School Committee and the laity took an unusually large share in dealing with the question. Catholic Members of Parliament had made repeated requests to receive an authoritative ruling on how they should regard the Bill. Lord Howard of Glossop organized a lay meeting to oppose acceptance of the measure; he also opened a crisis fund, to finance Catholic Voluntary Schools which withdrew from state aid. In March 1870, the Catholic laity pubished a Declaration pointing to the dangers of secularization. 'A system of popular education founded on the secular principle instead of being unsectarian would be sectarian in the most obnoxious sense to the community generally, and it would be especially unjust to Roman Catholics who under such a system would be compelled to support schools contrary to the plain dictates of their consciences.' They therefore urged that 'the Denominational principle at present existing' be 'supplemented and developed so as to

[36] Ibid. 5.

[37] Birmingham Diocesan Archives, B.4796, Ullathorne to the Vicar General, 23 Feb. 1870.

[38] Gordon Wheeler, 'The Archdiocese of Westminster', in *The English Catholics, 1850–1950*, ed. Beck, 158.

meet existing requirements'.[39] In the event, most Catholic schools in receipt of grants continued to receive them. There were some cases—as when the schools at Abergavenny were transferred to the care of nuns in 1873, as Bishop Brown discovered when he visited—where schools failed to qualify through failing to attain the required standards.[40] Ullathorne's own views on the propriety of Catholics sitting on the new School Boards underwent a change. He was originally favourable, accepting the best he could find in a system he distrusted. 'It is certain that the School Boards system is full of danger to the Religious Education of England, and most especially to our Catholic schools,' he wrote in a paper on the question, written as the new system went into effect early in the 1870s (and now among his papers at Stone). Yet Catholics could join the Boards without actually implying 'approbation of the system, or cooperation in any acts against which such a Catholic member may vote'. The London School Board, which he had especially observed, had so far 'acted with perfect fairness.' He therefore concluded that the presence of Catholics on School Boards constituted in fact 'the only securities we possess for the safety of our Catholic children', and that their withdrawal 'would diminish the check which at this time hinders a more rapid and dangerous development of the system.'[41] By 1876, however, as he wrote to Manning in that year, his views had changed. He then argued for Catholic withdrawal, because the Boards were 'in their nature un-Catholic'. He added 'Their constitution, object and aim is to establish and maintain schools and propagate a system of education in antagonism with Catholic education, and with all definite religious education.' He now believed, he wrote, that the Catholics would 'hold a far stronger position in the face of these Boards and of the whole system, if we had nothing whatever to do with them'. Then, he said, 'we should not be compromised in them'.[42] It was a return to the position

---

[39] Westminster Dioc. Archives, B1/177, *Proposed Declaration of the Catholic Laity* (1870), 7, 8.

[40] Downside Archives, VII.A.3.a *Abbots' Papers* (File marked '1871–1880'), Bishop T. J. Brown to the Provincial of the Benedictines, 31 Jan. 1873.

[41] St. Dominic's Convent, Stone, Ullathorne Papers, Box X, Paper on School Boards (n.d.).

[42] Ibid. Box X, Ullathorne to Manning, 29 Sept. 1876.

over Catholic education that he had always maintained. But by then about a half of the clergy were co-operating with the system. At the end of the century, 328 of the 680 Catholic Elementary Schools were grant aided.[43] In 1884 the Bishop of Salford, Vaughan, founded the Voluntary Schools Association in an attempt to co-ordinate Catholic attempts to rectify some of the deficiencies, from the point of view of denominational education, in the 1870 Act.

The last two decades of the century therefore saw a growing Catholic campaign to secure satisfactory legislation to meet the claims of Vaughan's Association—a campaign which quite rapidly spread throughout the dioceses of England. It impelled the Catholics increasingly into public life—following, anyway, Manning's own inclination to participate in public bodies for reforming and philanthropic objectives. Manning was appointed to Sir Richard Cross's Commission, which reported in 1888 on the working of the 1870 Act. In 1885 he and fourteen bishops had published a series of Resolutions condemning 'mixed education' and upholding, once again, the denominational principle. 'While we heartily unite in the universal desire that all children shall be suitably educated,' they resolved, 'we maintain that the State cannot, without violation of the natural and divine law, compel parents to educate their children in a system which is opposed to their conscience and religion; and we declare that the Catholics of this country cannot accept for themselves any system of Education which is divorced from their Religion.'[44] The introduction of compulsory primary education had enhanced the urgency of their claims, and the bishops therefore also urged Catholics 'to support candidates for parliament who agree to these principles'.[45] The denominational content of the instruction given in Catholic schools was also heightened, and in 1888 the bishops gave detailed instructions to the clergy and the Catholic teachers. Priests were to conduct catechism classes in school hours; the clergy were to 'superintend and

---

[43] A. C. F. Beales, 'The Struggle for the Schools', in *The English Catholics, 1850–1950*, ed. Beck, 380.

[44] Westminster Dioc, Archives. B1/177, 'Resolutions of the Catholic Bishops of England on Education' (31 Oct. 1885), III.

[45] Ibid. VII.

test the religious instruction given to Pupil-Teachers by Masters and Mistresses of the Schools'; there were to be annual Retreats for teachers and pupils; teachers were to attend mass on Sundays with their pupils; 'objects and pictures of piety' were to be placed in the classrooms.[46] With a Conservative administration in office, the prospects for concessions grew and in the 1890s the bishops involved themselves with actual legislative proposals. In 1895 they drew up an 'Education Manifesto' and a draft Bill for the attention of politicians, providing equality with the local government schools. 'The electorate must be persuaded and convinced, that all Denominational schools, faithfully complying with the requirements of the Education Department, have a right to receive an equal proportionate share with the Board Schools of all public moneys, whether paid from the rates or the taxes, for educational purposes.' The question, they declared, 'should be made a test question at the polls.'[47] When, in March 1896, Sir John Gorst introduced an Education Bill, the bishops suggested amendments in the form of a published *Declaration*. It pointed out that 'although the Bill was to be welcomed as embodying the principle of the necessity of doctrinal instruction in all public Elementary Schools, yet its provisions fell short of giving equal maintenance to the Voluntary Schools'.[48] With the setting up of a joint committee with the Catholic School Committee, the bishops then planned a more satisfactory measure. The failure of Gorst's Bill in 1896 was followed by successful legislation in 1897. This abolished the rating of the Voluntary Schools and was welcomed by the bishops as a large step in the right direction. They still claimed equality in the distribution of grants, and Cardinal Vaughan dedicated his last years to that end.[49] It was finally achieved in 1902: a measure agreeable to the Catholics despite some misgivings about the numbers of Local Government representatives on the management boards of Voluntary Schools in

[46] Ibid. ACTA, Meeting of the Bishops in Low Week, 1888 (10 April), IV. 2.
[47] Westminster Dioc. Archives, ACTA, Low Week Meeting of the Bishops, 1895 (23 April), VII.
[48] Ibid. ACTA, Low Week Meeting of the Bishops, 1896, I. 3.
[49] See chapter 8.

receipt of aid in the integrated system.[50] In his report to Propaganda on the Act, Vaughan pointed to the leading features. It had, he wrote, 'placed elementary, secondary and technical education in the hands of local authorities, and it gives them the power to coordinate the various steps in Education.' The Catholics retained possession of their school buildings; the Local Authority had the right to nominate two managers to each school, though these did not have to be Catholics; but 'we secure equal and full payment for all our teachers out of public money, and a right to teach our religion, in return for undertaking to erect our own buildings, and to keep them in repair'.[51] It was a very satisfactory conclusion, achieved, furthermore, without too great a measure of public involvement. Yet the continual hostility of the Liberal Party to denominational education meant that, in practical terms if not by wish, the Catholic bishops and the Conservatives had a bond of unity. The leaders of the Church of England found themselves in the same position, and for the same reason.

Relations with the government over education were confined to the primary level. In this area, the expansion of Catholic schools was very impressive—especially in view of the limited financial resources, in a century which also required a massive programme of church building and the provision and endowment of Catholic charitable and philanthropic institutions. The constituency was also a poor one. 'In the manufacturing and mining districts, where the Irish Catholics are most congregated, the number of substantial Catholics is comparatively few', as Ullathorne wrote in 1857; 'And it is an undeniable fact that, whatever the Irish labourer may give, when well urged, towards the building and support of his Church, he gives very little to the school.'[52] Yet the expansion was enormous, eliciting heroic qualities from the hard-pressed clergy in the slums. In London, at the start of the century, there were a mere four Catholic charity schools. First Wiseman, and then Manning, transformed the educational scene in the metropolis, with the appeals for funds made in

[50] Westminster Dioc. Archives, ACTA, Low Week Meeting of the Bishops, 1902 (8th April), I.

[51] Westminster Dioc. Archives, Vaughan Papers, 230 a. Vaughan to the Cardinal Prefect of Propaganda (Jan. 1903) [Draft copy].

[52] *Notes on the Education Question*, 9.

their Pastoral Letters—funds for schools, as Wiseman put it in 1864, 'into which the spirit of irreligion shall never creep, nor any tampering be allowed with the Faith of our Fathers'.[53] Manning's Diocesan Fund for Education, and his educational Pastorals, were the first work of his period as Archbishop, his earliest priority.[54] As the century advanced it became almost axiomatic that where a church was established there must be a Catholic school also: a situation which exactly paralleled the educational expansion of the Church of England in the nineteenth century. The Protestant Dissenters did not, in general, set up schools, and appealed instead to the state to provide undenominational schools in which the 'common Christianity' formula of non-sectarian religious instruction should be given. Early in the century there were a few Catholics who were attracted to the 'common Christianity' notion. They were those most noted for their adhesion to an English vision of Catholicism—particularly Charles Butler, whose support for the idea of educating Catholic and Protestant children in the same school, with common Bible instruction, led him to encourage the establishment of such a venture at Shadwell in 1816. The Catholics withdrew from the school after Bishop Poynter ruled against it.[55] In his evidence to the parliamentary Select Committee on Education in 1816, Butler maintained that secular and religious instruction could be separated in the schools.[56] It was precisely this view which the Catholic educational programme of the nineteenth century, inspired by the leading advocates of Ultramontanism, was intended to deny. The influence of the new religious orders was important in this, and so was the educational emphasis imparted to the Church by the arrival of the converts. Fr. Faber set up schools for boys and girls when he founded his community of St. Wilfrid at Cotton Hall in 1846;[57] and, again, in 1850, after he had moved to London to establish a branch of the Oratory, he founded a school for a thousand poor boys

---

[53] *Pastoral Letter of H. E. Cardinal Wiseman Enjoining the Collection for the Building of Churches and Schools in the Archdiocese*, London 1864, 20.
[54] See chapter 6.
[55] Bernard Ward, *The Eve of Catholic Emancipation*, II. 163.
[56] Ibid. II. 164.
[57] Chapman, *Father Faber*, 154.

in Holborn.[58] And Newman, in 1859, set up the Oratory School in Birmingham—a venture whose early existence was imperilled when all the staff resigned in protest about the authority apparently being exercised by the school matron.[59] Under the headmastership of Newman's old friend, Fr. Ambrose St. John, and a new staff of laymen, the school flourished. The educational expansion of the nineteenth century was also witnessed in the provision of secondary schools.

The first of these had been established around the turn of the century, as the Revolution in France dispersed the English seminarists and schoolboys overseas. Many arrived in England, seeking to re-found their colleges in the land from which they had once been exiled by the penal laws. The Catholic Relief Act of 1791 had actually (in Clause XV) prohibited the foundation of Catholic schools—but this was interpreted as applying only to schools concerned exclusively with the training of priests. Catholic foundations and re-foundations therefore followed, and were not challenged at law; but it always made their authorities nervous about their endowments, since legal protection could not be guaranteed. It also perpetuated the custom, established *ex necessitate* in the overseas colleges, of educating lay and ecclesiastical students together. The legal uncertainty of Catholic educational endowments was underlined in the fate of the Douai claims. In 1816 Bishop Poynter gained a sum of compensation from the French Government in settlement of the seizure of the College property and assets during the Revolution. The money was duly paid to commissioners of the British Government, who declined to hand it on to the English Catholics because of legal queries about the 'superstitious' uses to which it might be put. About £120,000 was thought to be involved, and in 1826 the British Government decided to keep it. The money was spent on the building of Brighton Pavilion.

The resettlement of the continental colleges provided, together with the Jesuit College at Stonyhurst in Lancashire, the first effective Catholic secondary education for boys in England. Douai itself was divided. One group of professors

---

[58] Ibid. 239.
[59] Reynolds, *Three Cardinals*, 163.

and students went north, settling for fourteen years at Crook Hall, and then founded the college at Ushaw in Co. Durham, in 1808, with Thomas Eyre as President. Although it was also the seminary for ecclesiastical students trained for the priesthood in the Northern District, Ushaw did not regard itself as a formal diocesan seminary, and retained a fiercely-guarded independence of the northern bishops. This led to disputes over jurisdiction which were not settled until the new rules governing the colleges in England were approved by Propaganda in 1863. Under the reforming presidency of Mgr. Charles Newsham, the college studies were in 1838 adapted to the requirements of the degree course at London University, and it was therefore at Ushaw that the first Catholic students in England since the Reformation qualified for degrees.[60] The other half of Douai moved to St. Edmund's Old Hall, at Ware in Hertfordshire, in 1793. An existing Catholic academy, founded in 1769 by Bishop Thomas Talbot, was converted by Bishop Douglass to receive them. St. Edmund's had an erratic start, partly because the President, Poynter, became coadjutor to Douglass in 1803 and spent much of his time in London.[61] There were also two purely English foundations: Challoner's Sedgley Park, and Oscott in the Midland District. Stonyhurst began in 1794 when Weld provided a house for the Jesuits exiled first from St. Omers and then from Liège. Despite the excellence of the education at the College, it was unpopular with the Vicars Apostolic, and in 1819 a defence was compiled against what he called 'the violent opposition which has been made to it', by Charles Plowden, which Milner forwarded to Propaganda. Plowden attributed the prejudice against Jesuit education to 'the real ignorance of its opponents'.[62] The Benedictines of St. Lawrence's, Dieuleward, were at Ampleforth from 1802, and in 1814 the Benedictines opened the school at Downside.

Over the nature and jurisdiction of the colleges which were also seminaries—Ushaw, Oscott, and St. Edmund's Old Hall—there developed one of the most prolonged and divisive of

[60] Milburn, *A History of Ushaw College*, 167–8, 173.

[61] Bernard Ward, *History of St. Edmund's College, Old Hall*, 180.

[62] Propaganda, *Scritture Riferite nei Congressi, Anglia* (1818–22), 390 (22 Sept. 1819), Memorial sent to Cardinal Fontana by Milner.

the episcopal disputes of the century.[63] The education of lay and ecclesiastical students together was not, of course, restricted to the Catholics. It was, until the establishment of Theological Colleges in the second half of the nineteenth century, the procedure also adopted for the Church of England—in the universities of Oxford, Cambridge, and Durham. It was always unsatisfactory for the Catholics; but the cost of founding and endowing diocesan seminaries on the Tridentine basis, together with the relatively small numbers of those being trained for the priesthood in each District (or diocese after 1850), meant that the old practice of united lay and ecclesiastical education was retained. Sometimes those who found the arrangements really intolerable attempted a separate training of the clergy—Manning's unsuccessful seminary at Hammersmith, Vaughan's partially successful pastoral college at Salford. Education at the Catholic colleges did not really differ very significantly from that in an ordinary English public school. A seminarist of St. Edmund's in the early nineteenth century recalled: 'We were all mixed with future Lords, Earls, and Dukes, and other lay students, who, at the end of each vacation, used to return full of London news and London pleasures.'[64] Half a century later, in 1860, Manning complained about the conditions in the college—'smoking goes on', with 'a good deal of drinking by the boys, too'. But his evidence was partisan: he was defending the position of Vaughan as Vice-President, against a hostile atmosphere in which the Oblates—of whom Vaughan was one—'are hated as "sneaks"'.[65] In his second report to Rome on the state of the Church in England, in 1847, Fr. Luigi Gentili wrote of the College seminarists—'They live with the lay boys who learn music, fencing, dancing, gymnastics and other things that are required for the world.'[66] Ullathorne, a few years later, also reported unfavourably to Rome on the mixture of lay and ecclesiastical students. It led to 'a secular tone'. He added: 'the Church in England will not be in a normal state until the higher ecclesiastical studies, at least, are

---

[63] See chapter 3.
[64] Bernard Ward, *History of St. Edmund's College*, 193.
[65] Purcell, *Manning*, II. 124–5.
[66] Leetham, *Luigi Gentili. A Sower for the Second Spring*, 286.

conducted in seminaries exclusively devoted to ecclesiastical training'.[67]

The colleges were at the very top end of the Catholic secondary schools; they provided an education for the gentry, and, as with their Protestant counterparts, for the aspirant higher bourgeoisie later in the century. The general expansion of Catholic education in the century also led to the establishment of secondary schools for the middle classes—the counterparts of the Anglican Woodard schools and the ancient grammar schools. A feature of the second half of the century, these schools got particular encouragement from the bishops —who were also often themselves direct founders or restorers of secondary establishments, like Ullathorne's Cotton College (1873) and Vaughan's St. Bede's (1875), and sometimes they were major patrons, like Brown with St. Edward's at Liverpool (1842). Night schools and technical and commercial schools and institutes were also encouraged by the bishops, especially at their Low Week meeting in 1888, when Manning urged them to attend to these areas of education.[68] In 1850 a training college for teachers was set up at Hammersmith, with a grant from the Privy Council Committee, intended to provide for the boys' primary schools; and in 1855, at the suggestion of the Poor School Committee, a training school for female teachers was established by Notre Dame nuns. The training of teachers for the secondary schools of the second half of the century was urgently considered by a conference of Catholic Colleges in January 1896. The same conference also agreed to hold an annual 'consultative conference of Head Masters of Catholic Colleges', and proceeded to elect a standing committee to watch over the development of Catholic secondary education.[69] In the following year, 1897, the bishops called for the larger dioceses to form educational associations and for the smaller dioceses to be grouped together into joint associations, eleven in all, to enhance the

---

[67] Birmingham Dioc. Archives. B.3915, 'Draft Letter to the Cardinal [Prefect of Propaganda] about the Decrees of the Third Synod of Westminster concerning the government of the English Colleges and Seminaries' (n.d., but 1859).

[68] Westminster Dioc. Archives, ACTA, Meeting of the Bishops in Low Week, 1888 (10 April), VIII.

[69] Westminster Dioc. Archives, Vaughan Papers, 388, 'Conference of Catholic Colleges, January, 1896', VOTA, II.

co-ordination of the expanding network of Catholic educational facilities.[70]

Because most of the finance available to the bishops went into the system of primary schools for the Catholic poor, secondary education came to be dominated by the religious orders—a situation challenged by Vaughan when he was Bishop of Salford, in 1875, over the Jesuit school opened in Manchester without his consent.[71] Apart from the early foundations at Ampleforth, Downside, and Stonyhurst, there was the Dominican school at Hinckley (1823), the Rosminians' Ratcliffe College (1847), the Jesuits' Mount St. Mary's (1842), and Beaumont (1861). The De La Salle Brothers opened schools at Clapham (1855), and at Southwark (1860); and within twenty years establishments had been set up by the Xaverians, Augustinians, the Marists, the Brothers of Mercy, and the Salesians.[72] The religious orders also predominated in the provision of education for girls. An early advance was made in the nineteenth century with the return of religious orders of women from the continent. Augustinians, Dominicans, Franciscans, Poor Clares, and Benedictines all founded schools, and so did the new orders, with their arrival in the mid-century: the Sacred Heart nuns, the Institute of Charity Sisters, the Sisters of Charity of St Paul, the Notre Dame nuns, the Sisters of the Faithful Virgin, the Sisters of the Christian Retreat, the Sisters of the Immaculate Conception, and the Sisters of the Assumption. New English orders also set up girls' schools—the Sisters of the Infant Jesus, Mother Margaret Hallahan's Dominican sisters, and the Sisters of the Holy Child. By 1850, already, there were over fifty religious orders of women conducting schools.[73] The Daughters of Mary Ward were leaders in the provision of secondary schools for girls in the second half of the century. So were some of the new orders—the Religious of the Cross, La Retraite, the Dames of Christian Instruction, the Ladies of Mary, the

---

[70] Ibid. Vaughan Papers 54a. Draft Circular of Vaughan to the Bishops (1 July 1897).

[71] See chapter 8.

[72] W. J. Battersby, 'Secondary Education for Boys', in *The English Catholics*, ed. Beck, 328, 331.

[73] W. J. Battersby, 'Educational Work of the Religious Orders of Women', in op. cit. 340.

Dames of Nazareth, and the nuns of the Most Holy Sacrament. Anti-clerical legislation in France, in the 1890s, led to the arrival of more teaching orders—the Sisters of the Christian Schools of Mercy in 1894 and the Bernadines in 1897.[74] The two most numerous orders were the Ursulines, who came in 1851, and the Sisters of Charity of St. Vincent de Paul, whose arrival in 1857 was followed by an expansive programme of girls' schools, which made them the most numerous of all the congregations in England. Although Vaughan remarked to Rome, in 1903, that the Catholics 'cannot expect to supply enough Secondary and Technical schools to meet the wants of a small and scattered Catholic population',[75] the achievement was still very impressive. In terms of the education offered to girls, in fact, at all levels, the Catholic schools provided very much better and more extensive facilities than the education available for females generally in nineteenth-century England.

There were, apart from education, two other leading issues which brought the Catholics and the government into contact: institutional chaplaincies, and charitable trusts. The question of army chaplains for Catholic soldiers, recognized and salaried by the state, was entrusted, on the Catholic side, to Thomas Grant, Bishop of Southwark. He came from an army background, and was actually born in France, in 1816, where his father was serving as a sergeant in the 71st Highlanders. The family travelled wherever the regiment went, and it was on a voyage returning to England from Canada, when he was ten years old, that the death of his mother occurred—in melancholy circumstances which deeply affected the boy. He not unnaturally never forgot the dreadful sight of the sailors throwing sand into her coffin to make it sink before it was lowered into the waves.[76] His trauma induced a great moral seriousness which led him, shortly afterwards, to discover a vocation to the priesthood. He entered Ushaw, with the encouragement of Dr Briggs (later Bishop of the Northern District) at the age of thirteen, in 1829. There he

---

[74] Ibid. 356.

[75] Westminster Dioc. Archives, Vaughan Papers, 230 a. Draft for Propaganda (Jan. 1903).

[76] O'Meara, *Thomas Grant, First Bishop of Southwark*, 6.

was a notably accomplished student, going on to complete his studies at the English College in Rome in 1836. He was ordained there in 1841, and became Secretary to Cardinal Acton, so acquiring the knowledge which made him the foremost canon lawyer in the English Church. In 1844 he became Rector of the English College, and increased his administrative and diplomatic experience as agent of the Vicars Apostolic. In 1851 he became Bishop of Southwark in the restored Hierarchy and returned to the country from which he had been absent for so long. Under his direction the diocese expanded its missions and institutions, Grant himself devoting particular care to the orphanage at Norwood, founded by the Sisters of the Faithful Virgin three years after their arrival from France in 1848. The orphanage was 'the chief external monument of Dr Grant's episcopacy'.[77] It was an episcopacy also punctuated by differences with Wiseman. Grant's personal sanctity and retiring nature never allowed these to cast long shadows, however. His was a Roman spirituality, acquired, like Wiseman's, at the English College. He practised daily confession, encouraged devotions to the Virgin throughout the diocese, and carried a relic of the True Cross on his person. As an act of humility he adopted the disconcerting practice of keeping his eyes lowered. Sometimes he was discovered in acts of self-mortification—'as when a nun came upon him unawares and found him shaking the pepper-castor over an orange that had been carefully sugared for him, and on another occasion when he was caught emptying a salt-cellar into his tea-cup at breakfast'.[78] Perhaps he should have relaxed his self-imposed visual disciplines. He died in Rome during the Vatican Council, in June 1870. There was universal sorrow. 'A great light is put out in our little Church in England,' Ullathorne wrote; 'a saint has departured from this world.'[79] Pius IX concurred. 'Another saint in paradise', he said on hearing of Grant's death.[80]

With his family background, Grant was the obvious person to be charged with the welfare of Catholic soldiers in the

---

[77] O'Meara, 89.
[78] Ibid. 267.
[79] *Letters of Archbishop Ullathorne*, 243.
[80] O'Meara, 397.

Crimean War. Irish Catholics were extremely numerous in some regiments—though Grant can hardly be said to have harboured particularly Irish sympathies. 'They abuse the Government till they get something, and then they frustrate it if they can', he wrote of the Irish.[81] Catholic assistant chaplains were appointed during the war. Grant also arranged, in 1854, for some of his Sisters of Mercy from Bermondsey, and some of the Sisters of the Faithful Virgin from Norwood, to join Florence Nightingale's staff in the Crimea. It was at the Scutari hospital, in a large room made available by Miss Nightingale, that the Catholic nuns celebrated the Definition of the Immaculate Conception 'with festal pomp'.[82] At the start, there were some among the bishops who regarded Grant's ability to negotiate with the government over army chaplains with some scepticism. Grant himself had heard that a feeling existed that it was 'embarrassing to the Government to treat with me', and believed that some of the laity, too, thought that a bishop was the wrong person to be concerned in such delicate issues so soon after the uproar over the Hierarchy.[83] 'If your Eminence finds that the Government is willing to hear our complaints privately, but is afraid (probably on account of the strong feelings of the Queen) to treat through yourself, it would be desirable to allow some other bishop to be a medium of communication with them,' he wrote to Wiseman in April 1853; 'The acts of the Archbishop will always commit his colleagues, but the agency of another bishop may be changed or disavowed at any time,' he concluded.[84] Though doubtful of his own suitability for the role he had defined, he was persuaded to undertake it—and with success. In June 1858, a permanent body of Catholic army chaplains was nominated by the government, on a basis of complete equality, both in rank and salary, with the Protestant chaplains. An immediate difficulty—over the licensing of the chaplains on a centralized rather than a diocesan basis—was

[81] Ibid. 141.
[82] Ibid. 129.
[83] Westminster Dioc. Archives, Wiseman Papers, Bishops' Letters R79/4, Grant to Wiseman, 9 April 1853.
[84] Westminster Dioc. Archives, Wiseman Papers, Bishops' Letters R79/4, Grant to Wiseman, 18 April 1853.

overcome after reference to Rome. General Peel, for the government, assured Grant that 'he was anxious to carry out the concessions made by Government in the way that was most likely to be agreeable' to the 'feelings' of the Catholics.[85] By 1862 there were eighteen full-time and sixty-three assistant Catholic chaplains in the Army.

The concession of chaplains in workhouses and prisons came next. In 1859 the Poor Law Board ruled that Catholic children in workhouses should not be instructed in Protestantism, and priests were formally admitted to the workhouses to give Catholic instruction. Legislation in 1862 allowed Catholic children to be removed to Catholic orphanages which had passed inspection by the Poor Law Board, and provided for their subsequent maintenance to be met out of the poor rate. Frederick Lucas and *The Tablet* had been campaigning for these sorts of reforms since 1853. In 1863 the Government provided for salaried Catholic chaplains in the prisons—a change Grant reported to Propaganda with a justifiable sense of accomplishment, for it was another area in which he had been concerned with presenting the case to the government.[86] The Act was also a response to the increased numbers of Catholics in prison; a result of Irish immigration. In 1862 there were between 3,000 and 4,000 Catholic prisoners in gaol, and some 1,500 more in convict prisons.[87] The Reformatory and Industrial Schools Acts, in 1866, allowed Catholic institutions which passed inspection to receive rate-aid, and to take Catholic children transferred to them by the Poor Law guardians. These were, altogether, a very successful series of reforms, which built confidence between the Church and the authorities and which safeguarded the faith of enormous numbers of Catholics.

But there were other political episodes of the 1850s and 1860s which perpetuated Catholic suspicions of the Protestant state. English antipathy to the Temporal sovereignty

---

[85] Ibid. R79/4, Grant to Wiseman, 28 July 1858.

[86] Propaganda, *Scritture* 16 (1861-3), 670, Grant to the Cardinal Prefect 9 Aug. 1862 [in Italian]. A printed copy of the new regulations drawn up by the prison authorities is enclosed.

[87] G. I. T. Machin, *Politics and the Churches in Great Britain, 1832 to 1868*, Oxford 1977, 305.

of the Papacy, which reached a peak during Garibaldi's visit in 1864, had for years been simmering through publicity in the Protestant press given to the Mortara case. This involved a Jewish boy of seven, who had been taken away from parents in Bologna on the grounds that he had been baptized (when a small infant, by a Christian servant in his parents' employment) and brought up in the Catholic religion. The case of Edgar Mortara soon became a European scandal, in a campaign of carefully contrived vilification got up by liberal and Protestant newspapers.[88] The question of a parliamentary inspectorate of convents also excited suspicions of the Catholics for the government. Protestant campaigners created the impression, through lurid appeals to the sinister life of the cloister, and to claims that unwilling young girls were imprisoned behind convent walls, that Catholic conventual institutions were a violation of common liberty. In 1853 there began a series of attempts in Parliament to secure official inquiries into the condition of the convents and other Catholic institutions, and this movement, which came to be led by C. N. Newdegate, the MP for North Warwickshire, eventually succeeded in the Royal Commission of Inquiry into Maynooth (1853–55),[89] and in the passing of Newdegate's motion for a Select Committee on 'Conventual and Monastic Institutions' in 1870—in the period of anti-Catholic hostility attendant upon the Vatican Council. The Committee's report, in 1871, showed—as was only to have been expected—that the requirements of the Catholic Emancipation Act for the suppression of such institutions had not been complied with in any case since the Act was passed.[90] Early in the 1850s Ullathorne had written two pamphlets to defend the convents against the charges popularly made against them.[91] Another area of encroachment derived from civil registration. The Marriage Act of 1836 had, of course, been beneficial to Catholics, since it

[88] Norman, *The Catholic Church and Ireland in the Age of Rebellion, 1859–1873*, 41-3.
[89] John Healey, *Maynooth College, Its Centenary History*, Dublin 1895, 462-78.
[90] *Parliamentary Papers*, 1871, vii, *Report* viii. For details of Newdegate's campaigns, see Arnstein, *Protestant versus Catholic in Mid-Victorian England. Mr. Newdegate and the Nuns*, 149-62.
[91] Cuthbert Butler, *Ullathorne*, I. 169.

legalized marriage in their own churches, provided they were conducted in the presence of a civil registrar, and so ended the obligation to be married in the Protestant parish church. But the Act of 1840 (3 & 4 Vict. c. 92) had provided that all non-parochial registers of births, deaths, and marriages should be deposited with the office of the Registrar General. A few Catholic priests sent theirs to London, alongside the eight thousand or so kept by the Protestant Dissenters—but most did not. In 1855 the Registrar General asked Wiseman to make other Catholic registers available, a move, as he pointed out, which would facilitate their 'being accepted as evidence in courts of justice'.[92] Fears of control of Catholic parochial affairs by the Protestant state made the Catholics cautious of complying. But it was the question of charitable Trusts which, above all others, generated these sorts of suspicions. The huge multiplication of Catholic charitable institutions in the middle years of the century made this a pressing and far-reaching question for the hierarchy.

The Irish Catholic bishops had led the way here, by rejecting the Charitable Bequest Act of 1844. Though intended to safeguard Catholic bequests, the Act was represented, by Archbishop John MacHale of Tuam, and by Frederick Lucas,[93] as an attempt by Parliament to control the Church. In England, the Bill was welcomed by the leading Catholic aristocracy: by Lord Beaumont, Lord Arundel and Surrey, and Lord Camoys. Legislation about charitable trusts in England was anyway overdue: some codification and regularization of the laws relating to trusts were clearly necessary. Many were obsolete. Catholic trusts were, in the existing state of the law, liable to confiscation or re-application as 'superstitious'. As agent of the English bishops in Rome, Grant had in 1849 been instructed to elicit the views of Propaganda on possible legislation, and he had asked Wiseman to produce a statement on 'the present state of the law, and the position of our trusts' which, 'either because of their illegal form or because of past neglect, require some special provision'.[94] As a result of a

[92] Westminster Dioc. Archives, Wiseman Papers, W3/33/77, 20 Oct. 1855.

[93] Edward Lucas, *The Life of Frederick Lucas M.P.*, London 1886, I. 164.

[94] Westminster Dioc. Archives, Wiseman Papers, Bishops' Letters 137/1/8, Grant to Wiseman, 13 Dec. 1849.

Royal Commission of Inquiry into Charities, an Act was passed in 1853 setting up a permanent body of Commissioners to register and administer charitable trusts. Ullathorne reported from Rome, in December of that year, that all were 'very anxious' about the new legislation.[95] Wiseman circularized the bishops to get both their opinions of the Act and also an account of the state of Catholic charities in their dioceses. Most replied, as did Bishop Thomas Joseph Brown from Newport, that the effect of the Charitable Bequests Act 'will be most serious': that 'in the hands of parties hostile to us, they may, with greatest probability, produce confiscation of property destined for Catholic purposes, and the total ruin of interests dependent thereon'. He favoured 'any scheme of opposition that may be approved of' by Rome and the bishops—'even though it brought upon myself loss of personal liberty'.[96] Bishop Alexander Goss of Liverpool, in his reply, pointed out that the bishops should not themselves become involved in promoting parliamentary action for a Catholic Bill—'in order that they may be free to act in evading its provisions if found detrimental'. The centre of Catholic objection to the Act lay in its retention of the doctrine of superstitious uses—that Catholic Charitable Bequests could not have the protection of law if they required masses for the soul of the departed. Goss actually believed that obligations to say such masses 'have been incurred on insufficient grounds', and suggested that the Holy See should cancel all existing obligations, so overcoming the difficulties of English law, and restore masses where a suitable obligation existed, on the authority of the Church itself, rather than that of a testator.[97] Manning, who had been asked by Wiseman to examine the Act, believed that the framers intended 'to draw all trust property under the cognizance of law, and to exclude the free and discretionary power of administrators by defining the particular cases'.[98] This was a correct interpretation, and it was, of course, meant to act as a protection. Manning was

[95] Ibid. 130/1, Ullathorne to Wiseman, 20 Dec. 1853.

[96] Ibid. R79/6, Brown to Wiseman, 15 Dec. 1853.

[97] Westminster Dioc. Archives, Wiseman Papers, Bishops' Letters R79/6, Goss to Wiseman, 25 Nov. 1853.

[98] Ibid. R79/5, Manning to Wiseman, 15 Jan. 1854.

optimistic, and, as reported by Bishop Wareing of Northampton, in October 1854, 'he seemed to think that we had no
reason to fear any attempt on the part of government to act
in an ungenerous or persecuting spirit towards us'.[99] In March
1854, Propaganda ruled that each of the bishops should be
left free to act individually over the operation of the Charitable Trusts Act: this had been elicited by differences of view
among them over whether they should register Catholic
charities with the Commissioners. Ullathorne favoured joint
episcopal action, before any approach was made to the
government.[100] Differences over the question merged with
the general division within the Hierarchy associated with
Wiseman's tendency to treat the bishops in a consultative
capacity only. In 1856 Errington reported an opinion that
Propaganda's Letter of March 1854 was 'not intended to be
final, but as it were proposals', and that the Cardinal Prefect
awaited further initiatives from the English bishops.[101] The
legal provision for registration of all trusts, made following a
Parliamentary Inquiry of 1860, sharpened the differences
within the Hierarchy, as the question itself became more
urgent. Wiseman declined to register the trusts, in the belief
that their existence would be hazarded; Errington and most
of the other bishops favoured registration. 'To submit the
accounts to a Commission', as Manning wrote to Talbot in
1861, 'is to recognize the *altum dominium* of the state.'[102]
In November 1861, there was a test case, brought forward
by Ullathorne. This was Blundell's Trust, heard before the
Master of the Rolls: four legacies were considered, and it was
ruled that all masses for the dead were in the eye of the law
superstitious, and that no legacy for them could hold. As
Wiseman wrote: 'Unless the Holy See shall rule to the contrary I feel I must suffer anything rather than allow a submission to such a law.'[103] He also supposed that 'Lay Catholics
will be ready enough to pounce on any disputed funds and

[99] Ibid. R91/9, Wareing to Wiseman, 10 Oct. 1854.
[100] Ibid. R91/9, Ullathorne to Wiseman, 6 Oct. 1854.
[101] Westminster Dioc. Archives, Wiseman Papers, Bishops' Letters 130/1,
Errington to Wiseman, 15 Feb. 1856.
[102] Purcell, *Manning*, II. 127.
[103] Cardinal Gasquet, 'Unpublished Letters of Cardinal Wiseman to Dr Manning' in *Dublin Review*, Oct.–Dec. 1921, 171 (23 Nov. 1861).

they will be easily swallowed up in litigation.'[104] At the Low Week meeting of the Hierarchy in 1861 the differences of view between Wiseman and the bishops over charitable bequests proved unresolvable. Clifford and Ullathorne drew up a statement of the general opinion, for presentation at a special meeting held in May—at which Wiseman was not present. They then addressed their case in favour of compliance with the law to Rome. In August 1862, Propaganda ruled that registration would jeopardize Catholic bequests. Wiseman had won. Reforms in the second half of the century partially removed the doctrine of superstitious uses from the law and the question of Catholic charities and bequests was solved along with them. The Declaration against Transubstantiation, as a qualification for civic offices, was abolished in 1867. In the same year the Religious Disabilities Removals Act removed further restrictions on Catholics in public life, and also repealed that clause of the Catholic Emancipation Act which prohibited civic dignitaries from appearing in Catholic places of worship wearing their insignia of office. The law of mortmain—regulating the bequest of property to ecclesiastical corporations—was changed in 1888, although the leading provision of the old law remained.

However much issues like education or charitable bequests may have impelled the Catholic leadership into relations with the government, the Church remained independent of political action as such—demonstrating a feature of English Christianity in the nineteenth century which also characterized the Church of England but not important sections of Protestant Dissent. There had, early in the century, been some signs that the Catholics might ally themselves to radical politics, just as the Dissenters were doing. From the 1780s there was a stream of common sympathy between those Catholics seeking relief measures from Parliament, and the Dissenters, who were seeking a comparable adjustment of the Constitution to secure rights against the Established Church. This led to some actual political co-operation in the rising popular politics of the provincial cities.[105] The Dissenters' campaign against the

---

[104] Ibid. 172 (7 Dec. 1861).
[105] Bossy, *The English Catholic Community, 1570–1850*, 352.

educational clauses of Graham's Factory Act, in 1843—itself
rather a catalyst in emergent liberal politics—drew in the
Catholics. The militancy of the Dissenters was really directed
against the whole constitutional position of the State Church,
and it was precisely this radicalism which appealed to Lucas,
who used *The Tablet* to swing Catholic opinion behind the
Dissenters' campaign.[106] The Vicars Apostolic produced a
petition against the legislation, regarding it, as did the Dissenters, as an unfair expenditure of public money in support
of the educational claims of the Anglicans. Catholics were
less active in most of the other political enterprises launched
by the agencies of the militant Dissenters, and as the demand
for state non-sectarian education rose to the front of the
Dissenters' campaign, with the foundation of the Education
League in 1869, the Catholics detached themselves altogether.
Some Catholics took part in local agitations against the payment of Church Rate—another of the formative political
influences which lay behind the consolidation of popular
politics in the 1850s and 1860s. But their petitions against the
rate were much less numerous than those of the Protestant
Dissenters, perhaps because many lived in large cities where
the rate had already lapsed through local agreement.[107] One
Catholic opponent, at Rugeley in Staffordshire, got placards
against the rates on especially favourable terms from his
Protestant printers: 'as they are also themselves round enemies of the Establishment and do this work cheap'.[108]

The old political sympathy between the Catholics and the
Whigs, revised into support for liberal-radicalism, was perpetuated in the career of Frederick Lucas. Born in 1812, the
son of a London Quaker, a corn merchant, Lucas had been
educated by the Quakers at Darlington and then at London
University. He had, therefore, a thoroughly Dissenting pedi-
gree. He entered the legal profession and was called to the Bar
in 1835. The political atmosphere of the 1830s was wholly
conducive to him, with the expectation of reform, and he
became a professed disciple of Benthamism. Then, in 1839,

[106] Lucas, *The Life of Frederick Lucas M.P.*, I. 121.
[107] Machin, 307.
[108] Westminster Dioc. Archives, Wiseman Papers, W3/33/56, Whitgrave to (?)
Searle, 17 Sept. 1855.

and apparently on impulse, he suddenly became a Catholic. His religious convictions were turned upside down; his political beliefs remained the same. He had been interested in politics, in fact, while 'still a mere lad',[109] and his entire life was political. In the first number of the famous Catholic paper he founded in 1840, *The Tablet*, he claimed Whig allegiance, but, as the politics of the paper were to show, it was a Whiggery deeply infiltrated with radicalism. After a visit to Ireland in 1843 he was converted to Repeal and became increasingly absorbed by Irish Catholic politics—*The Tablet* itself moved to Dublin in 1850, and in 1852 Lucas was elected to parliament for Meath. The encouragement he gave to the political action of the Irish priests was a considerable embarrassment to Archbishop Cullen, and was watched nervously by the bishops of England. Lucas called the politics of the priests 'an inestimable jewel',[110] but in 1854 Cullen secured the approval of Rome for *Decrees* which drastically curtailed clerical participation in politics. As it happened, and as was only to be expected in Ireland, the *Decrees* had a very limited effect.[111] Lucas appealed against them, unsuccessfully, in Rome, and then died unexpectedly, at the age of forty-three, in 1855. His influence was in Ireland rather than in England; but even in England he furthered, for a time, a tradition of Catholic political radicalism. His successor in that was perhaps T. P. O'Connor, one of the MPs for Liverpool elected in 1880, whose United Irish League of Great Britain organized the Irish vote in industrial areas and then, in 1885, adhered it to the Home Rule cause. The electoral strength of the Irish has sometimes been exaggerated, however. High mobility of the immigrant workers, and their limited education, resulted in large numbers never registering as voters.[112] O'Connor was a radical and his support of Charles Bradlaugh's campaign to secure the admission of freethinkers to Parliament, early in the 1880s, was characteristically radical;[113] but it offended many of his Catholic co-religionists and may have limited his

---

[109] Lucas, I. 21.   [110] Lucas, II. 33.

[111] Norman, *The Catholic Church and Ireland in the Age of Rebellion*, 28.

[112] M. A. G. O'Tuathaigh, 'The Irish in Nineteenth Century Britain: Problems of Integration', in *Trans. Royal Hist. Soc.*, Fifth Series, 31 (1981), 171.

[113] Conor Cruise O'Brien, *Parnell and his Party, 1880–1890*, Oxford 1957, 50.

influence. O'Connor's main movement was also too sectional-
ized, too concerned with Irish affairs, to affect the leadership
of the Catholic Church in England; just as Manning found
few echoes for his Irish interests in the rest of the Hierarchy.
Most of the bishops were more concerned with the censure of
Fenianism than they were with Irish reform: they regarded it
as a secret society which came *ipso facto* under the ban of
the Church, an English Mazzinianism. There was widespread
sympathy for the Fenians among the Irish in the English
cities, and Ullathorne's Pastoral against them, in 1869, elicited
a lengthy campaign of vituperation in the Fenian press.[114]
Ullathorne was anyway a Conservative in politics, though he
abstained from public political expressions or actions. The
drift was towards Conservative support in mid-century Catholic leadership: in 1851 the Ecclesiastical Titles Act had
broken the old sympathy for the Whigs, and the Whig–Liberal
hostility to the Temporal Sovereignty of the Papacy led to
Wiseman's support of the Tories in 1858—a support given,
as Disraeli said, 'without solicitation'.[115] Wiseman's normal
condition, however, was one of non-partisanship. 'In our
body there exist all possible shades of political opinions', he
told the Malines Congress in 1863; 'we have men professing
the most decided conservative principles; we have others who
preach their liberal ideas as far as is consistent with moral and
social maxims.'[116] But all, he said, 'make their prosecution
of such sacred purposes independent of any party differences'.[117] The Catholic Institute was, by its constitution, forbidden to take part in politics, and so, by convention, was
the Catholic Poor School Committee. Manning disliked the
laity taking up Catholic questions with the government, except under direction from the Hierarchy, and professed, anyway, to employ his own personal influence with ministries:
'one of the results of the Archbishop's line of action was that
the Catholic laity abstained from public action in furtherance of Catholic interests'.[118] The move away from the Whigs

[114] Cuthbert Butler, *Ullathorne*, II. 142.
[115] Wilfrid Ward, *Wiseman*, II. 449.
[116] *The Religious and Social Position of Catholics in England*, 58.
[117] Ibid. 57.
[118] Purchell, *Manning*, II. 383.

produced the first Catholic Conservative Member of Parliament in 1859, when Sir John Pope-Hennessy was elected. The Duke of Norfolk, the leading Catholic layman in the last three decades of the century, was also a Conservative. Catholics in the constituencies still tended to support Liberal candidates: they were much less affected than the bishops and the lay leaders were by the priority of the Education question and the support of the Conservative Party for denominational schools. When, in the November general election of 1885, Parnell directed the Irish voters in England to support Conservative candidates it was the hope of securing a Home Rule solution from Salisbury, rather than because of educational issues, which prompted the tactic. The position was always liable to become destabilized, and there exists in the archives at Downside an interesting letter of Lord Ripon's, sent in 1880 to Fr. Bulbeck, seeking to influence Catholics not to support the Conservatives because of the Education issue or out of antipathy to Gladstone because of his pamphlet against the Vatican Council. Ripon was the most significant political figure to become a Catholic in the second half of the century. He had been attracted to the Christian Socialism of F. D. Maurice and retained an element of social radicalism within his Liberalism. In 1874 he became a Catholic: something of a revolutionary change for one who was Grand Master of the English Freemasons. He had served in the Cabinets of Palmerston and Gladstone, and was to become Viceroy of India. In 1880, as he wrote in the letter, he had 'observed with great regret that there is a tendency among some Catholics in different parts of the country, who have hitherto always supported the Liberal Party, to change sides at the present Election'. He also declared: 'I have felt ever since I became a Catholic that it is a great advantage to our interests as Catholics that there should be men of our Faith attached to both our great political parties, so that, whichever party may be in power, we should have friends at court.' His point in 1880 was that Catholic defection from the Liberals could result, should they win, as he hoped they would—and as they did—in a degree of political vindictiveness towards their interests. He also claimed that, as far as the Education question was concerned, 'the alarms which the Conservatives are trying to excite on this subject are baseless'. He did not believe that the Liberals would upset the 1870 Act—a belief in which the Gladstone administration proved him correct— and earnestly enjoined them all to follow his own policy: 'to keep everything connected with our schools out of the battle-field of politics'.[119] But it was a policy which became imposs-ible when the Radicals and Nonconformists made education a leading political issue, in the 1890s. The Hierarchy con-tinued to be unavoidably attached to the Conservatives in consequence.

There was one exception, both to the general convention of avoiding party allegiances, and to the actual politics es-poused. In 1885 Bishop Edward Bagshawe of Nottingham canvassed the idea of a distinct political party for Catholics. He got very little support. Bagshawe was, anyway, noted for his political radicalism. In 1886 he announced that he would withdraw the sacraments from any Catholics in his diocese who joined the Primrose League—the Conservative society founded to honour the memory of Disraeli. 'The scandal is great, and it will shake the confidence of our people in the Episcopate', Manning wrote in near despair to Bishop Clifford.[120] And again he wrote: 'I am forced unwillingly to say that if the Bishop of Nottingham persists in the impru-dent action of the last three years, we shall be compelled to take action upon it.' The matter involved 'the relation of the Church to the public opinion and the Government of the country'.[121] Ullathorne, who had himself been addressed as to whether the Primrose League was 'one of those secret so-cieties which come under the condemnation of the Church',[122] and who, of course, said that it was not, spoke twice to Bagshawe. In the event no suspensions of the sacraments were made and the matter passed off.

Bagshawe's was also the closest Catholic approximation to the social reformist mood of Anglicanism in the last three

[119] Downside Archives, VII.A.3.a, Abbot's Papers (File marked '1871–1880'), Ripon to Bulbeck, 27 March 1880.
[120] Bristol Record Office 35721, Clifton Dioc. Archives, Clifford Papers, Manning to Clifford, 16 March 1886.
[121] Ibid., Manning to Clifford, 22 March 1886.
[122] Birmingham Dioc. Archives, B.8882, Letter of Ullathorne, 8 Oct. 1885.

decades of the nineteenth century—to the rejection of *laissez-faire* orthodoxy and to the political radicalism found in the Anglican Christian Social Union, established in 1889 by Gore, Westcott, and Scott Holland. The atmosphere of social radicalism was also present in Manning, though in a less systematic degree.[123] Lucas had anticipated some of these attitudes during the Irish Famine, in the later 1840s, when he had criticized the application of classical Political Economy to the condition of Ireland, especially the scheme of public works conducted by the government as a form of relief: the works were deliberately intended to be non-productive and so avoid state interference in normal economic relationships.[124] The publication of Leo XIII's *Rerum Novarum* (1891) in the English Catholic press, with its limited encouragement of a more reformist attitude to economic relationships, did little to foster in English Catholicism the spirit which was making such advances within the Anglican intelligentsia. Bagshawe, alone, was a sort of Catholic equivalent; his critique of Political Economy was very similar to Westcott's. In 1883 and 1884 he published two Pastoral Letters in favour of collectivism, and these, re-issued in a consolidated form as *Mercy and Justice to the Poor*, in 1885, were markedly similar to the Anglican writings of these years. A lot of his evidence for social conditions came from the Congregationalist tract, *The Bitter Cry of Outcast London* (1883), which had influenced both William Booth and the founders of the Christian Social Union. 'There can be no doubt that in many of the received usages of business and modes of making money prevalent in modern times, by which such enormous fortunes are accumulated in the hands of a few, while the multitudes are ever more and more impoverished, there is very much which is contrary to justice no less than to mercy,' Bagshawe wrote. The needs of labour were 'taken advantage of by capitalists and employers to deprive them unjustly of the greater part of the just fruit of their toil', while 'the sacred rights of property' were 'loudly invoked by the moneyed classes' to protect themselves against change.[125] State intervention was

---

[123] See chapter 6.
[124] Lucas, I. 231.
[125] Edward G. Bagshawe, *Mercy and Justice to the Poor*, London 1885, 7.

required: 'I do not think that the right and duty of the state, and of its citizens, are so limited as political economists appear to suppose.'[126] Christianity teaches, he contended, 'that the poor and the helpless are not really free in their contracts, but need protection against the extortions of the rich; that labour has its just remuneration, and that its right to receive it should be protected by the community'.[127] There can be no doubt that in the expression of such opinions, Bagshawe showed himself to be the closest among the Catholic leaders to the most dynamic social thinking of the day, but his influence within Catholicism was negligible—and, because he was a *Catholic* bishop, it was negligible outside Catholicism, too. There was a streak of poor judgement in him, witnessed in the Primrose League anathema, which, quite as much as his actual radicalism, isolated his influence. One of his own laymen in the diocese of Nottingham, with allusion to the political and social positions catalogued in the *Syllabus of Errors*, articulated what must have been the general Catholic response: 'If the authority of a Catholic Bishop is to be quoted in favour of such radical views, it will be well that the higher authority of the Holy See be consulted.'[128] Such a problem did not exist for the Anglican social radicals, since there was no authority in their Church to whom an appeal could anyway be directed. Catholic Christian Socialism therefore developed rather slowly. The ancient universities, where social idealism flourished among the young, were still restricted for Catholic students through the ban maintained by the Hierarchy. Catholic youth were insulated against the views which fired so many of their Anglican contemporaries. The Catholic Social Guild, 'a kind of Catholic Christian Social Union',[129] was not founded until 1909 although it was preceded by a philanthropic and faintly radical body which had undertaken Catholic relief work. The first Catholic Socialist Society was not founded until 1906.

---

[126] Ibid. 15.

[127] Ibid. 17.

[128] Edwin De Lisle, *Pastoral Politics. A Reply to Dr Bagshawe, Catholic Bishop of Nottingham*, London 1885, 5.

[129] Peter d'A. Jones, *The Christian Socialist Revival, 1877–1914*, Princeton 1968, 29.

Most Catholic social consciousness during the second half of the nineteenth century issued in charitable and 'Rescue' work—the latter, directed primarily to linking social improvement with denominational preservation, and so pastoral rather than radical in style and intention, was especially associated with Vaughan's work at Salford in the 1880s.[130] The new religious orders, of the mid-century, were particularly sensitive to the poverty of many Catholics. 'The ignorance and vice of these people are such as to beggar description,' Gentili reported to Rosmini from rural Leicestershire in 1841; 'and the destitution is such that I cannot think of it without tears of compassion.' There were many who on 'Sundays do not go to any church, because they have no decent clothes to wear'.[131] It has to be remembered that he wrote at a time of exceptional social suffering—in the 'Hungry 'Forties'. One response was Temperance reform—later associated with Manning's *League of the Cross* (1872). At this time, it was largely due to the inspiration of Father Theobald Mathew, the great reformer from Cork who campaigned in England during 1843. He experienced a good deal of success in the northern cities. In London, however, there were difficulties: 'availing themselves of the stupid prejudice against "the Popish priest", which was felt most strongly by the lowest class of their besotted customers, some crafty publicans in Bermondsey, in Westminster, and in other parts of the metropolis, who were afraid of losing their unhappy slaves, organized several attempts to interrupt the proceedings of his meetings, to upset the platform, or to create disturbance and confusion'.[132] Catholic concern to provide charitable assistance to the poor certainly equalled Anglican, and in view of the proportionately and qualitatively different resources available, perhaps exceeded it. At the level of the Catholic aristocracy and gentry there were some especially noted for philanthropic largesse: Ambrose Phillipps de Lisle, for example, or John Talbot, sixteenth Earl of Shrewsbury. The latter lived in great simplicity at Alton Towers in Staffordshire, in order to devote his resources to Catholic good works and to

[130] See chapter 8.
[131] Leetham, *Luigi Gentili*, 138-9.
[132] J. F. Maguire, *Father Mathew. A Biography*, London 1863, 282.

church building. 'No servant in the house had his room so poor as was the private room of the Earl,' Ullathorne once wrote; 'It was as poor as my convent cell could be.'[133] Most funds for Catholic welfare, however, were collected by the local clergy from the poor themselves, so creating, in effect, a sort of organized network of self-help. At times of particular social distress, too, the Catholic bishops often appealed for extra financial assistance for the poor. Thus a strike among the iron workers of South Wales, in 1873, elicited a Circular Letter from Bishop Brown addressed 'to the affluent and to those whose resources will enable them to exercise charity for the relief of the corporal necessities of others'. He reported thousands of families as being 'destitute'. 'The resources of the clergy are taxed far beyond their strength,' he continued, 'for their incomes, which were at all times precarious, (being dependent on the poor Irish, who constitute the members of most of my missions), have now almost entirely ceased, and their congregations, consisting almost wholly of labourers, are besieging their doors in hundreds asking for the necessaries of life.'[134] Anglican parsons, whose relations with the working classes were rather less intimate, encountered such problems on a more modest scale.

[133] Ullathorne, *Letters*, 26.
[134] Downside Archives, VII.A.3.a, Abbots' Papers (File marked '1871–1880'), *The Distress in the Iron District of the Diocese of Newport and Menevia*, by Bishop T. J. Brown, Jan. 1873.

5

Church Expansion

'Catholicity in England is proceeding at a railroad pace': even the exaggerated language of Ambrose Phillipps de Lisle was not, for once, inappropriate.[1] He wrote in 1840. By then the physical signs of Catholic advance were becoming very clear in England. Pugin, in that year, was engaged in building no less than seventeen Catholic churches; and in 1841 St. Chad's in Birmingham, the first Catholic church intended to serve as a cathedral to be built in England since the Reformation, was opened with magnificent ceremonial made all the more impressive by the fortuitous discovery of the relics of the saint himself—'which had been stored away by Mr. Fitzherbert of Swynnerton and forgotton'.[2] In 1848 another cathedral was completed, St. George's in Southwark, built by Pugin upon a site which had, in 1780, been a centre of the anti-Catholic Gordon Riots. Two hundred and forty priests attended the opening, and fourteen bishops. Wiseman preached the sermon and Sir John Acton was thurifer. 'Something very strange is passing over this land, by the very surprise, by the very commotion, which it excites', Newman declared in one of his most famous sermons—preached at the first Provincial Synod of Westminster to the restored Hierarchy of England, in 1852. 'It is the coming in of a Second Spring; it is a restoration in the moral world.'[3] Now some of his 'Second Spring' was rhetorical embellishment, the justifiable exultation of those who had crossed to Rome and landed more safely upon her shores than they could have expected; it was the relief of ancient families whose recusancy was at last no longer the whispered tradition of the rural English catacombs. Catholic

    [1] Louis Allen, 'Letters of Phillipps de Lisle to Montalembert', in *Dublin Review* 228, no. 463 (1954), 57.
    [2] Gwynn, *The Second Spring, 1818-1852*, 134.
    [3] Newman, *Sermons Preached on Various Occasions*, 195-7, ('The Second Spring', 13 July 1852).

expansion in nineteenth-century England was English in its roots. 'I listen, and I hear the sound of voices, grave and musical', Newman said on that moving occasion in 1852; 'renewing the old chant, with which Augustine greeted Ethelbert in the free air upon the Kentish strand.'[4]

Everywhere the signs of revival were evident to observer and participant. In his first two years in London, Wiseman recorded the establishment of seven new religious communities of women and three of men; two Catholic orphanages were opened, a secondary school for boys, and eleven new missions. Devotional and charitable associations were spread among the laity by the clergy. 'I think I can safely say that in a year or little more', Wiseman wrote in 1850, '15,000 persons have been reclaimed by the Retreats given in courts and alleys'—among the slums of the working classes.[5] With the possible exception of the Western and Eastern Districts, where advance was in places rather unencouraging, each area—each diocese after 1850—disclosed comparable signs of the Catholic renewal. During Ullathorne's period as Bishop of Birmingham, for example, 44 new missions were established, 67 new churches were built, over a hundred elementary schools were set up, the number of priests increased from 86 to 200, and the religious communities of women rose from 7 to 36.[6] Not all the expansion was entirely beneficial: the pressure to increase the number of priests resulted in the occasional ordination of those who were not of the highest intellectual or pastoral capacity. In the Diocese of Nottingham, some 25 of the 82 secular clergy were said to be unsatisfactory by the closing years of the century: 11 of these had been hastily ordained at the diocesan seminary because of the urgency of the pastoral need.[7] Yet the overall picture was one of great hope and optimism—too much optimism at times. 'The Anglican Church is in the greatest possible decline, and the sect which is the most expanding is that of the Methodists,' according

[4] Ibid. 204.

[5] Wilfrid Ward, *The Life and Times of Cardinal Wiseman*, I. 516.

[6] Cuthbert Butler, *The Life and Times of Bishop Ullathorne, 1806–1889*, II. 192.

[7] Holmes, *More Roman than Rome: English Catholicism in the Nineteenth Century*, 174.

to a Report drawn up on the state of the English Church by Propaganda in the 1830s, in the belief that Catholicism could step into the place soon to be vacated by the ailing national church.[8] 'The general progress of Religion in England, through the Grace of God, is such that it causes great fear to the Protestants,' according to an address of 1835, drawn up for the Pope and also preserved in the archives of Propaganda.[9] And indeed it was true that one measure of the rising confidence of English Catholicism was the enhanced level of anti-Catholicism is elicited in response. The Reformation Society, a particularly militant national agency of Protestant extremism, organized resistance to the missionary activity of the new Catholic orders: the three Catholic Chapels opened in 1837 by Phillipps de Lisle in rural Leicestershire attracted the Society's hostility and there were 'No Popery' meetings at Ashby de la Zouch. After one such assembly, Father Gentili 'was pelted with mud, and his cassock covered from top to bottom with filth'.[10] In Staffordshire Father Barberi's preaching, in 1842; obliged the Protestant ministers to start house-to-house visiting with, as he explained, 'the sole object of exhorting the people not to come near me'.[11] The Maynooth Grant question in 1845 and the Restoration of the Hierarchy in 1850, of course, prompted great national demonstrations of anti-Catholicism, and anti-Catholic rioting continued in the provinces during periodic outbursts in the 1850s and 1860s. Most of these disturbances derived from traditional English suspicions about the political loyalty of Catholics and a loathing of the supposed idolatry of Catholic devotional practices, but in areas of heavy Irish immigration there was the addition of antipathy to an immigrant labour force, with its potential to depress wages and living-standards. There was anti-Catholic rioting at Birkenhead in November 1850, and in June 1852 the Stockport riots, in which two Catholic chapels were sacked and desecrated by a Protestant

[8] Propaganda, *Scritture* 9 (1834–41), *Missioni di Europa; Inghilterra*, 1834 [in Italian], 1.

[9] Ibid., *Esposizione vera e fidele dello stato della Missione in Inghilterra*, 1835 [in Italian], 100.

[10] Purcell, *Life and Letters of Ambrose Phillipps de Lisle*, I. 111.

[11] Urban Young, *Dominic Barberi in England. A new series of Letters*, London, 1935, 83.

mob, became one of the most infamous civil disturbances of the century. The rioting of the 1850s was sometimes inspired by Alessandro Gavazzi, a former Catholic monk from Naples, who addressed hundreds of meetings on an anti-Popery platform. Rioting in the 1860s often attended the anti-Catholic addresses and demonstrations of William Murphy. At Portsmouth in June 1866, at Birmingham in June 1867—where the police had to use their sabres on the crowds—and in May 1868—when a hundred houses and two Catholic Churches were destroyed by the mob—Murphy's preaching drew Protestant gatherings into violent confrontations. Finally, in 1871, he was attacked by a Catholic mob and received mortal injuries.[12] The general trend, despite all this, was towards an acceptance of Catholicism. Gentili probably encountered more sympathy than hostility in the villages of rural Leicestershire: the Catholic missioners 'were regarded by the labourers and the poor as friends and benefactors'.[13] In his address to the Catholic Congress at Malines, in 1863, Fr. Hermann, Prior of the Discalced Carmelites in London, remarked on the 'day by day' improvement in public attitudes to the Catholics—'and this in proportion as the happy effect of Emancipation introduces Catholics, more or less, into every branch of public employment'. He added: 'prejudices are dying out'.[14] But it was a slow process. That Catholics were conscious of it, however, greatly assisted their sense that a new age lay ahead for their work and missionary enterprise. In 1851 Newman delivered a series of lectures in Birmingham on the *Present Position of Catholics in England*— ignored by the press at the time—which comprised a lengthy critique of the traditional Protestant view of Catholicism. He said, as if in conclusion, 'We live in a happier age than our forefathers; at least, let us trust that the habits of society and the self-interest of classes and of sects will render it impossible that blind prejudice and brute passion should ever

[12] Norman, *Anti-Catholicism in Victorian England*, 18; John Denvir, *The Irish in Britain. From the Earliest Times to the Fall and Death of Parnell*, London 1892, 262.

[13] Purcell, *Ambrose Phillipps de Lisle*, I. 111.

[14] *Catholicism in England. An Address delivered 3rd September, AD 1863, at the Catholic Congress at Malines by Father Hermann, Prior of the Discalced Carmelites in London*, London 1864, 13.

make innocence and helplessness their sport and prey, as they did in the seventeenth century.'[15] And these words were spoken within a few months of the 'No-Popery' demonstrations consequent upon the restoration of the Hierarchy. Catholic England was very conscious of its new presence in the life of the nation.

The statistics of expansion were impressive. According to the Catholic Directory there were in 1850, the year of the restored Hierarchy, 587 churches in England and Wales, and 788 clergy; in the London District there were 104 churches and chapels and 168 clergy.[16] In 1870, the year of the Vatican Council, there were 1151 churches and 1528 clergy; in the Westminster Diocese, there were 126 churches and 246 clergy.[17] It should be noticed, however, that many of the churches comprised in the figure of 1151 were actually *private* chapels, belonging to religious houses or landed estates, and that those registered for marriages, about 660, were really the 'parochial' churches. In 1900 there were 1529 churches in England and Wales, with 2812 clergy; in Westminster there were 153 churches and 415 clergy.[18] The figures for 1900 excluded churches not open to the public. In the religious census held in March 1851—of the number of persons attending public worship in the various churches of the country—there were estimated to be 252,783 Roman Catholics. This was actually less than the size of the Irish immigrant population— to the surprise of *The Times*, which could scarcely believe that the 'Papal Agression' uproar it had inspired in the preceding year rested on so slender a numerical threat.[19] The figures already illustrated the problem of 'leakage', if not from the faith, at least from regular attendance at mass. There were, in 1851, 519,959 persons who were of Irish birth in the

[15] J. H. Newman, *Lectures on the Present Position of Catholics in England, Addressed to the Brothers of the Oratory in the Summer of 1851*, London (new edn.) 1892, 269.

[16] *The Catholic Directory and Ecclesiastical Register, 1850*, London 1850, 41.

[17] *The Catholic Directory, Ecclesiastical Register, and Almanac, 1870*, London 1870, 288.

[18] *The Catholic Directory, 1900*, London 1900, 410.

[19] Owen Chadwick, *The Victorian Church*, Part I, London 1966, 367. For an analysis of the Catholic census returns, and the tables of attendance broken down regionally, see Philip Hughes, 'The English Catholics in 1850', in Beck, *The English Catholics, 1850–1950*, 42–53; 80–5.

country. Catholics formed 3.5 per cent of all worshippers in England on that March Sunday of 1851. The actual number of Catholics in the country must have been nearer to 700,000.[20] In Liverpool, for example, 38,123 Catholics went to mass, but the same census revealed that there were 83,813 Irish-born in the city, a high proportion of whom must have been Catholics.[21] The local distribution of Catholics, altered in the mid-century by the Irish influx, remained fairly stable during the second half of the century.[22] Figures for the expansion of Catholic schools and religious houses, like those for churches and clergy, showed a remarkable expansion. In 1850 there were two religious houses of men, and seventeen of women, in the London District; in 1900 the corresponding totals were thirty-three and forty-nine. Between 1850 and 1874 the number of Catholic schools in the country rose from 99 to 1,484. To an age fascinated by the statistics of growth these were all indications of an astonishing achievement, proportionately comparable, indeed, to the multiplication of religious institutions within the Protestant Established Church in these decades, but accomplished without the financial resources of the Church of England. Most of the expense was carried by the poor of the Catholic parishes, in what was an impressive demonstration of the vigour of the 'voluntary system' in nineteenth-century religion.

To the later observer, as often to contemporaries, it was the converts who seemed most to symbolize Catholic advance. In fact, of course, they were statistically a small part of the expansion—most of which came from the Irish immigration, from the conformity to Catholicism produced by mixed marriages, and from a continuation of the 'natural' growth of the traditional Catholicism which had already been evident in the later years of the eighteenth century.[23] Even the conversions were not due either to the example or to the evangelizing of the English Catholics. 'Not one of these people was converted by the sermons or instructions of any of our

[20] Hughes, ibid. 44.　　　　[21] Ibid. 52.

[22] Gwynn, 'Growth of the Catholic Community', ibid. 411.

[23] For a catalogue of some of the converts, see W. G. Gorman, *Converts to Rome. A biographical list of the more notable Converts to the Catholic Church in the United Kingdom during the last sixty years* (new edn.), London 1910.

clergy,' as Gentili noticed in one of his reports to Rome in 1847; 'Nearly all came after reading the Fathers or our books; it was not because of our efforts.'[24] Most came through disillusionment with the Church of England, in an era when Church Reform, carried out by a legislature which was also divesting itself of its religious exclusivity, was disclosing unacceptable features of erastianism. Some, including the earliest, were attracted by the 'medievalism' of contemporary aesthetic romanticism, and by travel in Catholic countries, where they were drawn to the popular devotional atmosphere of the faith, and to its universality. Thus the 'Cambridge converts' of the 1820s—Kenelm Digby, whose conversion while an undergraduate at Trinity 'caused some sensation' in the College,[25] Ambrose Phillipps (later known as Phillipps de Lisle), also at Trinity, and George Spencer. Digby and Phillipps had to travel twenty-five miles each Sunday on horseback to hear mass at Ware in Hertfordshire, the nearest Catholic place of worship to Cambridge in those days.

Ambrose Phillipps de Lisle was born in 1809 of a Leicestershire family, and first acquired a knowledge of Catholicism when he was taught as a boy by the Abbé Giraud, a French *émigré* priest. He was 'a born ritualist',[26] who, after visiting French churches in 1823, set up a Catholic-style altar in the Protestant Church at Shepshed on his family's estates. He had religious visions as a child. In 1825 he became a Catholic, and at Trinity College, in the company of Digby, he fostered discussion of religious differences between Anglicanism and Catholicism. After leaving Cambridge because of ill-health, in 1828, he travelled to Rome and there met Fr. Dominic Barberi. He remained a layman, and became a great benefactor of English Catholicism, founding a Trappist monastery and encouraging mission work by the new orders. He was also a leader of the Christian Reunion movement. In 1838 he became one of the founders of the Camden Society, and it was, in fact, through cultural and artistic interests, as much as through theological knowledge, that his Catholicism achieved its form and influence. He disliked the 'paganism' in the classical and baroque architecture of Rome,[27] was inspired by

[24] Leetham, *Luigi Gentili. A Sower for the Second Spring*, 284.
[25] Gwynn, *The Second Spring*, 20.   [26] Ibid. 21.
[27] Purcell, *Ambrose Phillipps de Lisle*, I. 37.

the 'gothick' ideal, and became a leading opponent of the attempt made by Ultramontane Catholics to introduce the art and devotional styles of the Italian Church to England.[28] He died in 1878.

It is sometimes too easily supposed that the converts were all Ultramontanists, like Manning, Ward, and Faber, more Catholic than the Catholics they had joined; but for every one whose new faith expressed itself in that way there was probably another, like Newman, Pugin, or Phillipps de Lisle, whose Catholicism was more nearly attuned to an English style. George Spencer probably belonged to the first category, however. He was the youngest child of Earl Spencer, born in 1799, whose brother was Lord Althorp, the Whig Chancellor in 1830. He too was at Trinity, after Eton, and then travelled in Europe, where he first encountered Catholicism. He was not at first moved by it, and in 1824, having no other career open to him, he received the holy orders of the national Church, having, at the time, 'very vague notions as to religious belief'.[29] His conversion was largely due to his friendship with Phillipps de Lisle, whom he met in 1829. It occurred in 1830, when he was incumbent of the living of Great Brington, and was, according to his sister, Lady Lyttleton, 'altogether a bad business'.[30] Spencer himself resigned his Anglican parish with the words: 'There goes £3,000 a year.'[31] He departed to Rome, to study at the English College under Wiseman, and there met Digby and Fr. Dominic Barberi. Ordained in 1832, he returned to England as a mission priest in Walsall and West Bromwich. In 1839 Bishop Walsh moved him to Oscott, where he taught until in 1847 (as Fr. Ignatius) he was received as a Passionist. He joined Fr. Dominic at Aston, becoming Provincial of the Passionists on Barberi's death in 1849. As a notable missioner, he travelled extensively in England and Ireland, and, though still giving missions, became rector of St. Anne's Retreat, Sutton, Lancashire, in 1863. He died the following year.

It was the Oxford Movement which produced the numerically significant waves of conversion, with Newman's, in

[28] Ibid. I. 313.   [29] Ibid. I. 39.

[30] Urban Young, *Life of Father Ignatius Spencer*, London 1933, 45.

[31] Gwynn, *The Second Spring*, 34.

1845, as marker. On his reception, masses of thanksgiving were offered up in the churches of Rome, France, Germany and Belgium. It sent a *frisson* of alarm through English Protestantism, leading some to suppose that the Church of England really was liable to disintegration. Disraeli was later to observe, however, that 'he would only begin to worry when he heard that the grocers were becoming converts'.[32] It was actually Pugin who established the first personal link between the Catholics and the Oxford men; after visiting Oxford in 1840 he maintained a correspondence with Oakley, Faber, Ward, Dalgairns and Bloxam. He transmitted his optimistic assessment of the possibility of large-scale conversion to Wiseman at Oscott.[33] This optimism fell upon well-prepared ground, for Wiseman had already, when in Rome as Rector of the English College, become convinced that the Oxford Movement presaged a re-Catholicizing of England. But it was Ambrose Phillipps de Lisle who was the most influential exponent of the belief that Oxford indicated a return of England to Roman allegiance. While Newman was composing Tract XC, in January and February 1841, Phillipps de Lisle wrote enthusiastically to his friends about the impending revolution of religious attitudes. He also visited Oxford, and met Bloxam. To the Earl of Shrewsbury he wrote, in January 1841, 'the Catholick movement at Oxford I certainly regard as the brightest symptom of England's reconversion, but thank God it is not the only one'. He added—deriving evidence from Gentili's work in Leicestershire—'there is a general movement amongst the lower classes'.[34] To Montalembert he wrote, in October of that year, 'I am fully persuaded that there is no point of the globe at the present moment in which a more important work is going on for the glory of the Catholick Church, than that which is in progress at Oxford.'[35] His optimism, based on slender evidence, actually increased in the following year. 'The devotion of the glorious Mother of God is rapidly increasing, great numbers of Anglicans now

[32] *Letters of Herbert Cardinal Vaughan to Lady Herbert of Lea, 1867 to 1903*, ed. Shane Leslie, London 1942, ix.

[33] Wilfrid Ward, *Wiseman*, I. 372.

[34] Purcell, *Ambrose Phillipps de Lisle*, I. 107.

[35] Allen, 62.

keep her blessed picture with extreme reverence, putting flowers before it, especially on her principal feasts, many recite her little office; a Fellow of Exeter College at Oxford burst into tears when speaking of the Dear Mother of Our Saviour', he wrote to Cardinal Acton.[36] In December 1842, de Lisle felt able to affirm: 'There are now hundreds of young men of our best families determined on becoming Catholick, many of whom only wait to see whether their Church can be at once reunited, and failing that to quit her communion to join that of the one true fold of our Blessed Lord, for which they evidently sigh . . .'[37] Even the more cautious Gentili was impressed, when visiting Oxford with Phillipps de Lisle in 1842, with his reception by the High Church enthusiasts. 'Dr. Gentili wore *his religious habit* all the time,' Phillipps de Lisle recorded excitedly; '*which was much approved of in Oxford*.' These sorts of views were transmitted to Rome by Wiseman and were adopted by Pius IX, who became even more impatient with the English Church for not seeming to respond to the opportunities of mass conversion. With each new reception into the Church, anticipations were heightened. Conversion itself was actually something of a heroic act, in the circumstances of English popular prejudice against Catholicism, leaving many of the converts without livelihood or professional standing—and this, too, added to the sense that a truly momentous change was taking place. When, in December 1842, the Revd. Bernard Smith, formerly a Fellow of Magdalen College, Oxford, was received into the Church, the Bishop of Lincoln was so incensed that he endeavoured to have him imprisoned for deserting his benefice of Leadenham in Lincolnshire.[38] It was Smith who visited Newman at Littlemore in 1845, to determine whether he was ready to take the same step. Not all the conversions were of High Churchmen, nor were all stable. The Revd. Richard Waldo Sibthorp was, according to his biographer, never a Tractarian, nor was he 'wafted utlimately to Rome on the crest of the Tractarian wave'.[39] Converted in 1841, he returned to the

[36] Purcell, *Ambrose Phillipps de Lisle*, I. 237.
[37] Allen, 198.
[38] Wilfrid Ward, *Wiseman*, I. 412.
[39] J. Fowler, *Richard Waldo Sibthorp. A Biography*, London 1880, 56-7.

Church of England in 1843 because of 'mental disquiet',[40] but was again re-converted in 1865. For those Anglican clergy who remained converts, which was most, and who sought to exchange their orders for those of the Catholic priesthood, the Collegio Pio was founded in the English College buildings in Rome, largely through the work of Talbot—himself a convert —in 1852. Louis English became the first Rector. In 1898 it was reorganized under the more familiar name of the Beda.[41]

The exaggerations of prospects made by a few of the Catholic observers of the Oxford Movement, especially since they acquired credence in Rome, fostered internal Catholic divisions in England, and contributed to one of the leading features of English Catholicism in the nineteenth century—the antipathy between converts and 'Old Catholics'. It is a feature which is itself easily exaggerated. Nevertheless, the sense that the traditional Catholic leaders were unduly unresponsive to the waves of conversion contained some substance. 'The English Catholics *as a body* are utterly unprepared and unfit for the great occasion,' Phillipps de Lisle complained in 1841: 'It is impossible to conceive a set of men more stupidly perverse than they in general are—instead of meeting the Catholick movement of our Anglican Brethren with courtesy, charity, or tact, they indulge in the bitterest sneers.'[42] The truth was that many 'Old Catholics' did not regard the Oxford men as sincere: they could not believe that the traditional antipathy of the Protestant Church could so easily be exchanged for genuine Catholicism. Lingard always felt like that, and warned Wiseman against trusting the Oxford divines. The *Orthodox Journal* was suspicious of the converts, and Lucas's *Tablet* was openly hostile. Some, like the Earl of Shrewsbury, and Kenelm Digby—who belonged to an earlier period of conversions—believed the Oxford men actually held others back from reception into the Church by holding out the deceptive promise of a re-Catholicizing of Anglicanism itself. Fr. Joseph Rathbone, the Catholic priest at Cowes, published a pamphlet in 1841 entitled *Are the Puseyites sincere?* and supplied a decidely negative answer. The scorn

[40] Ibid. 75.
[41] Michael E. Williams, *The Venerable English College, Rome*, 139.
[42] Allen, 62-3.

expressed by some of the converts for the educational and cultural capabilities of the 'Old Catholics' exacerbated matters considerably. The *Rambler*, after its foundation in 1848, was critical of the intellectual levels achieved by traditional Catholics, inspiring some very disagreeable controversy. Since the journal was in the hands of converts, it was widely supposed that its tone and conclusions, on this issue, represented their general view. And in some ways it actually did. Lucas used *The Tablet* for a pretty constant vituperation of the Catholic aristocracy—mostly for political reasons, but to some extent because he believed that they were uneducated. 'This appearance of want of education', Bernard Ward once noticed in an aside, 'was emphasized by the prevalent custom among Catholics of not sounding the letter H—a custom which was probably due in the first instance to their foreign education.'[43] The 'Old Catholics', for their part, sometimes regarded the Oxford converts as affected. The reception of the converts, therefore—the most potent symbol of Catholic advance in the nineteenth century—was not without its internal disadvantages. 'When a Catholic meets a Protestant in controversy,' W. G. Ward observed to Jowett in 1858, 'it is like a barbarian meeting a civilized man.'[44]

The euphoric hopes inspired by the Oxford movement were also expressed in the 'Crusade of Prayer', for the conversion of England, started in 1838, as part of a wider European movement of Catholic prayers for the unity of Christendom. Spencer and Phillipps de Lisle were prominent among those sponsoring the prayers for the conversion of England. Some of the English bishops were sceptical—Baines, Briggs, and Griffiths, especially, were fearful of arousing Protestant hostility and also doubtful about the realistic prospects of mass conversions. Baines's hesitancy advanced to actual opposition: he devoted the whole of his 1840 Lenten Pastoral to a series of objections to the thesis that England was about to be converted. He also attacked the converts for introducing new devotional practices, and forbade the clergy from using the prayers for the conversion of England. In prevailing

---

[43] Bernard Ward, *The Sequel to Catholic Emancipation*, I. 5 (fn.).
[44] Wilfrid Ward, *William George Ward and the Catholic Revival*, 75.

circumstances, he contended, such a conversion was 'morally impossible'. Baines expressed himself with characteristic vigour; the main burden of his analysis was accurate enough, however. Rome, attentive to Wiseman, was exceedingly displeased, and an inquiry into the Pastoral was instigated at Propaganda. In March 1840, Baines wrote to Propaganda explaining the force and pervasiveness of anti-Catholic sentiment in England.[45] He was summoned to Rome to give an explanation. His lengthy statement, drawn up when in Rome for Propaganda, and now preserved in its archives, gave detailed reasons for his opposition to the Crusade of Prayer.[46] It was to no avail. In December Cardinal Fransoni's inquiry reported adversely, and after being threatened with deprivation of his Vicariate, Baines submitted. In March 1841, he published a retraction.[47] Many shared his opinions, however. In a lecture of 1850 in a series called 'The spirit and genius of St. Philip', Faber declared that there were 'no signs of the conversion of England'.[48]

Those who saw an imminent expansion of the Church through mass conversions were also those who tended to be attracted to the idea of a Reunion of the Catholic and the Anglican Churches. Even Wiseman was initially quite favourable to it—though he later changed his mind, principally because of a crucial difference of opinion about the nature of the Church itself which opened up between himself and Phillipps de Lisle—the leading contender of Reunion. Phillipps de Lisle believed the Church of England was a 'branch' of the Catholic Church which was in schism; Wiseman, who had always attacked the 'branch' idea anyway, did not regard the Church of England as a Church at all. Phillipps de Lisle was impervious to the problem: 'he regarded himself as a prophet sent as it were by God to proclaim the coming of things invisible to the grosser eye'.[49] In fact the notion was not entirely new: in 1824 Bishop James Doyle, of Kildare and

[45] Propaganda, *Scritture* 9 (1834-41), 773, Baines to the Cardinal Fransoni, 23 March, 1840 [in Italian].
[46] Ibid. 1101 (15 Aug. 1840) [in Italian]. 1086 is a copy of Baines's *Pastoral* (24 Feb. 1840).
[47] Bernard Ward, *Sequel*, I. 217.
[48] Raleigh Addington, *The Idea of the Oratory*, London 1966, 165.
[49] Purcell, *Ambrose Phillipps de Lisle*, I. 349.

Leighlin in Ireland had suggested a scheme for the union of the Protestant and Catholic Churches. But his was, at least within the Catholic leadership, an isolated voice.[50] In 1841 de Lisle told Shrewsbury, 'the leading men in the Anglican Church are determined to reunite their Church to the Holy See'. He gave a detailed assessment, remarkable for its detachment from realities. 'The Archbishop of Canterbury and the Bishop of Oxford approve of the design,' and even those bishops who held back 'see that they cannot much longer resist the movement'. He concluded, 'you may rest assured that the reunion of the Churches is certain'.[51] In 1842 he met Newman in Oxford, and was somehow confirmed in his diagnosis. Newman, he recorded, 'has the intellect of the cherubim', and, like the others of the High Church Party, he believed, was working for 'the Reunion of Xtendom'—not by leaving the Church of England, but by transforming it inwardly to authentic Catholicity.[52] Events did not change Phillipps de Lisle's assessment; but Newman's attitude to Reunion, once he was safely within the Catholic fold, was hostile. Not only were there many 'indirect proofs' of the invalidity of Anglican orders, he wrote to Phillipps de Lisle in 1857, in the course of a correspondence about Reunion, but there were reasons for '*wishing* them invalid'. He wrote 'I mean the ineffable sacrilege offered to our Lord in the Blessed Sacrament, if the Anglican clergy are priests . . . it seems to me impossible that God should allow this almost universal sacrilege for three hundred years.' He recounted how a priest of the Birmingham Oratory, visiting a parish some twenty or thirty miles away, and awaiting his return train, had watched the unconsumed consecrated Communion bread thrown out of the window of a Protestant Church for the birds. 'I recollect how shocked Hurrell Froude was, at the Anglican chapel at Rome, at seeing the consecrated wine put back into the bottle.'[53] In the year of this exchange, however, the Association for the Promotion of the Unity of Christendom (APUC) was founded by Phillipps de Lisle and Pugin on

[50] Fitzpatrick, *The Life, Times and Correspondence of the Right Rev. Dr. Doyle*, I. 320.
[51] Purcell, *Ambrose Phillipps de Lisle*, I. 217.
[52] Ibid. I. 258.   [53] Ibid. I. 371.

the Catholic side, by Bishop Forbes of Brechin, in the Scottish Episcopal Church, and Frederick George Lee, another Anglican.[54] In letters to Barnabò in Rome, seeking approval of the APUC, Phillipps de Lisle displayed his usual disproportionate enthusiasm, claiming two thousand priests and ten bishops of the Anglican church as committed to the scheme. To the doubtless astonished Barnabò he added 'this party of the Anglican Church humbly desires ecclesiastical reunion of the National Church of the whole British Empire with the Holy Catholic Mother, by embracing without any ambiguity all the articles defined in the sacred Council of Trent and the whole orthodox Faith, also the latest definition of the Immaculate Conception.'[55] Barnabò rejected de Lisle's offer of a gold chalice, evidently regarding it as a bribe to secure a favourable opinion on the APUC. Manning and Ward were already denouncing the whole enterprise to Rome, and *The Tablet* was directing lay opinion against it. Catholics, in general, were again unable to imagine that the Anglicans involved were sincere. In September 1864, Cardinal Patrizi, of the Holy Inquisition, addressed the English bishops on the dangers inherent in the APUC, and in November of the following year he instructed the faithful not to join it. Rome's objection was to the principle, implicit in the APUC's view of the Church, that the Catholic, Orthodox, and Anglican bodies were of equal validity. De Lisle and Bishop Moriarty of Kerry—the only Catholic episcopal advocate of the APUC—were then awkwardly placed. An address was sent to Cardinal Patrizi by 198 Anglican clergy, regretting the censure of the APUC. But both this, and Phillipps de Lisle's correspondence with Wiseman,[56] failed to alter the situation. For Manning, who succeeded Wiseman at this time, the question of Reunion was solely a matter of submission to Rome. 'The unity of the Church is absolute and indivisible', he wrote in his Pastoral of 1866; 'the Church has never lost its unity.'[57] Phillipps de Lisle's

---

[54] For an account of the APUC, see Cuthbert Butler, *Ullathorne*, I. 334–468.

[55] Purcell, *Ambrose Phillipps de Lisle*, I. 376 (May 1857).

[56] These letters are preserved in the Vaughan Papers in the Westminster Diocesan Archives, B25 (9 items for the years 1864–5, sent by Wilfrid Ward to Vaughan in 1896).

[57] Purcell, *Life of Cardinal Manning, Archbishop of Westminster*, II. 285.

view was quite the contrary. 'Every day convinces me more and more that God's Design is a fusion of Churches, not a mere picking up of a few men one by one,' he told Bishop Clifford in April of the same year.[58] Nor did he ever lose this vision, despite the hostility of Rome. In 1874 he congratulated Gladstone on his opposition to Disraeli's Public Worship Regulation Act on the grounds that Reunion would only be possible if the Anglican Church could express its Catholic inheritance.[59]

This aspect of Church extension—the plan of Reunion—was resuscitated in 1893 by Lord Halifax and the Abbé Fernand Portal.[60] As President of the English Church Union, the agency of the 'Anglo-Catholic' wing of the Church of England, Halifax persuaded Portal that the differences between the two Churches were merely historical rather than doctrinal or hierocratic. Portal then published *Les Ordinations anglicanes*, a work which acquired immense publicity in France and throughout Europe and which, while not actually endorsing the validity of Anglican orders, was clearly sympathetic to Anglican claims. He put the matter to Rome. But Propaganda had not shifted ground since the controversy over the APUC. Sympathetic lobbying attracted the support of Leo XIII, however, and in 1895 it took the combined energies of Vaughan, Gasquet, and Merry del Val to secure an International Commission of theologians, which reported, in the following year, against the case made out by Halifax and Portal. In July 1896, the cardinals of the Holy Office delivered a unanimous judgement against the validity of Anglican Orders. In September Pope Leo XIII published *Apostolicae Curae*, in which they were declared 'null and void'—a judgement which was 'now and for ever in the future valid and in force.'[61] The second phase of the Reunion question was at an end.[62]

The Irish immigration was the leading feature of Catholic

[58] Bristol Record Office, 35721, Clifford Papers, Phillipps de Lisle to Clifford, 7 April 1866.

[59] Purcell, *Ambrose Phillipps de Lisle*, II. 87.

[60] See chapter 8.

[61] *Apostolicae Curae*, London (CTS), 1967, 24.

[62] For an account of these proceedings, see Snead-Cox, *The Life of Cardinal Vaughan*, II. 141–223.

expansion in the nineteenth century. Indeed, as Denis Gwynn remarked, 'Any statistical study of the Catholic Church in England and Wales during the past century is therefore largely a study of the Irish immigrants and their descendants.'[63] During the Famine years, of the later 1840s, the existing volume of Irish immigration was suddenly increased, and although not all the Irish who arrived were Catholics—for there were quite sizeable groups of Protestants from North-east Ulster in some English cities—most were. It is also important to realize, as Professor Bossy has pointed out, that Catholic growth in England was 'continuous and self-generating', quite independently of the Irish,[64] and that the main features of the changes that occurred in the Church would anyway have happened, if less rapidly and often less decisively.[65] But for all that, the sheer weight of the Irish numbers made the Church, in many urban areas, the Church of the Irish. When Faber opened the Oratory Chapel in London, in 1849, his first problem, as it happened, was the infestation of fleas left by the Irish worshippers—'Brother Chad catches them by handfulls,' Faber wrote: 'The Irish are swamping us; they are rude and unruly and after many complaints the Catholic tradesmen are leaving us.'[66] To the English Catholics the Irish were thus sometimes a practical problem—especially to the ex-Anglicans, with their bourgeois or gentry susceptibilities. In some places, such as Birmingham, informal segregation took place; there the Irish attended St. Chad's Cathedral, and the English Catholics resorted to St. Peter's Church. In South Wales, in the 1850s, the Italian priest Fr. Signini was obliged to compile his own Irish phrase-book in order to hear confessions.[67] As Bishop Brown reported after visiting the Catholic church in Abergavenny in 1873: 'instead of good religious instruction on Sundays, there is only a weekly scolding of the Irish'.[68] Faced with these conditions, and perhaps also reflecting more

[63] Denis Gwynn, 'The Irish Immigration', in Beck, ed., *The English Catholics, 1850–1950*, 282.
[64] Bossy, *The English Catholic Community, 1570–1850*, London 1966, 306.
[65] Ibid. 309.
[66] Chapman, *Father Faber*, 233.
[67] Gwynn, 'The Irish Immigration', in Beck, 268.
[68] Downside Archives, VII.A.3.a, Abbots' Papers (File marked '1871–1880'), Bishop T. J. Brown to the Provincial of the Benedictines, 31 Jan. 1873.

deeply-felt prejudices against the Irish, some English Catholics were soon regretting the enhanced membership of their Church. Phillipps de Lisle was not unique in his distaste for the link of Catholicism and national politics among the Irish, another cause of their poor reputation in England. Of the Famine he wrote, 'God has visited that wretched and untameable race with those chastisements which are inseparably the lot of all Catholick Nations that disgrace the Name of the Church.'[69] When the Irish conveyed their national politics to the English cities, there were additional complications for the clergy. Fenianism was censured by the Church as a secret oath-bound society, and pronouncements about it, especially by Ullathorne in 1868 and 1869, divided the Irish congregations and caused a great deal of internal hostility.[70] The condition of the 'rough' Irish was often, of course, exaggerated, especially by those who had no previous experience of proletarian or peasant mores. The Irish were actually a revitalizing force in many churches, and, despite their poverty, in the first generation, often made financial contributions to support the clergy which must have involved real personal sacrifice. They also elicited evangelistic and philanthropic qualities among the English Catholics that might otherwise have remained undeveloped—and produced, in the process, some of the most impressive spiritual work of the century. In the cities, where half of the Irish settled, 'many', as John Denvir remarked in his contemporary survey of the Irish in Britain, 'sank into a condition of wretchedness it is appalling to contemplate'.[71] 'One may depend upon seeing mainly Celtic faces, if ever one penetrates into a district which is particularly noted for its filth and decay,' Engels observed in 1844: 'The Irish have also brought with them filth and intemperance.'[72]

[69] Allen, 'Letters of Phillipps de Lisle to Montalembert', in the *Dublin Review* 228, no. 463 (1954), 318 (Jan. 1849).

[70] See *Letters of Archbishop Ullathorne*, ed. by the Dominican nuns of Stone Convent, 206.

[71] John Denvir, *The Irish in Britain*, 157. (Denvir was an Irish Catholic journalist from Liverpool who became first editor of the *Catholic Times*. He studied the Irish electorate as Chief Organizer of T. P. O'Connor's United Irish League of Great Britain.) See also J. A. Jackson, *The Irish in Britain*, London, 1963.

[72] Frederick Engels, *The Condition of the Working Class in England* (trans. and ed. W. O. Henderson and W. H. Challoner), Oxford 1958, 105.

There was an early response among the Catholic clergy to the drink problem. 'You will rejoice to hear of the great work going on here among the Irish poor through the Temperance movement,' Frederick Oakeley wrote to Talbot from London in 1861; 'It has been taken up with great speed.'[73] Schools were another means of elevating Irish life. Faber explained in 1852 that the ragged school set up by the London Oratorians was 'because we felt that the one work of those who wish to raise the condition of the Irish Catholics in London was education'.[74] A large part of the Catholic educational programme in the nineteenth century was similarly motivated. Gentili, who accused Wiseman of neglecting the Irish, felt a special mission to the Irish poor. With the flood of immigration during the Famine years, he directed his itinerant missions especially to the Irish. After 1845 he travelled with Father Moses Furlong, a Liverpool Irishman, in the cities of Yorkshire and Lancashire with a special commission from Rosmini. Barberi, too, was much concerned with the immigrants. Nor did they lack the attention of Protestant proselytizers—whose conversions, at least in London (—where their work has been studied by Dr Gilley—) were comparatively few, and were often of men of rather low quality.[75] Clerical philanthropic action among the Irish immigrants, in fact, coupled with the Church's ban on inter-marriage with Protestants, helped to retain a sense of Irish separateness. 'In short', Dr O'Tauthaigh has concluded, 'the Catholic Church was a crucial force inhibiting, indeed actively discouraging, the assimilation of the Irish immigrants in the working class culture of the native majority.'[76]

The actual size of the Irish-born population can be determined from the decennial census returns. At the end of the eighteenth century, for which period there are no accurate figures, the number of Irish in England was evidently insignificant; in 1841, however, just before the Famine influx,

[73] English College, Rome, Talbot Papers, 552, Oakely to Talbot, 24 Jan. 1861.

[74] Raleigh Addington, *Faber, Poet and Priest. Selected Letters, 1833-1863*, London 1974, 242.

[75] Gilley, 'Protestant London, No Popery and the Irish Poor, II (1850-1860)', in *Recusant History*, 11 (1971-2), 32.

[76] M. A. G. O'Tuathaigh, 'The Irish in Nineteenth Century Britain: Problems of Integration', 168.

there were (in the year of the first reliable figures) 284,128 Irish-born, or 1.9 per cent of the total population. The numbers then rose sharply to 1861, when they reached 3.5 per cent of the population, and then declined slowly to 1.7 per cent in 1901. Distribution was unequal—in 1881, for example, when the Irish-born were 1.5 per cent of the overall population, they were actually 12.8 per cent of the population of Liverpool, 7.5 per cent of the population of Manchester, and 3.3 per cent of the population of London.[77] Most came from rural Ireland and were quite unused to city conditions: hence the symptoms of *anomie* and personal dislocation described by Engels. It was the Catholic Church which, in most cases, retained their sense of identity and integrity. As an unskilled labour force they sank at once to the lowest levels of social expectation, and it was the Church, again, which, through its schools and charitable institutions, set many upon the first slow steps in upward social mobility. 'Leakage' from the faith was also largely an Irish phenomenon; but it was on a much less significant scale, proportionately to the numerical strength of the different churches, than lapses by English Protestants from the Protestant denominations.

An important feature of the Catholic advance of the nineteenth century was the revival of monasticism, and it was the foundation of Mount St. Bernard by Phillipps de Lisle, the first Cistercian house to be built in England since the reformation, which indicated the new confidence of the Church in the re-establishment of its traditional institutions. Monasticism, especially, had featured luridly in the popular depictions of the anti-Catholic tradition in England. To Phillipps de Lisle, therefore, as Ullathorne remarked upon his death in 1878, had belonged the honour of 'boldly bringing the Catholic religion into open view, at a time when others had not the courage or generosity of these things'.[78] He had seen monasticism as the means by which the conversion of England could be initiated. Land was purchased in Charnwood Forest in 1835 for presentation to the Cistercians. There was quite a lot of opposition from Catholics themselves to the scheme; some believing it would inflame Protestant prejudices; some

---

[77] Denvir, 386.   [78] *Letters of Archbishop Ullathorne*, 373.

regarding monasticism as (in the circumstances of the progressive new age of the nineteenth century) an inappropriate means of conversion, and preferring mission churches to be built instead; some arguing that schools should be built with the money. 'I am apt to think that a society of brothers of Christian Instruction, with almshouses for the poor old people, would be more *useful* than a regular monkery,' Shrewsbury told de Lisle in 1836.[79] Bishop Walsh 'desired that the monks should on no account appear in public wearing their habits and cowls, and he suggested that the place should not be openly called a Trappist monastery but an "agricultural and philanthropic community"'.[80] Both opinions illustrate the approximation of some English Catholics to the prevailing attitudes of their fellow-countrymen. Purcell's description of the eventual building of the monastery reflected the romantic appeal of monasticism to the gothic taste. As the monks got to work, 'they cleared the ground in a very short time, and soon were enabled to leave their poor cottage with its ruinous roof, through which the snow fell upon them as they lay at night on their bed of straw'.[81] The temporary chapel was opened by Bishop Walsh in 1837, and the main buildings were completed under Pugin's direction in 1844. Crowds of the curious were by then a familiar sight at the monastery. 'All go away edified and delighted', Phillipps de Lisle noted, 'with prejudices diminished if not removed, not only in reference to Monasticism, but the Catholick religion in general.'[82] The foundation was also intended, by Phillipps de Lisle, to take pastoral charge of his Leicestershire villages, but the monks disappointed him, after a short while, by declaring that parochial duties were against Cistercian custom. In 1849, the monastery was placed under the General Chapter of the Cistercian Congregation of Strict Observance in France, and in 1857, after lengthy representations in Rome, this affiliation to the French Order was regularized upon satisfactory terms.[83]

[79] Purcell, *Ambrose Phillipps de Lisle*, I. 69.
[80] Gwynn, *The Second Spring*, 69.
[81] Purcell, *Ambrose Phillipps de Lisle*, I. 75.   [82] Ibid. I. 81.
[83] Propaganda, *Scritture* 14 (1855–7), 1080, Abbot of Mount St. Bernards to the Cardinal Prefect, 29 May 1857 [in English].

The century also saw the expansion and consolidation of the other regular orders of the Church in England. The Jesuits, the strongest order in the first half of the century—operating within the twelve districts into which the Society had divided the country—became even more influential in the second half. The Benedictines were the most numerous of the orders; the Dominicans re-established themselves in 1850 at Woodchester; the Franciscans, also, began again in England in 1850, and in 1873 an English Province was formally established; the Cistercians had returned in 1837 due to the work of Phillipps de Lisle. The growth of the religious orders of women was helped by early nineteenth-century modifications to the rules of enclosure which enabled the nuns to undertake charitable and educational work in the secular missions.[84] The most impressive work here was perhaps done by the Sisters of Charity—whom Manning encouraged—the largest of the orders of women. Most notable among these orders were the Dominican foundations of Mother Margaret Hallahan. Born in London of Irish Catholic parents in 1803, Margaret Hallahan was educated by the Abbé Carron, an *émigré* priest, at his school in Somers Town, and then, following the death of her parents when she was eleven, she entered domestic service. For twenty years she lived with households in London, Margate, and Belgium. It was in Margate that she felt called to the spiritual life; but it was not until she was in Bruges, in 1835, that she became a Dominican Tertiary. In 1842 she returned to England, to Coventry, where she met Ullathorne —who had arrived as missionary priest in the city in the previous year—and became his sacristan.[85] She also set up a school for two hundred girls. In 1845 she took full Dominican vows and founded a Dominican house. The next year, when Ullathorne became Vicar Apostolic of the Western District, Mother Hallahan moved her Dominicans to Bristol with him, and there, at Clifton, began the building of the convent.[86] When Ullathorne left for Birmingham, in 1848, she was left

---

[84] Edward Cruise, 'Development of the Religious Orders', in Beck (ed.), *The English Catholics, 1850–1950*, 443–5.

[85] See chapter 4.

[86] For details of the later development of the convent at Clifton, see Propaganda, *Scritture* 14 (1855–7), 549.

with uncompleted buildings and without her sponsor and friend: in 1852, therefore, she founded a second house at Stone, in Staffordshire, within Ullathorne's new diocese of Birmingham. The convent at Stone was opened in 1853. It was a very impressive record, and Mother Hallahan's life of devoted service to the Catholic revival in England—witnessed not in the centres of Catholic activity, but in the quiet culti-vation of the interior life and of educational works—was one of noted personal sanctity. At her convent in Stone there may still be seen a glass case containing relics of her self-mortification: a hair-shirt, a small cross of spiked nails to be worn next to the body, and other items intended to turn her mind away from earthly comfort. She died agonizingly in 1868: 'all this is a special judgement on me for my sins', she said.[87]

The new orders also made a great impact on the Catholic advance of the nineteenth century—not so much because of the extent of their work (which was not so great as the ordi-nary parochial duties undertaken by the other regulars) but because of the new techniques of evangelization which they pioneered in England, and because they were a sign of the triumph of the Ultramontanist spirit. The Passionists came with Blessed Dominic Barberi in 1842, the Redemptorists in 1843 with two Fathers from Belgium who were settled in Falmouth by Bishop Baines, and the Oratorians in 1847, when Newman founded the Birmingham house. Wiseman turned to the new orders to help in the work of evangelizing the poor in London; he recognized at once the value of their special gift for conducting local evangelistic missions—an innovation which was to be a tremendous stimulus to the Catholic revival. Father Luigi Gentili and Father Dominic Barberi were to become the two greatest and most well-known missioners and retreat-leaders of the century: the former was a Rosminian, the latter a Passionist. The phenomenon ap-peared in the United States at the same time. There, also, European priests were attracted to the challenge of working for Catholic conversions among the poor of the predomi-nantly Protestant cultures. There, too, revivalism conducted

[87] Drane, *Life of Mother Margaret Mary Hallahan*, 521.

by the new orders was based upon missions within the parishes. It was unlike the Protestant revivalism of the period—a more well-known phenomenon—which was not related to formal ecclesiastical structures and was often, indeed, antipathetic to them. In 1832 the Redemptorists arrived in America.[88] In London, Wiseman found on his arrival that there was not a single community of men—'There were two Jesuits *en garçon* in a house; that was all,' he remarked.[89] He introduced the Redemptorists (at Clapham) and the Marists (at Spitalfields), and took a leading part in bringing the Passionists to Aston Hall. There were, however, some disappointments, for Wiseman was soon found complaining that the new orders stuck rather rigidly to their own rules and often declined to undertake regular parochial duties.[90] Phillipps de Lisle experienced a contrary problem. He had brought the Rosminians to his Leicestershire villages to serve the churches which his Cistercians at Mount St. Bernards would not attend to. But Phillipps de Lisle was soon complaining that Gentili, his Rosminian missioner, was so attentive to the villages and their pastoral needs that the chapel at Grace Dieu, his own house, was neglected.[91] The Rosminians came under Fr. Giovanni Battista Pagani, Vice-Provincial in England of the Institute of Charity, and in the early years they undertook educational work at Prior Park in Bath. In 1840 they started a mission at Loughborough instead, and it was to Loughborough that Gentili was sent in 1842, following his differences with Phillipps de Lisle. Of all the new orders, the work of the Brothers of Charity was perhaps the most successful. In July 1846, Pagani reported at length to Propaganda on the extent and nature of their labours in England, and it is quite clear, from the document—now in the archives of Propaganda—that a new enthusiasm for Catholicism was being generated among the people to whom they went as evangelists, preaching missions and conducting retreats. The Church was being carried into the market place for the first time since the repeal

---

[88] Jay P. Dolan, *Catholic Revivalism. The American Experience, 1830–1900*, Notre Dame, 1978, 19.

[89] Wilfrid Ward, *Wiseman*, II. 116.

[90] Ibid. II. 120.

[91] Leetham, *Luigi Gentili*, 142.

of the penal laws. Pagani was especially appreciative of Gentili's missions—to Huddersfield, when Bishop Briggs gave particular support;[92] to York, where 'all attended the meditations with diligence';[93] and to Newcastle, and Sunderland. Another hand has written on the margin of the document 'Soli Deo honor et gloria'; even at Propaganda they were impressed with the work.[94]

The Oratorians were established by Newman in Birmingham in February 1848. The Rule of St. Philip Neri was almost perfectly suited to the Oxford converts, used, as they were, to communal collegiate living. It was the 'common life' that attracted Newman to the Rule.[95] In 1846 he had gone off to Rome with Ambrose St. John and had been given rooms at Propaganda while he sought some means of expressing his new Catholic vocation. Soon he was studying the Oratorian Rule—which 'seemed more adapted than any other for Oxford and Cambridge men'.[96] In a letter to Cardinal Fransoni in which he laid out his plans for introducing the Oratory to England, however, Newman projected an evangelizing role of converting the large industrial towns from the base at Birmingham. In November 1847 a Papal Brief established the English house, with Newman as Superior. It was stated in the document that the Oratory was to concern itself principally with the educated and upper classes. The house itself, Maryvale, opened in February 1848, and almost immediately the original six Fathers were joined by Faber's Wilfridians, of whom there were seventeen. Differences soon developed between Newman and Faber, and with the departure of the latter, to set up the London Oratory in 1849, it became clear that different emphases within Catholicism were expressing themselves: the London Oratory became increasingly associated with Ultramontane ecclesiasticism and with the new devotions. The two houses thereafter diverged, particularly in 1855 as a result of a quarrel, leading to appeals to Rome, as

[92] Propaganda, *Scritture* 11 (1846–7), 89, Gio. Baptiste Pagani to the Cardinal Prefect, 14 July 1846 [in Italian].
[93] Ibid. 92.
[94] Ibid. 94.
[95] Addington, *The Idea of the Oratory*, 125.
[96] Ibid. 107.

to whether it was proper for the Oratorians to hear the confessions of nuns. More substantial divergences resulted over educational work, which came to predominate at Birmingham with the establishment of the Oratory School in 1859. Faber believed too much emphasis on education was a departure from St. Philip's intentions. Newman's educational priorities also became clear—and were resisted—in his plans for an Oratory at Oxford. Despite these differences, it could still be remarked, by the historian of the Order, that 'probably there are no other Oratorian houses in the world which so closely resemble each other' as Birmingham and London.[97] Amongst the other foundations of the new orders in England there should also be special mention of the Salesians, in view of their work for poor children and young people. The Order was begun in Turin by St. John Bosco in 1868. His thoughts had been directed towards England by the vision of Blessed Dominic Savio—a boy who saw 'the English people groping in a fog which was eventually dispelled by the Pope bearing a torch representing the light of Faith'.[98] The English house of the Salesians was started in Battersea in 1887, at the suggestion of St. John Bosco himself.

Of the two most prominent missioners of the new orders in England, Fr. Luigi Gentili was the most well-known at the time of his death in 1848; indeed, he was probably better known than any Catholic except Wiseman or Newman.[99] He was responsible for hundreds of conversions and his example enormously enhanced the morale of the English Catholics— and that despite the reservations of some of the 'Old Catholic' element about the influence of the new orders. Educated in Rome, he entered the legal profession and pursued a talented and markedly secular career until 1829. He then met Antonio Rosmini and soon decided to enter his new order, the Institute of Charity. From the very beginning he seems to have thought of missionary work in England, and the inclinations were encouraged by meetings with Spencer and Phillipps de Lisle in Rome. In 1831 he began training at Domodossala, the headquarters of the Institute, under Rosmini himself, and

---

[97] Addington, *The Idea of the Oratory*, 149.
[98] Cruise, in Beck 460.
[99] Leetham, *Luigi Gentili*, 1.

in 1835 finally arrived in England at the invitation of Bishop Baines, to join the staff of Prior Park. His Italianism was always part of his appeal. He spoke good English, but with a broken accent—this 'foreign touch was an added attraction' for some.[100] Other features of his Italianism were perhaps less alluring. The two French brothers at Prior Park 'complained that when they first came to England Gentili had said it was effeminate to shave more than twice a week.'[101] Together with the other Italian Rosminians at Prior Park—Pagani, Rinolfi, and Signini—he did not even eat English food: the memorial to their years at the College was a field of garlic. Yet he made friends among the English easily enough, and especially close relations grew up with Pugin and Ullathorne. His view of English society, however, was very critical. He wrote back to Italy of the appalling conditions of poverty and the apparent indifference of the gentry. 'People shout at you that they are free', he wrote in 1835, 'but they are slaves to a nobility that wallows in opulence.'[102] He was personally ascetic, eating little, drinking no alcohol, and staying awake for hours at night in prayer. Prayer was the centre of his action for evangelization. 'This is the first step we must take,' he told Spencer in 1836, when considering the conversion of England—'sanctify ourselves.'[103] Hence, also, his promotion of the new devotions, and the use, which he encouraged, of scapulars, holy medals, public processions, Benediction, weekly communion, the Forty Hours Devotion, Missions, and retreats—all things which externalized and witnessed to inner conversion and personal religious discipline. His first retreat in England was for the boys and staff of Prior Park, in Passion Week, 1836. It was based on the model of St. Ignatius of Loyola and conducted in conditions of drama and anticipation; 'the windows of the Chapel were darkened' and Gentili 'really let himself go'.[104] The result was a series of complaints from the boys' parents. His influence was gradually curtailed; the exuberance of the Italianate spirit of

---

[100] James McHugh, *Father Gentili, Priest and Missionary*, Dublin 1958, 65.
[101] Leetham, *Luigi Gentili*, 71.
[102] Ibid. 62.
[103] Ibid. 69.
[104] Ibid. 70.

triumphalism had to be introduced more circumspectly. Half the boys in the school were withdrawn, and in 1837 Baines felt obliged to get rid of Gentili himself. He became confessor to the Augustinian nuns at Spettisbury. The first phase of his work in England was at an end. This disappointing start proved merely the preparation for Gentili's greatest and enduring work however. For after an interlude at Grace Dieu, and in the Leicestershire villages, acting as chaplain to Phillipps de Lisle—where in 1842 it was estimated he made a thousand conversions—and at Loughborough, in the new Rosminian house, Gentili began his remarkable and final career as an itinerant missioner. He directed his preaching to the working-class poor of the industrial cities. The Leicestershire work had well prepared him for this. There he had combined Italian-style emotional preaching with the mass-meeting techniques of the Methodist tradition; many Dissenters were among his converts in consequence of the resulting popular appeal. During the course of his provincial missions, after 1844, he made over three thousand conversions, and in 1846 was released from all other work by Rosmini in order to become a full-time evangelist with Father Moses Furlong. His refusal to charge fees for baptisms, his opposition to pew-rents, and his disregard of the convention that required the poor to dress in good clothes to go to Church, added to his popular appeal. In his last four years of life, he preached 51 missions, gave 15 clergy retreats and 21 retreats for the religious, and delivered an enormous number of sermons.[105] His was the first popular preaching of Catholicism to the English masses, and elicited extraordinary scenes of religious enthusiasm, with crowded churches and confessionals.[106] Some of the more traditionalist Catholics were shocked by the Italian excesses. At York, in November 1845, there were shouts of 'blasphemy!' from some Catholics when Gentili spoke of the honours due to the Virgin.[107] The London mission, in May 1846, was unlike the provincial ones; there was a more restrained atmosphere and

---

[105] Claude Leetham, 'Gentili's Reports to Rome', in *The Wiseman Review*, 498 (Winter, 1963-4), 395.

[106] Denis Gwynn, *Father Luigi Gentili and his mission (1801-1848)*, 204-6.

[107] Leetham, *Luigi Gentili*, 237.

fewer conversions. The provincial successes were repeated in Ireland, however, in 1846, during two different missionary tours. So greatly did Rome come to value his knowledge of religious conditions in England, derived from these travels and labours, and confirmed by Pagani's Reports to Propaganda in 1846,[108] that Gentili was in 1847 commissioned by Cardinal Fransoni to write a series of statements about the English Catholic Church. He compiled five lengthy reports which, though critical of the English clergy and of the leadership of the Church,[109] were in no sense an attempt to intrigue against the Vicars Apostolic, as some supposed at the time.[110] Even his friend Ullathorne seems to have regarded the Reports as 'first crude impressions', and observed—'Accustomed to the impulsive and demonstrative style of his Italian countrymen, he did not for a long time comprehend the quiet energy and unobtrusive plodding character of Englishmen.'[111] Worn out by his travel and his constant work of conversion, Gentili died of fever on a visit to Dublin in September 1848. His tomb, at Omeath in Co. Louth, where his coffin is exposed for veneration, continues to attract crowds of faithful, who cover it with intercession papers and flowers.[112]

Blessed Dominic Barberi,[113] the other great missioner of the new orders, was the man who received Newman into the Church in 1845. Newman, indeed, said of him—'His very look had about it something holy.'[114] Barberi was born near Viterbo in 1792. Lacking any formal education, he worked as a shepherd on his uncle's farm until in 1814 he was entered as a novice Passionist at Santa Maria di Pugliano. He was then aged twenty-two, and already had mystical experiences—one of which suggested work in England, to help in restoring the English people to Catholic unity. Between 1829 and 1831 he was teaching in Rome, and was then for a time Rector of the new Passionist house at Lucca. In 1840 he went to work in

---

[108] Propaganda, *Scritture* 11 (1846–7), 87.
[109] See chapter 2.
[110] Leetham, 'Gentili's Reports to Rome', 396–7.
[111] Ullathorne, *History of the Restoration of the Catholic Hierarchy in England*, 22.
[112] MacHugh, 9.
[113] Beatified in 1963. He does not seem to have yet been raised to sainthood.
[114] Denis Gwynn, *Father Dominic Barberi*, London 1947, 211.

Belgium for the Order, and then, finally, in 1841, he arrived in England. During the next eight years, until his death, he worked as a missioner from the Passionist houses at Aston Hall and Stone in Staffordshire. As Gentili had discovered, there was some opposition from the Protestant clergy to 'the stuttering Papist'; stones were thrown at him in the streets.[115] 'My hope is', he wrote, 'that the little building at Stone will be the grain of mustard seed which, blessed by God, will become a great tree.'[116] There were in fact over fifty conversions a year at Stone, and during the 1840s he gave numerous missions and retreats in the Midland counties of England. 'The real obstacles to be overcome', he correctly observed of the religious condition of the English people, 'are the extreme ignorance and even indifference to their salvation which they display.'[117] His own contribution to the evangelization of England was both noble and effective. But he died unexpectedly in 1849, at the Railway Hotel in Reading. When his coffin was opened nearly forty years later, in 1886, his body was found to be incorrupt.

The work of the new orders for the extension of Catholicism in England also helped the spread of the new devotional practices, much favoured by the Ultramontanist clergy, by Wiseman, and by many of the converts who had been trained for their Catholic vocations in Rome. The devotions and new styles of public worship were the external sign of the triumphant emergence of Catholicism from the confinement of the penal years. Both Gentili and Barberi encouraged the veneration of the Virgin, and preached the doctrine of the Immaculate Conception—which was not formally declared to be part of the dogmatic teaching of the Church until 1854. Amongst many Catholic leaders there was also an attempt to reform Church music. Phillipps de Lisle published liturgical books; the *Little Gradual* in 1847, the *Supplementum ad Graduale* in 1862, and in 1868 an edition of nine Gregorian masses. Like Pugin, he did much to foster the revival of plainsong in Church use. 'At the present day in our English Catholic Chapels and Churches', he wrote, 'the antient Church

[115] Ibid. 150.
[116] Gwynn, *Father Dominic Barberi*, 168.
[117] Young, *Dominic Barberi in England*, 75 (May 1842).

musick has been almost totally abandoned, and instead of it has been substituted a light and indecorous style of singing far more calculated to express the feelings of earthly passion than the grave and solemn effusions of true Christian devotion.'[118] Faber thought similarly, though he had no illusions about the superiority, as some imagined it, of continental Catholic music in church. From Belgium in 1839 he reported: 'Here the organ is drowned with innumerable fiddles, there is a leader of the band in a box as at the opera, and instead of the boys in white a row of meretricious looking females, talking, nodding and looking about in the intervals.'[119] It was like Pugin's *Contrasts* in reverse; the Protestant choirs of Faber's Anglicanism were much to be preferred to Catholic singing. Faber's Italianate style as a Catholic, however, contrasted with Phillipps de Lisle's gothicism. The London Oratory became the chief English centre of 'Italian' worship—dividing the London Catholics into its adherents and those of 'Old Catholic' religious taste who were known, after Challoner's great work of 1740, as 'Garden of the Soul Catholics'. At times opposition to the new devotional and liturgical practices—symbolized in the conflict over the use of Gothic or Roman vestments—became extremely divisive; when Pugin heard of the votive candles burned before an image of the Virgin in the Chapel of the Oratory he said: 'What a degradation for religion! Why, it is worse than the Socialists.'[120] Similar shocked opinion was elicited by the publication of the series of works entitled *Lives of the Modern Saints*— translations of Italian and Spanish originals. They were full of ecclesiastical miracles and Latin folk belief in the supernatural gifts of the saints, and more or less exactly corresponded to the spiritual outlook of Faber—who was largely responsible for the series. After heated criticism of the *Life* of St. Gertrude, and the widespread opposition to the publication of the *Life* of St. Rose of Lima, the series, which had the initial support of both Walsh and Wiseman—as well as of Newman—was briefly suspended. The volumes, as Faber acknowledged, were 'meeting with dreadful opposition,

[118] Purcell, *Ambrose Phillipps de Lisle*, II. 189.
[119] Chapman, 41.
[120] Ibid. 230.

especially from Catholics'.[121] Walsh was obliged to object even
to some parts of the *Life* of St. Philip Neri 'because some old
Catholic priests found it too popish', as Faber complained.[122]
From a broader perspective, however, it may be seen that the
new devotions, the popularization in England of continental
uses, came to furnish a common spiritual culture 'accessible
and acceptable to many Old Catholics and ex-Anglicans, as
well as to the Irish proletariat—and transcending differences
of class'.[123] It was one of the weaknesses of Anglicanism in
the nineteenth century that its public worship contrived no
such bridge between the social sections.

It is in fact possible to regard Faber as 'the guiding spirit of
Victorian popular Catholicism'.[124] Frederick William Faber
was born in 1814, of a prosperous Yorkshire family; his
father, an Anglican clergyman, had been Secretary to Shute
Barrington, Bishop of Durham. Educated in the Lake District,
where his lonely wanderings inspired a permanent romanticism, he went on to Shrewsbury School in 1825, and to Harrow
in 1827. As a 'born mystic'[125] his life in neither institution
can have been entirely satisfactory. He was an Evangelical. In
1833 he went up to Balliol, heard Newman's sermons in the
University Church, and was attracted as so many other young
men were. In 1836 he became a Fellow of University College,
Oxford, but was never really successful as a don, and in 1843
he accepted the College living of Elton in Huntingdonshire.
He had been ordained a priest of the Church of England in
1839. The day after his induction at Elton, however, he departed to Italy, with introductions supplied by Wiseman to
Acton and Grant, regarding the journey as something of a religious pilgrimage. The mysterious seeds of his future Catholic
life were already germinating in his soul. He visited the Chiesa
Nuova in Rome, and was deeply moved by the shrine of St.
Philip Neri's bed, preserved in a glass case. He fell avidly upon
the works about the lives of Italian saints of the Counter-
Reformation. In a private audience, arranged by Cardinal

[121] Ibid. 191. See also Bernard Ward, *Sequel*, II. 243.
[122] Chapman, 191.
[123] Sheridan Gilley, 'Vulgar Piety and the Brompton Oratory, 1850–1860', 15.
[124] Ibid. 16.
[125] Chapman, 9.

Acton, the Pope told him not to wait for the Anglican Church to move, but to regard the salvation of his own soul. Back in Elton his inner transformation was disclosed in the conversion of his household into a kind of monastic community. As a bachelor, Faber was surrounded by menservants, and village boys, and these now began spiritual exercises together, and listened to readings from the Italian saints. The Protestant Parish Church 'began to look something like a Catholic Church'.[126] Then, following Newman's secession in 1845, Faber was received into the Catholic faith, together with six boys and one woman of his parish. He moved to Birmingham with the boys, intending to start a proper monastery near St. Chad's Cathedral. A further visit was made to Rome, to seek advice as to procedure; he returned with enormous numbers of devotional books, medals, statues, and rosaries. His little community, in 1846, now numbered twelve. Later that year they moved to Cotton Hall at Cheadle and formally established the Community of St. Wilfrid. Faber, who began to suffer from Bright's disease at almost this time, was ordained by Wiseman at Oscott in 1847. In 1848 the Wilfridians moved into Newman's house at Maryvale and joined the Oratorians. 'You should consider us as giving ourselves over to you in the spirit of surrender', he told Newman at the time.[127] But there were, of course, difficulties. Faber's rather dramatic personality and Newman's oversensitivity did not promise well for a single community, and in 1849 Faber set up the London Oratory in a converted liquor shop in King William Street. The six priests, two novices, and three lay brothers who went with him were looked after, as Faber said, by 'floods of devout Irish charwomen'.[128] In 1852 a site was purchased at Brompton for new buildings and, despite obstruction by the local Anglican clergy, the splendid Church was completed, and the first mass offered at Brompton, in 1854. But Faber, increasingly ill, spent much of his time at Sydenham, where the Oratory had built a country house in 1852.

Faber was known in his day as a writer of popular devotional works, and of hymns (the first book was published

[126] Ibid. 96.
[127] Raleigh Addington, *Faber, Poet and Priest*, 165 (Jan. 1848).
[128] Chapman, 220.

in 1849) which are still among the most loved among English congregations, both Catholic and Protestant. There was a strong current of emotion and sentimentality in Faber which is not to modern taste; but as an influence for the self-confidence and advance of Catholic practice in the difficult conditions of Victorian England, Faber's writings were of quite outstanding importance. Some Catholics were surprised by the simplicity of his own veneration of the saints; of his reference to the Virgin as 'mamma'. His was an exaggerated piety, full of all the sharp light of the Italian originals. But it was inspiring. Some found his love of Mary too great. In *All For Jesus* (1853), his most popular book, he wrote that it was impossible 'to have enough devotion to her'.[129] 'The Son has transferred to the Mother what is His', he added; 'She is more than all creation beside, more worthy, more beautiful, more mighty, more loved of God.'[130] This book was intended to help Catholics to sanctify themselves in ordinary vocations, in their daily lives. By 1869 it had sold 100,000 copies, and was one of the acknowledged spiritual classics of the century. 'It sounds like a trumpet and penetrates like a fire', Ullathorne remarked on its publication.[131] To the later judgement of others it has seemed that Faber had 'a perhaps slightly un-original literary talent'.[132] In 1854 he was awarded a Doctorate of Divinity by Pius IX. By then his health was in sad and advancing decline, and his later extended years were full of pain. He died in 1863; his last words exhorted the clergy to spread devotions to the Immaculate Conception. 'No one could hear him speak of the love and service of God without being attracted to it,' Manning wrote in his final tribute.[133]

The great nineteenth-century expansion of the Church provided the occasion for the differences between the Ultramontane and the 'English' Catholics to be expressed in an extensive controversy over Church buildings, furnishings, and liturgical practices. The disputes acquired particular point

[129] Frederick William Faber, *All For Jesus: or, The Easy Ways of Divine Love*, London (4th edn.), 1854, 152.
[130] Ibid. 342.
[131] Raleigh Addington, *Faber, Poet and Priest*, 251.
[132] Mathew, 204.
[133] Manning, *Miscellanies*, 'Father Faber' (Jan. 1864).

and urgency because the sudden increase in church building required numerous local decisions about architectural style, and the Ultramontanes' preference for 'Roman' or 'Italian' buildings came into a series of direct collisions with the 'English' Catholics' insistence on Gothic. The matter was at once raised to ideological dimensions: opponents of the Gothic style regarded it as symptomizing a sort of Gallicanism, an emphasis on the national character of the Church in England—'the emblem and advocate of a past ceremonial and extinct nationalism', as the *Rambler* put it.[134] The new Italianate style of worship and ecclesiastical ceremonial and clerical dress, legitimized though not actually first introduced by Wiseman, needed—so the Ultramontanes contended— 'Roman' buildings. In contrast to the Gothic models coming into vogue, they promoted the *Instructions for Ecclesiastical Fabrics and Furniture* of St. Charles Borromeo. The revival of Gothic itself was not the work of Catholics, of course—at least in England. In the eighteenth century, when few churches had anyway been constructed, the Gothic style was in general considered as amusing and sometimes engagingly eccentric: the fancy of rich men who built follies on their property. As an ecclesiastical style, Gothic was safe as an antiquated survival, but decidedly 'Popish'; such churches as were built were usually Classical. Of the 214 churches constructed under the terms of the Commission set up by Parliament in 1818—for the worship of the State Church[135]—174 were Gothic.[136] It has often been contended that Gothic churches were built because they were cheaper than classical ones.[137] Had that actually been the case, it would have provided material rather than ideological reasons for the Catholics, who were extremely poor, to have opted for the Gothic style. But the matter is certainly not clear. Enormous numbers of Dissenting chapels were built in the first years of the century in the Classical style—in Welsh valleys and less fashionable parts of

---

[134] *Rambler*, New Series, I (May 1859), 'The Development of Gothic Architecture'. 78.
[135] Norman, *Church and Society in England, 1770-1970*, 53-4.
[136] Kenneth Clark, *The Gothic Revival*, London, 1975 edn., 95.
[137] Basil F. L. Clarke, *Church Builders of the Nineteenth Century. A Study of the Gothic Revival in England*, London, 1969 edn., 30.

large English cities—and the wealth available to local groups of Dissenters cannot have been great, even if the large Dissenting entrepreneurs were able to make better provision in the major centres. When Pugin was called in to design the new chapel at Ushaw in 1840, both sides in the resulting controversy between Gothic and Classical styles claimed that theirs was the less expensive to build.[138] Early Catholic support for the Gothic revival appears to have followed the existing trend, and in response to the 'general intellectual and cultural stimulus'[139] which the revival supplied in England. Bishop John Milner, who built a Gothic Catholic Chapel in Winchester (1792) was an 'important figure in the Gothic Revival'. His chapel, according to Lord Clark, 'is usually considered the first instance of Gothic applied to ecclesiastical architecture during the Revival, and which is certainly the first chapel built in that style from what we may call Gothic Revival motives'.[140] Like Pugin later, Milner believed that a link existed between the Gothic style and true principles of Catholic doctrine. Yet Milner, unlike Pugin, was more sympathetic to Roman than to 'Old Catholic' views of the Church. The redivision of ideological identification, which left the Gothic style as the symbol of the anti-Ultramontanes, awaited the arrival of Wiseman and some of the converts. An important step, however, was made by Kenelm Digby, friend of Ambrose Phillipps de Lisle, and one of the luminaries of 'Gothic' literature. Digby was Irish, born in 1797, of a Protestant Ascendancy family. As a child he was influenced by the poetry of Sir Walter Scott and developed a passion for the middle ages—for chivalry. In 1815 he went to Trinity College, Cambridge, and in 1825 became a Catholic. His *Broad Stone of Honour*, first published in 1822, was enlarged and in part rewritten in order to show that the virtues of chivalry and the Catholic faith were interrelated, and that chivalry had declined as a consequence of the Protestant Reformation. The book went through a number of editions and was both widely read and extremely influential in cultivating

---

[138] Milburn, *A History of Ushaw College*, 177.

[139] David Watkin, *The Triumph of the Classical. Cambridge Architecture, 1804–1834*, Cambridge 1977, 2.

[140] Clark, 101–2.

nineteenth-century ideals of virtue.[141] Digby's medievalism was inherently English and national in tone; it went well with the Englishness of Catholicism as understood by so many of those who began to turn to the Gothic style in building as a physical embodiment of their hostility to Ultramontanism.

The Gothic Revival within English Catholicism was also expressed in the manner of worship. Just as the Church was emerging from its quiet, undemonstrative, 'Garden of the Soul' worship, the new influences divided the Catholics: some developed 'Gothic', and some 'Roman' liturgical practices and dress. Gregorian Chant—first introduced, together with a surpliced choir, at Grace Dieu by Phillipps de Lisle—became the devotional badge of the 'English' Catholics. 'Till the old Gregorian music is restored, nothing can be done', Pugin said;[142] he once observed to Phillipps de Lisle 'A man may be judged by his feelings on Plain Chaunt.'[143] The Ultramontanes were equally persuaded that the new Roman devotions and the rather dramatic musical styles which went with them were important for bringing the English Church closer to the centre of unity, to the practices of the Roman churches. The first rupture between the two attitudes actually took place over the matter of vestments. Should the clergy use the Roman chasuble and appurtenances at Mass, or the revived Gothic vestments? In 1839 Propaganda—at the insistence of the English Jesuits or of Bishop Baines (as Phillipps de Lisle at once supposed[144]) —issued a formal instruction to Bishop Walsh that Gothic vestments were not to be used. The question was ideological, not practical or aesthetic, on both sides. 'I regard the censure as a death-blow to the Catholic cause in England', Phillipps de Lisle wrote to Shrewsbury, 'all the rights and privileges of a National Church are to be stamped out for ever.' He added that Propaganda showed more respect to 'Ethiopian Negroes'.[145] Pugin said the ban was 'the result of some diabolical falsehoods and misrepresentations made at

[141] Mark Girouard, *The Return to Camelot. Chivalry and the English Gentleman*, London 1981, 56.

[142] Denis Gwynn, *Lord Shrewsbury, Pugin, and the Catholic Revival*, London 1946, 75.   [143] Trappes-Lomax, *Pugin. A Mediaeval Victorian*, 221.

[144] Gwynn, *Lord Shrewsbury*, 71.

[145] Purcell, *Ambrose Phillipps de Lisle*, II. 219.

Rome by our adversaries.'[146] Propaganda had in fact made very careful enquiries, asking the Vicars Apostolic to send them detailed and illustrated information about liturgical dress in England. The replies still exist in the Archives of Propaganda, spaced over the following year. Walsh himself included (rather good) pen drawings of both types of vestments, Roman and Gothic, together with their accessories.[147] Baines sent a (not so good) coloured drawing of a priest in a Gothic chasuble.[148]

It is important to realize that, like Pugin, Wiseman, as leader of the Ultramontanes, saw a close connection between good art and sound Catholic faith. He, too, believed that art was the evidence of the moral condition of men and the external revelation of the truth or falsehood of ideals. Pugin did not divide the Catholic body because of the nature of his personal exclusivity, therefore: exclusivity existed on both sides and was inspired by a very similar vision. Wiseman looked for 'the foundation of a religious school of design and art in England'.[149] This could only come about, however, 'by the formation of a school of religious artists',[150] whose work would be 'the fruit of their constant conversation with things spiritual and holy'.[151] He later added: 'what is called the Pre-Raphaelite school has arisen, and made progress, which may one day, under religious influences, which it clearly wants, become the germ of a truly Christian school of art'.[152] The reservation is important. The religious symbolism in the art and design of the Pre-Raphaelites reflected an idealized medievalism which was inherently Catholic and religious, but the Pre-Raphaelite artists themselves were not—at least in any conventional sense. Rossetti 'entered no church except to see the treasure in it', and 'seemed to believe in no orthodox God'.[153] Morris 'found the vital secret of Gothic not in

[146] Gwynn, *Lord Shrewsbury*, 71.

[147] Propaganda, *Scritture* 9 (1834–41), 762, Walsh to Propaganda, 21 Nov. 1839 [in French].

[148] Ibid., Baines to Propaganda, 11 Oct. 1840 [in Italian].

[149] *Essays on Various Subjects by His Eminence Cardinal Wiseman*, III, 356, 'Christian Art' (from *Dublin Review*, June 1847).

[150] Ibid. III, 369.   [151] Ibid. III, 370.

[152] Ibid. III, 380 fn.

[153] Frances Winwar, *The Rossettis and their Circle*, London 1934, 187.

Christianity but in Socialism'.[154] Holman Hunt, the most overtly religious painter of the school, employed Biblical rather than ecclesiological symbolism in his iconography: he was a thoroughly and obviously Protestant painter.

In 1859 the *Rambler* observed 'The Gothic movement has progressed beyond the limit at which its first authors wished it to stay.'[155] The man largely responsible for that was Pugin. His father, a noted architectural draughtsman, was an immigrant from Freiburg im Breisgau, a lapsed Catholic. Augustus Welby Pugin, born in London, in 1812, was brought up as an Anglican and sent to Christ's Hospital. Even as a boy he had absorbed a 'Gothic' atmosphere: 'tales of chivalry and romance delighted him',[156] and in 1826 he began to make a particular study of castles. In 1830 he set up in the same profession as his father and, after a faltering start, ending in a business failure, he established a successful practice near Salisbury. His conversion, in 1834, was without evident external influence—he had never even met a Catholic priest. Some supposed that his attraction to Catholicism was to be attributed to his 'admiration of architectural excellence', but Pugin himself denied it; he was converted, he said, ' by the most powerful reasons, and that after long and earnest examinations'.[157] It was a remarkable conversion, likely to affect his professional life adversely. The Oxford movement conversions were still a decade away and it was, in 1834, still regarded as a sign of some peculiarity in a man that he should find attraction to the Catholic Church. Pugin was, indeed, eccentric in many ways, especially in his almost manic application to work. But the exaggerated peculiarities of his last years were not typical of his whole, and short, life. In his forty years, he married three times. The result of his astonishing labour was enormous: numerous churches, the rebuilding of Oscott, St. Chad's Cathedral in Birmingham, the co-operation with Sir Charles Barry in the new Palace of Westminster, work at Alton Towers for the Earl of Shrewsbury and at Grace Dieu for Phillipps de Lisle. From 1837 to 1839 he also

---

[154] William Gaunt, *The Pre-Raphaelite Tragedy*, London, 1975 edn., 173.
[155] *Rambler*, New Series, I (May 1859), 78.
[156] Benjamin Ferrey, *Recollections of A. N. Welby Pugin*, London 1861, 35.
[157] Ibid. 104–5.

lectured at Oscott, as Professor of Ecclesiastical Art and Antiquities. In 1841 he started to build 'The Grange' at Ramsgate, and lived there for the remainder of his life, enjoying his love of the sea and also being able to live near his aunt. Next to the house he began to build St. Augustine's Church, at his own expense. It was intended as a little masterpiece of his style and is, indeed, a gem of the Gothic revival. Begun in 1846, the Church was unfinished at his death, six years later, and still does not, to this day, have the steeple which he originally intended as a welcoming sign to ships at sea as they neared the harbour of Ramsgate. It was in this church that he was buried, in 1852, after a last terrible year clouded by insanity. The marble effigy upon the alcove tomb was 'wrapped in a mantle of medieval shape'.[158] His achievements had been quite extraordinary. He had set the Gothic Revival upon a new course; he had covered the land with actual examples of his architectural dogmas; he had given Catholicism itself a new respectability through the prominence of his ideas in an important area of cultural life. Nor was he without public recognition in the non-Catholic world. In 1851 he was appointed by the Crown as a Commissioner of Fine Arts for the Great Exhibition, and on his death, in the following year, the Queen ordered that his surviving wife should receive a pension from the Civil List.

Pugin's life was also full of controversy, especially within Catholic society itself. His attachment of the case for the Gothic style to fundamental assertions about the nature of Catholicism widened and solidified the existing division between the 'Roman' party and the 'English' Catholics, until they were, as Bernard Ward remarked, 'deeply and even bitterly opposed to one another on questions of far deeper moment than that of mere taste in ecclesiastical ornament'.[159] 'He has the great fault of a man of genius, as well as the merit', Newman wrote in 1848; 'he is intolerant, and, if I might use a stronger word, a bigot.' This was only too true: 'The canons of Gothic architecture are to him points of faith, and every one is a heretic who would venture to question

---

[158] *A Short Guide to St. Augstine's Abbey Church, Ramsgate*, Ramsgate, 1968, 11.
[159] Bernard Ward, *Sequel*, I. 82.

them.'[160] Pugin himself denied that he was 'a fanatic for pointed design,'[161] but he was self-deceived. His execrations of classical and Italianate styles were very forthright. Both the Birmingham and the London Oratories had been built in the neo-classical style, (something to be expected of Faber, but which interestingly indicates one of the 'Roman' characteristics of Newman). To Pugin both churches were dreadful, especially the London Oratory, which was anyway well known for its Italian devotional practices. Pugin said the church was 'quite lamentable'; it was 'fitted up in a horrible manner'.[162] According to Faber, the Oratory was actually 'cursed' by Phillipps de Lisle.[163] In 1847 Pugin visited Italy and was appalled at the ecclesiastical structures of Rome: 'St. Peter's is far more ugly than I expected, and vilely constructed—a mass of imposition—bad taste of every kind seems to have run riot.'[164] He thought the Sistine Chapel 'a melancholy room, the Last Judgment is a painfully muscular dilineation of a glorious subject.'[165] Most notoriously of all, Pugin's dogmatism about the requirements of the Gothic style was expressed in his insistence on rood-screens. To the Ultramontanes, the revival of chancel screens was an unnecessary antiquarianism; worse, it symptomized a rejection of the Roman rites whose performance should be readily visible to the people. Hence Wiseman's opposition in 1840 to the rood-screen for St. Chad's Cathedral in Birmingham—opposition which had itself to be withdrawn because of Pugin's 'explosion of wrath'.[166] In his last book, *A Treatise on Chancel Screens and Rood Lofts* (1851), Pugin turned the scorn he had largely reserved for Protestants—at least in print—against the Romanizing opponents of his taste. There is a story of how Pugin was one day showing some Protestant friends the rood-screen in a church he had designed: he explained that inside the screen

---

[160] Ibid. II. 206 (5 June 1848). See also J. Patrick, 'Newman, Pugin and Gothic', in *Victorian Studies* (Winter, 1981).

[161] A. Welby Pugin, *An Apology for the Revival of Christian Architecture*, London 1843, 5.

[162] Trappes-Lomax, 224.

[163] Gwynn, *Lord Shrewsbury*, 121.

[164] Ferrey, 225.

[165] Ibid. 226.

[166] Gwynn, *The Second Spring*, 133.

was 'the holy of holies', adding 'never is the sanctuary entered by any save those in sacred orders'. At that moment Bishop Wiseman appeared in the sanctuary accompanied by two ladies, whom he was also showing round the church. Pugin is said to have retired in tears.[167]

His essential position was a simple one. It was that good architecture and design result from sound faith and morals, and conversely, that wrong interior beliefs produce corrupt styles. The middle ages, the age of true Catholic faith, inspired Gothic: Gothic was the only authentic 'Christian' art. As Pugin observed in *Contrasts*, his most famous book— though a book which made a financial loss on its publication in 1836, it made Pugin's reputation—'from Christianity has arisen an architecture so glorious, so sublime, so perfect, that all the productions of ancient paganism sink, when compared before it, to a level with the false and corrupt systems from which they originated'.[168] In his *Apology for the Revival of Christian Architecture* (1843), Pugin declared, 'We must turn to the principles from which all styles have originated', in order to assess their merit. Classical buildings, he argued, were 'perfect expressions of imperfect systems'. He added: 'but I claim for Christian art a merit and perfection, which it is impossible to attain even in the Mosaic dispensation, much less in the errors of polytheism'.[169] But around him, in the actual buildings of the English Catholics of his day, he saw debased neo-classicism and the performance of 'theatrical' liturgy. 'Everything in modern chapels is bad—vestments, music, altars', he declared (in 1839).[170] The Catholic clergy 'apparently reject tradition and authority', so that 'men of devout minds are scandalized with the foreign trumpery that is introduced on the most solemn occasions'.[171] As he remarked in *Contrasts*, 'Before true taste and Christian feelings can be revived, all the present and popular ideas on the subject must be utterly changed.'[172] This attempt at re-education,

---

[167] Trappes-Lomax, 222. The story is sometimes told of St. Barnabas, Nottingham, sometimes of St. Chad's Birmingham—see Fothergill, *Nicholas Wiseman*, 136.

[168] A. W. N. Pugin, *Contrasts*, London 1836, 2.

[169] Pugin, *An Apology*, 4–5.

[170] Gwynn, *The Second Spring*, 90.

[171] Pugin, *An Apology*, 24.

[172] Pugin, *Contrasts*, 16.

however, simply precipitated differences with the Ultramontanes. It was a sad irony, for Pugin's point of view, that his
ideas were more readily taken up by Protestantism—which he
called 'a sort of disease or fungus'[173]—than they were within
the Catholic body. In large parts of the north of England 'Old
Catholics' preferred the neo-classical style to the Gothic. The
Camden Society, founded in 1839 by John Mason Neale and
Benjamin Webb (and which, within a few years, had the
patronage of two Anglican archbishops and sixteen bishops),
promoted the interests of Gothic taste and 'ecclesiology'—
the word was actually coined by the Society—more effectively within the Anglican Church than Pugin had managed
within the Catholic. His was, nevertheless, a very impressive
achievement. His stamp upon a central aspect of the English
Catholicism of the nineteenth century has surely proved
indelible.

[173] A. Welby Pugin, *Church and State; or Christian Liberty. An Earnest
Address on the Establishment of the Hierarchy*, London [1850], 1875, 7.

6

Cardinal Manning: Ultramontanist Confidence

'The public school-life of Harrow in which all are equal and dukes are fags', Manning recalled in an autobiographical note of 1880, 'is a great leveller, not in a bad sense, but in teaching human equality and the inequality of merit rather than rank'.[1] He was seeking the origin of one of his most well-known convictions: that the needs of working people should be the priority of political life. But this early recollection was actually an unusual exercise for Manning, for he regarded his life as marked—as Christian lives often are marked—by discontinuities. Reading his own letters, written when he was still a member of the Church of England, in a reflective moment during 1887, he recalled that it was 'like returning to an extinct world'.[2] The barriers he set up across the road he travelled, to divide off each segment of the past, were the feature of his existence which most impressed his own judgement of events. The first barrier, and in the end the most momentous for his future life, was the death of his wife in 1837: her memory was sealed away so completely 'that on his death, Catholics with one or two exceptions, as well as the general public, knew nothing about his married life'.[3] Many years later, when he was a Cardinal, Manning received a letter from the churchwardens at Lavington about the decayed state of his wife's grave; but he had no wish to restore it. 'It is best so; let it be', he replied: 'Time effaces all things.'[4] The greatest division of his life, of course, was his conversion to Catholicism, in 1851. In personal relationships, too, men, like events, were isolated in his regard and often treated separately from preceding experience. Thus Gladstone, with whom Manning had once been so intimate a correspondent,

---

[1] Purcell, *The Life of Cardinal Manning, Archbishop of Westminster*, **II.** 629.
[2] Leslie, *Henry Edward Manning. His Life and Labours*, Preface, x.
[3] Purcell, I. 105.
[4] Ibid. I. 124.

and with whom he had shared so many religious convictions, could write, in 1875: 'Our differences, my dear Archbishop, are indeed profound. We refer them, I suppose, in humble silence to a Higher Power.'[5] Affable and easily communicative as an Anglican, as a Catholic Manning—though still enjoying society—was personally withdrawn and reserved. It was as if his life had acquired a new solemnity; that it had been set aside by God for an austere service whose purpose somehow separated him from the commonplace distractions of ordinary men. His singularity and dedication were quite extraordinary: a life of sacrifice and vicarious suffering which even those closest to him in ecclesiastical affairs and daily business could perceive but were not allowed to share.

Yet it has to be declared at once that Manning's reputation has suffered as a result of his own biographer: E. S. Purcell, a Catholic journalist, editor of the *Westminster Gazette*, a friend of Manning's. His *Life of Cardinal Manning*, published in 1895, was intended to be an unadorned account of the whole man, weaknesses as well as strengths. It was to show the nuts and bolts of holiness—or, as Gladstone put it, 'a dividing of marrow and bone'.[6] When the book appeared there was something of a sensation. Herbert Vaughan, Manning's successor, described it as 'almost a crime'—'I do not recognize the portrait of him with whom I was in constant communication during forty years.'[7] That assessment could have been an indication, not of Purcell's inaccuracy, but of the effectiveness of Manning's personal reserve: but in fact the book had two characteristics which rendered its depiction of Manning unreliable. In the first place, Purcell emphasized *continuities* in his subject's life. The development of personality and of public career go hand-in-hand, young man to Anglican parson, Archdeacon to Roman Catholic Cardinal, so that the reader's impression is one of a single plan laid out by Manning and pursued through a lifetime. In the second place, Purcell decided to print in full the very close professional correspondence which Manning maintained for many years with Mgr. Talbot in Rome. There was nothing discreditable in that correspondence, but the necessary and frank details of business

---

[5] Ibid. II. 478.   [6] Leslie, ix.   [7] Ibid. xiii.

are laid bare: assessments of candidates for positions in the Church, descriptions of the errors of men and movements, attempts to procure favourable opinions on controversial matters from Rome, and so forth. Reproduced in conjunction with an overall thesis which elicited a single unfolding career, Anglican and Catholic, Purcell's effect was to portray Manning as an ambitious fixer. It is a very inaccurate impression, which was refined still further by Lytton Strachey: his view of Manning in *Eminent Victorians* has achieved almost universal acceptance. The Cardinal has emerged as characterized by—in Strachey's phrase—an 'appetite for supreme dominion'.[8] But the materials of reassessment are not to hand. The Manning–Talbot letters which Purcell reproduced are no longer to be found among the rest of his papers at the English College in Rome, and the surviving collected papers of Manning himself are not available.[9]

It was at Copped Hall, Hertfordshire, in July 1807, that Henry Edward Manning was born. He was the son of a London merchant who had entered Parliament in 1790. After two years at a school in Streatham conducted by a Welsh clergyman, and then another two at an establishment in Totteridge, he proceeded to Harrow in 1822. There his 'youthful fondness for dress and personal adornment was conspicuous',[10] and after a conventional enough sojourn in the school he arrived at Balliol in 1827. His political liberalism,

[8] Lytton Strachey, *Eminent Victorians* [1918], London, 1948 edn., 88.

[9] The Manning letters in the Talbot collection at Rome were almost certainly removed by Purcell. They may now be among the Manning Papers. These, however, would appear to be rather a decimated collection. Manning bequeathed his papers to the Oblates of St. Charles, in Bayswater, where they remained for many years. Professor McClelland used them when writing his *Cardinal Manning. His Public Life and Influence*, in 1962; and I had access to some of the correspondence of Manning and the Irish bishops when writing my *Catholic Church and Ireland in the Age of Rebellion* in 1964—in which some of them are reproduced. The Manning Papers are in the custody of the Revd. Professor A. Chapeau of the Université Catholique de L'Ouest, at Angers. He wrote (29 Aug. 1981) that 'They are not for public inspection, and the Superior of the Oblates has instructed me to say that permission to consult them cannot be granted.' In another communication (18 Sept. 1981), he wrote, 'the original "Manning Papers in the Care of the Oblates of St. Charles" do not exist any longer, having been destroyed, after other mishaps, finally during the blitz of 1940–44. It has been my work for the last thirty years to gather and reassemble all I could find of them.' Since permission to consult these papers has not been granted, they are not used in this present study.

[10] Purcell, I. 17.

though not especially distinctive, was first revealed in his successful offerings at the Oxford Union. It was clear that he
was becoming aware of his social success at Oxford—where he
was said to have been 'self-conscious even in his night-cap'.[11]
It was at the University that he first met Gladstone, then a
slightly junior contemporary, and, like Gladstone, he planned
a career in public life. His religious opinions were orthodox,
slightly Evangelical, and temperate. He was not attracted to
the group of enthusiasts who attached themselves to Newman
at Oriel. In 1830 he took his degree and returned to the family home in Hertfordshire, awaiting the opportunity to be
called by some patron to a seat in Parliament. His father had
always hoped that he might receive ordination in the Church
of England, but this was not among the avenues of vocation
which Manning himself intended to explore.

Patrons did not appear, however, and his father meanwhile
went bankrupt. So in 1831, at the age of twenty-four, he
became a supernumerary clerk at the Colonial Office—still,
apparently, hoping for some opening in the political field.
Disappointed in love, called by a new sense of Evangelical
urgency, and finding work at the Colonial Office exceedingly
irksome, he decided after all to heed the long-expressed wish
of his father: he returned to Oxford in 1832, and, at Merton,
prepared for Holy Orders. Manning was ordained in December
1832. He then became first curate, and later rector, of
Lavington in Sussex, and in 1833 married Caroline Sargent,
daughter of the patron of the benefice. Parochial life was
happy and ordinary: he took his duties seriously, and seems
to have enjoyed the rural existence.

There then occurred the first of those decisive breaks that
characterized Manning's life. In 1837 Caroline died. More
perhaps than most men would have been he was affected by
her departure: something died in him too. For months he sat
by her grave to compose his sermons; he could not share his
grief—it entered into his being and gnawed away at the internal flesh of his existing religious sense. Like many in his
situation, he applied the therapy of hard work: 'I feel the

[11] Ibid. I. 30.

absolute need of full employment.'[12] In his case, however, the labour intensified with the progression of time. Out of it all—as yet unperceived, and mysterious in the Divine economy—there was emerging the slow movement of religious consciousness that was, so many years later, to result in his conversion to the Catholic faith. It was an outcome that would have seemed incredible to Manning in 1837. Yet it was from that date that his serious religious interests began, when he started an extensive reading of the Fathers and of the Caroline divines, and, in 1838, he read some of the *Tracts* from Oxford. To his heightened spiritual senses, the new High Church attitudes proved attractive, though, unlike Hurrell Froude and some others of Newman's circle, Manning retained a respect for the Protestant Reformers. But his doctrine of the Church began to change. He saw it now as possessed of a spiritual integrity quite separate from the State. His increasing distaste for erastianism was made explicit in his assault—in a pamphlet—on the Ecclesiastical Commission set up by the government in 1838 to regulate the incomes of the State Church. In 1836 he had begun to correspond with Newman, and was asked by him to contribute to the *Library of the Fathers*—evidence, incidentally, that Manning's intellectual capacities were judged, at least by Newman, more generously than Purcell allowed. During this period, also, his communication with Gladstone on Church issues increased. With this quickening religious sense came promotion. In 1837 he became Rural Dean; as Secretary of the Diocesan Board in the Diocese of Chichester he became active in the cause of education; and in 1840 he was, at the age of thirty-four, made Archdeacon. In the winter of 1838 he journeyed to Rome with Gladstone, and met Wiseman for the first time. But the easy assumption of High Church opinions was then shaken, as it was for some others, by Newman's retirement to Littlemore in 1843. Manning was still secure enough in his adhesion to Anglicanism: his unease at Newman's approaching secession lay in the conviction, correct as it turned out, that the High Church party would be discredited. A 'No

---

[12] David Newsome, *The Parting of Friends. A Study of the Wilberforces and Henry Manning*, London 1966, 253.

Popery' sermon, which he preached at Oxford in November 1843, ended relations with Newman. Some have regarded his simultaneous espousal of both High Church and Protestant attitudes, at this moment, as a question of expediency—as an indication of his inherent fever of ambition. It is certainly true that he was widely spoken of as a future bishop, and this prospect must have been enhanced when in 1845 his brother-in-law, Samuel Wilberforce, became the Bishop of Oxford. The clue to Manning's double-espousal of Tractarian and Protestant opinions at this moment is not to be taken as an indication of time-serving expediency, however, but of his sense of duty. Manning really believed in the *via media*: he sought to hold men together by the avoidance of extremes. He stood out because he was more successful at this characteristic of Anglicanism than some others were. In 1842 he published *The Unity of the Church*, in which he unfolded the vision of a body that was both Catholic and Protestant. Yet he was further unsettled by Newman's conversion in 1845, and by Newman's last work as an Anglican, the *Essay on Development*, which appeared to vitiate some of the grounds of his own defence of the Church of England's position. Thereafter, he worked for synodical government in the Church; for a relaxation of State control. His social circle was also extending: he was known as a man of conciliation and moderation.

For Manning, the polished exterior life and the successful steps upon the ladder of promotion were not satisfactory. The spiritual intensity he had received at the time of his wife's demise was burning, still, with an illumination which showed up an unsettled interior life. A second visit to Rome, in 1848 —where he witnessed the Revolution—must have helped to focus a conclusion to which his mind was arriving, but which he dared not allow himself to recognize. The diary he kept during the visit showed how easily he worshipped in the Catholic churches of the city, how satisfying he found the spiritual life of the priests and regulars he met, and how *authentic* Catholic truth seemed to be.[13] He was received by the Pope. Unlike Newman and Ward, Manning had an extensive knowledge and experience both of Catholic practice and

[13] Purcell reproduces large parts of the diary; see I. 411 ff.

of Catholic doctrine before his conversion. But he could not bring himself to face the awful conclusion to which his emotions were directing him. For over two years more he agonized. By 1850, however, even in advance of the disruptive ecclesiastical events of that year, a serenity of mind had begun to descend upon Manning; he was now clear that the Anglican position could not be maintained, that the Church of England was not part of the Church, and that union with the voice of the universal Church was all that he desired. In view of the social limbo into which Catholics were cast in England at the time, especially after the 'Papal Aggression' episode of 1850, there can be no surer indication of Manning's innocence of ambition than his motivation at this second decisive break in the continuity of his life. Appalled by the Gorham Judgment of 1850, which re-emphasized in a particularly unadorned fashion the subservience of the Church to the State, and shocked by the national loathing of Catholic truth apparently manifested during the 'Papal Aggression', and after unsuccessfully appealing to Gladstone to join him, Manning slipped quietly into the Catholic faith. It was the 6 April, 1851. 'After all intellectual processes', he wrote, 'there remains a step which can be taken only by the will.'[14]

Manning's new life began with his ordination by Cardinal Wiseman in June: the rapidity of his admission to orders being itself an indication of Wiseman's acknowledgement both of Manning's understanding of Catholicism and of his position in the Church from which he had seceded. Manning was now forty-one years old. In December he left for Rome, to study at the *Accademia Ecclesiastica*—the school where Vatican diplomats were trained and which was known as the 'nursery of cardinals'. There he was later joined by Edward Howard, a former Guards officer, who was to serve most of his life on the Propaganda staff in Rome, and became a cardinal in 1877; and by Herbert Vaughan, who was to succeed him in the Archbishopric of Westminster. It is from this period that his close friendship with Vaughan dates. In 1854 Manning returned to England as a priest in the Diocese of Westminster, preaching frequently at the Jesuit Church in Farm Street and

[14] Purcell, I. 596.

holding his confessional there. Almost at once Wiseman began to depend upon him for various administrative services, and it was this reliance upon one so newly arrived within the Church, as much as suspicion about the nature and intentions of the Oblates of St. Charles, which aroused some early opposition to Manning's growing influence. The Oblates were founded in 1857, with Manning at their head, in the Church of St. Mary of the Angels in Bayswater; in the same year he was appointed Provost of the Chapter of Westminster. Manning's subsequent promotion to the Archbishopric, in 1865, was regarded by some as controversial and will be separately considered: as will the details of his work at Westminster. But the outline of the rest of his ecclesiastical life can be simply related.

In June 1865, in preparation for his work as Archbishop, Manning went into Retreat with the Passionists at Highgate. He saw the occasion, characteristically, as making a decisive break in his life. God, he wrote, in his private journal of the Retreat, 'has now called me to the greatest Cross of my life and to the greatest separation from the world'.[15] The work ahead seemed formidable and lonely. 'Walking on the terrace and looking down upon London in the broad sunlight has been very moving to me', he recorded: 'The Son of God would have wept over it.'[16]

The burden was initially lightened by the peaceful acceptance of his new dignity and authority by the English bishops, and by the Chapter of Westminster, many of whom, of course, had sought to prevent his appointment. 'I suppose by this time', Vaughan wrote to him, 'more than half of those who used to bite their lips on seeing you have humbly bent their knees, and forgotten their former thoughts.'[17] And they had, too. Manning went out of his way to make gestures of conciliation; he behaved tactfully and with moderation. Errington, the principal loser by Manning's appointment, wrote 'The decision of Rome being to us the manifestation of the will of God, we have the best grounds to trust that the welfare of the see has been most effectually provided for.'[18]

---

[15] Ibid. II. 162.   [16] Ibid. II. 168.
[17] Ibid. II. 245.   [18] Leslie, 160.

In 1868 Manning proposed that Errington should become the head of a restored Scottish Hierarchy: peace and union was the governing principle of the Archbishop's actions. At the Vatican Council, too, it was Manning's attempts to provide a peaceful acceptance of Infallibility that made him one of the most notable diplomatists. In 1875 he was made a Cardinal. But with the death of Pius IX in 1878, Manning's influence declined in Rome. Talbot's efforts on his behalf had ceased in 1869, and on visits to Rome in 1876 and 1878, even before the death of Pius IX, he had been unhappily aware of a new climate of opinion in which he was less at home. Leo XIII was more open to those English Catholics who were friendly to Newman. On his last visit to Rome, in 1883, he felt a degree of antagonism: 'It is clear to me that an attempt has been made to make them believe me to be despotic', he wrote.[19] His personal relations with Leo XIII, though not as intimate as those with Pius IX, were good, however. It was Manning's changed views about the Temporal Power, which became clear early in the 1880s, that separated him from the leading figures of the Roman Curia. He had ceased to believe, as they did, that the Pope could be restored by the armed intervention of the Powers.

In England, too, his position was an isolated one—just as his predecessor's had been. His social and philanthropic interests, though not as unattractive to the Catholic laity as some have contended,[20] were not particularly serviceable as bonds of union with those who harboured suspicions about the autocratic nature of his Ultramontanism. The bishops, with the exception of Cornthwaite and Vaughan, were not close to his thinking or his counsel. He worked hard and effectively, often preaching two or three times each Sunday; attended to the closest administrative detail; absorbed himself in devotions. When he died in 1892 there were unexpected scenes of popular grief—the silent file of people who moved past his body as it lay at Archbishop's House extended for three days along the length of the street. They were the poor and the uneducated and those who had sensed in the Cardinal some quality of eternity whose definition or content they

[19] Purcell, II. 579.
[20] Purcell, for example. See II. 714.

could not even begin to comprehend. The isolated man whom they honoured had adherents after all, and an enormous number of them. Trade Unionists carried their banners in his funeral procession. 'A great light of the Church has gone out', Leo XIII said when he heard of Manning's death. 'I feel that my own hour is at hand.'[21]

Manning had chosen to be a private man. It was not one of his natural characteristics: witness the social young clergyman of the Church of England days. Since he did not disclose his thoughts to others, they, for their part, sometimes imagined a degree of autocracy, an inhuman austerity, an emotional desiccation. His austerity has been greatly exaggerated, particularly by those who found his conversion to the Temperance cause, in 1867, and his subsequent refusal to drink wine even at his own table, a matter of hostile commentary. His appearance, too, was deceptively ascetic. He indeed lived simply. But he was, throughout his time at Westminster, a regular and good social entertainer; he was often at the Athenaeum; he told Irish jokes in a simulated Irish accent. He was not really that much like 'Cardinal Grandison' in Disraeli's *Lothair*, and he was not really, in Shane Leslie's expression, 'A Puritan under the purple'. His antipathy to the theatre was an expression of the moral seriousness very widespread within the Victorian intelligentsia. He voiced it rather stiffly, however. 'I have watched the Divorce Court, and have found that, I may say in a majority of cases, directly or indirectly, the co-respondents are of the theatrical world', he wrote; 'every theatre is a centre of all kinds of evil'.[22] What Archbishop Mathew called 'the atmosphere of Harrow and Balliol'[23] continued to attach to him throughout his life; and it is an interesting confirmation that when Manning gave Florence Nightingale his reasons for entering the Catholic Church, she pronounced that they 'were of the Oxford historical school'.[24] This suggests only, however, an intellectual consistency in Manning: the values 'of Harrow and Balliol' he had most emphatically rejected—they were, by the middle years of the

[21] Leslie, 495.
[22] Leslie, 455.
[23] Mathew, *Catholicism in England, 1535-1935*, 208.
[24] Leslie, 109.

nineteenth century, the harbingers of Rationalism and the dissolvents of religious truth. Manning's refusal to counten-ance the attendance of Catholics at Oxford and Cambridge was the sign of this; for the universities were becoming the centres of 'the stream which is evidently carrying English society every year more and more decidedly and perceptibly towards Worldliness and Rationalism'.[25] Yet Manning did not cut himself off from the intellectual society of his day. Indeed his membership of the Metaphysical Society, in the 1870s, shocked Newman precisely because the Society was full of agnostics and sceptics. Purcell believed that Manning was 'out of his depth' in the Society,[26] largely because on one or two occasions his arguments were confounded or he failed to appreciate the philosophical position of others. But, in the heightened critical atmosphere of the Society, his was not by any means a unique experience. He was more intellectually accomplished than some writers have supposed. It was Purcell, again, who established the conviction, repeated by others, that Manning was 'not a profound thinker, nor possessed of original ideas, nor deeply read'.[27] He was not, it is true, an original thinker—very few men are—but he was very widely read and could himself write with subtlety and depth, often beneath a deceptive appearance of simplicity. *The Eternal Priesthood*, published in 1883, ought to be regarded as a spiritual classic—even if the office of priesthood, as there described, represents an aspect of Ultramontanism now rec-ognised, at least by some, as belonging to an ecclesiastical outlook that has passed away.

Manning's great weakness, both as an administrator and as a pastor, was his inability to consult others. He regarded his sacred office as imposing a trust whose terms and applications only he could adequately determine. 'For him, it sufficed to consult the Divine Will', Purcell wrote, rather than 'the will of man'.[28] The result of this lack of effective counsel was a tendency 'to regard', as E. E. Reynolds observed, 'those

[25] Manning, 'The Work and Wants of the Catholic Church in England' (1863), in *Miscellanies*, I. 68.
[26] Purcell, II. 513.
[27] Ibid. I. 234.
[28] Ibid. II. 233.

who hinder him as wilfully obstructive, if not maliciously minded.'[29] It is a characteristic commonly met in great men. Dr Derek Holmes has written of Manning's tendency 'to identify his own opinions with the guidance of the Holy Spirit'.[30] And indeed he did so: that, too, is a quality frequently encountered in Christian leaders. Yet must there not be occasions when the opinions of men and the directions of the Holy Spirit coincide? Manning, who was conscious of the responsibility of getting weighty spiritual decisions made on behalf of others right, acted affirmatively; sometimes, no doubt, mistakenly. But he may only imprecisely be indicted for 'the narrowness of his mind'—another conclusion of Purcell.[31] He did not have a narrow mind, but a mind which was clear and decided about issues which others wished to leave opaque or undecided. The distinction, again clear to Manning, was obviously liable to slide away from vision in the heat of controversy. In all the assessments of Manning there is one which supervenes, however. Manning's spiritual priorities, his interior life, his devotion to the Blessed Sacrament—a feature of his daily discipline, in his private Chapel—his sense that the treasures of eternity lay round about their daily lives for those with eyes to discern them: these were the realities of his service as leader and guardian of English Catholicism in the second half of the nineteenth century. No one was more conscious of his own faults. Few have achieved his insights.

Yet Manning has gone down in the record as an ambitious man, as one who sought and procured his own succession to the Archbishopric of Westminster—that it was 'clear beyond doubt that he sought and furthered his own cause'.[32] The truth is probably rather mixed: Manning's overriding priority was the preservation and enhancement of the 'Roman' spirit that Wiseman had brought to English Catholicism. In him, as is well known, the battle for the Church was clearly drawn—between Ultramontanism and a slide into easy Catholic

---

[29] E. E. Reynolds, *Three Cardinals*, 146.
[30] Holmes, *More Roman than Rome*, 226.
[31] Purcell, II. 505.
[32] Gordon Wheeler, 'The Archdiocese of Westminster', in *The English Catholics, 1850–1950*, ed. Beck, 158.

acceptance of the surrounding English religious sense, pervaded as it increasingly seemed to be by Rationalism and Indifferentism. As Wiseman's illnesses grew longer in duration, early in the 1860s, the problem of his successor became a matter of urgency for Manning—who was, by then, co-equal with Mgr. Searle as the Cardinal's confidant. By a simple process of elimination, all the other possible candidates who could preserve the authentic 'Roman' note removed themselves from Manning's judgement. What survived the scrutiny —the realization appalled him—was only himself. Manning still did not act directly to secure his own succession; he criticized the leading candidates at a time when he was not, in the eyes of most, himself a likely candidate. When he alone received the approval of Rome, as guided by himself and several others, he accepted the logic of his own preceding actions and regarded his appointment as right. The motive was not ambition in the ordinary sense: it was a desire to protect what had been achieved in the Church from those whom he believed would prove less stalwart custodians. Whether this was a process of self-deception may only be estimated in the broader perspective of Manning's life and behaviour. The notion of Manning's overweening ambition was not an invention of Purcell's. Contemporaries who disliked Manning's early rise to influence with Wiseman were quick to attribute ambitious motivation. 'I hate that man', the President of Ushaw once said, 'he is such a forward piece.'[33] Searle spoke often of Manning's 'intrigues'—but the two men were unable to get on anyway, because of some sort of personality clash. Canon John Morris on one occasion wrote to Talbot that it 'would be quite impossible for two such men as Mgr. Manning and Mgr. Searle to live in the same house'.[34] Searle saw Manning as a rival for his influence over Wiseman. There was a tendency for the bishops to regard Manning as—in the opinion reported to Talbot by Vaughan—'extreme, exaggerated, and contentious',[35] and this opened up the suggestion that he was ambitious to wider contexts. In 1860, when writing to Talbot about the removal of Errington as Wiseman's coadjutor, the Bishop of

[33] Purcell, II. 77.
[34] English College, Rome, Talbot Papers, 510, Morris to Talbot, 26 June 1863.
[35] English College, Talbot Papers, 715, Vaughan to Talbot, 6 May, n.d.

Emmaus, Patterson, referred to 'a great and growing mistrust of Manning . . . founded on the belief that he is a schemer—a man fond of influence and power'. He also noted that the dispute between Manning and the Chapter of Westminster, over the diocesan seminary issue, had 'driven the Cardinal further in his defence than perhaps he originally meant to go'.[36] It is not difficult to see that, given the thesis that Manning was overwhelmingly ambitious, it would be a short step to Lytton Strachey's malicious conclusion that Manning stirred up quarrels between Wiseman and Errington precisely in order to secure his own promotion. Thus also Frederick Oakeley, the convert priest, writing to Talbot in 1861 about 'the ascendancy of Manning's policy in the Diocese' pointed out that it 'would undoubtedly render it impracticable for any future Archbishop to govern it, unless he were himself an Oblate'.[37] Manning was the only Oblate who could possibly have become Wiseman's successor, so the implication was unambiguous.

The man to whom most of these opinions were directed has shared, with Manning himself, the reputation of being an ambitious schemer. Mgr. George Talbot was a younger son of Lord Talbot of Malahide, in Co. Dublin; one of the converts in the tail that followed Newman into the Church. He became a Catholic in 1847 and was ordained by Wiseman—and, after a period as a priest in London, was sent to Rome as Wiseman's special representative. There he rapidly acquired the confidence of the Pope, who made him one of his Chamberlains. The views of English Catholicism and the English bishops which Pius IX (and to some extent the Curia) adopted were often those of Talbot. He maintained an enormous correspondence with various prelates and priests in England, and most of it has survived in the archives of the English College in Rome. The view that his was the only effective or decisive representation of English views at Rome, however, is inaccurate. The staff at Propaganda maintained their own regular communication with the bishops, and it was this, and not Talbot, which furnished the most authoritative information when decisions about the English Church had to be

---

[36] English College, Talbot Papers, 572, Patterson to Talbot, 20 May [1860].
[37] English College, Talbot Papers, 552, Oakeley to Talbot, 24 Jan. 1961.

made. But Talbot's opinions were not discounted. He *was* very influential. He had diplomatic skills and easily acquired the Roman manner of representing issues and people at the Holy See. As the letters printed in Purcell's book showed, he was frank and often realistic about men and their motives. Strachey's unpleasant portrait is a caricature of what English Protestantism had always supposed a Roman official to be like, and is to be assessed accordingly: 'He could mingle together astuteness and holiness without any difficulty; he could make innuendoes as naturally as an ordinary man makes statements of fact; he could apply flattery with so unsparing a hand that even Princes of the Church found it sufficient.'[38] In reality, Talbot was an effective ecclesiastical civil servant whose major defect was an overconfidence in the discretion of others: he was too candid in correspondence. Even Manning, in later years, described him as 'the most imprudent man that ever lived'.[39] But the sort of personal responses he sought in his letters were exactly those most needed by the Holy See in the manifestly delicate task of seeking to further 'Roman' influence in the English Church when making ecclesiastical appointments. Those English bishops who thought Talbot a slippery schemer were also those whose own internal disputes —themselves not unacquainted with personal antipathies— were referred to Rome because they could not agree among themselves. Talbot won the great personal respect and friendship of Pius IX, and when, in 1869, he was removed insane from Rome to an asylum at Passy, near Paris, it was the Pope who directed that his rooms at the Vatican should be left undisturbed, to be ready for his recovery. Talbot died in 1886, his mind still closed off from the world he had tried to serve.

Manning's succession to the Archbishopric of Westminster was because he was the only candidate the Holy See felt it could trust to continue the work of Wiseman. That was a conclusion which could well have been reached without any representations or any intrigue. During his visits to Rome to found the Oblates of St. Charles, in 1856 and 1857, Manning came to have a wide acquaintance with officials. 'These visits made me known to the chief official personages; the ruling

---

[38] Strachey, 73.   [39] Leslie, xii.

Cardinals at Propaganda, and brought me into intimate relations with the Pope', he later recalled: 'All this led to my becoming what I now am.'[40] Even before that, as a student at the *Accademia* the Pope had treated Manning, as Manning wrote, 'with a confidence greater than I ever had from an Anglican bishop'.[41] It should not have caused surprise that with Wiseman's decline in health, Manning's name should begin to be spoken of as his coadjutor—if Wiseman could be induced, as the Holy See wished, to name a successor. In 1862 Errington had been obliged to resign as coadjutor, in Pius IX's famous '*coup d'état* of the Lord God'. The matter of a new successor was raised in 1863, but Wiseman was unwilling to reopen all the contentious rivalries again, especially if Manning's was the name eventually brought forward. 'Everybody naturally expects him, and if it is done it will cause little surprise,' Vaughan wrote to Talbot about Manning's prospects.[42] But Vaughan was at Bayswater with Manning, his perspective was a limited one. Canon John Morris believed that Manning could be appointed coadjutor and effective ruler of the diocese, and that Wiseman should retire to Rome.[43] In the end nothing was done, and Manning's worst fear was realized: Wiseman died in 1865 without arranging his own successor. What then happened is well known. The Chapter of Westminster, after some delays, produced a *terna* for the Holy See consisting of three names: Clifford, Bishop of Clifton, Errington, Archbishop of Trebizond, and Grant, Bishop of Southwark. The withdrawal of the other two left Errington as the final choice—which, after consultation with the Hierarchy, was sent to Rome. In a joint letter to Barnabò, Grant and Clifford explained why, in their judgement, Errington's name alone ought to be considered. They wrote of his 'superior ecclesiastical knowledge', of his 'excellent administrative abilities', of his 'great firmness of character', and of the 'great personal sacrifices' he had made for the Church—'both in person and in purse'.[44] Errington himself,

---

[40] Purcell, II. 2. [41] Ibid. II. 43.

[42] English College Archives, Talbot Papers, 703, Vaughan to Talbot, 20 June 1863. [43] Ibid. 510, Morris to Talbot, 26 June 1863.

[44] Bristol Record Office, 35721, Clifford Papers, 'Heads of a Joint Letter from Bishop Grant and Bishop Clifford to the Cardinal Prefect of Propaganda' (n.d.).

aware that his last contacts with Rome had been, to say the least, unhappy (—there had been the personal row with the Pope about his resignation as coadjutor—) believed that circumstances had changed, and that his candidature was therefore in order. Canon Morris, Manning's friend in the Westminster Chapter, wrote his assessment to Talbot in March 1865, just after the meeting had agreed the *terna*. His opinions represented a minority view on the Chapter, of course: 'We want a Roman', he told Talbot, 'I do not mean by education, but in mind and feeling.' He ruled out Ullathorne, who, though 'an excellent Bishop' had 'all the faults of a self-educated man', and who also 'carried his idea of episcopal power and position very far'. Clifford was 'very silent on matters, and it appears to me that his reputation has been made by silence'. He added, however, 'Better to have his laugh than to have Dr. Ullathorne dropping his h's in London.' Of Errington, 'the position was how the Holy See would take his name'. Cornthwaite was 'the best Bishop in England'. He would have been glad to have him. Lastly came two names. 'The most prominent man in England is Dr. Manning, and it is he whom the Cardinal would have preferred as his successor,' he wrote; and then he added 'On the whole, after grave consideration, the man I hope that the Holy Father will send is the one to whom I write.'[45] At one point, indeed, Pius IX did think of Talbot. The British Government wanted Grant, with whom they had had dealings over the provision of Catholic army chaplains during the Crimean War, and an approach on the matter was made to Cardinal Antonelli.

Cardinal Barnabò, at Propaganda, was incensed with the Chapter of Westminster for sending Errington's name to Rome. Pius IX described it as 'an insult to the Pope'.[46] Manning's candidature was brought forward at this moment, as the only possible safe 'Roman' alternative. Barnabò was opposed to the idea. But Talbot worked hard for Manning's cause—the Pope himself later remarking on his diplomatic accomplishment in persuading him to accept his advice. 'Nevertheless', Talbot added, in sending this information on to

Manning, 'I believe your appointment was specially directed by the Holy Ghost.'[47] Fr. Robert Coffin, Manning's Confessor, who was in Rome at the time, also promoted Manning's candidature, and had an audience with the Pope in which the matter was discussed. (Coffin was an Oxford convert, one of Newman's original Oratorians, who left to become a Redemptorist. In 1882 he became the third Bishop of Southwark.) Manning was appointed Archbishop by direct Pontifical act in April 1865. 'The real motive why the Pope named you is because he thought you were the man to introduce a new spirit into the Church in England,' Talbot wrote to him. 'Your appointment has been a severe blow given to the club theory,' he continued; 'I mean the view that the Catholic body, as it is called in England, is a kind of club, and that the dignities in it ought to be the property of the Cliffords and other Catholic families.'[48] Manning's promotion, that is to say, was intended to diminish the influence of the Old Catholics. From the point of view of Rome, their influence was finally revealed in its true colours by the nomination of Clifford and Errington in the *terna*. This had always been Manning's own opinion. 'The present crisis is not one of men, but of policy', he had observed in February, when the Chapter had still to make their choice.[49] 'I have therefore never, as you once said people thought, "aimed at it", or desired it,' Manning wrote to Talbot after the event; 'If I had wished for my reward in this world, I should not have spoken out to the last syllable what I believe to be true.' It was an assessment whose verity will be decided, again, according to extraneous considerations. Manning believed he could support his contention: 'I have consciously offended Protestants, Anglicans, Gallican Catholics, National Catholics, and Worldly Catholics, and the Government and public opinion in England.'[50] Rome, in making appointments, preferred to choose those who had a wide base of support in their own countries: Manning could hardly have calculated his chances highly. Barnabò had wanted Ullathorne's succession—and had even, back in 1863, got Manning to suggest his name to the Pope as Wiseman's

[47] Ibid. II. 221.   [48] Ibid. II. 257.
[49] Leslie, 150.   [50] Purcell, II. 209.

coadjutor. Had the Chapter of Westminster not made all the English bishops seem unpalatable, by forwarding Errington's name with their consent, Manning would never have been chosen.

Since Manning therefore owed his archbishopric, and his leadership of English Catholicism, to his Ultramontanism, it will be well to give some assessment of it. In 1860, Patterson had remarked to Talbot that many in the English Church mistrusted Manning because his views were 'not thoroughly Catholic'.[51] What did he mean? Patterson himself did not elaborate; but he must have been conscious of a paradox. For Manning was thoroughly 'Roman'—Wiseman's chosen amanuensis and guide. What he must have meant was that Manning's very 'Roman' qualities were out of sympathy with conventional English Catholicism, in which case his remark was merely a commentary on the division between the two leading dispositions within the English Church. And yet, as his views on the Temporal Sovereignty of the Papacy were to show, there were some curious eccentricities in Manning's Romanism. In this, he was close to W. G. Ward,[52] whose opinions he consulted on visits to St. Edmund's College, Ware, after 1854 —visits whose frequency increased as the Oblates extended their influence in the College later in the decade. In 1860 Manning gave a series of sermons on the Temporal Power at St. Mary of the Angels. These contained some exaggerations of the basis of the Papal claims, including the prediction that the Temporal sovereignty would one day be defined as a dogma of faith.[53] A translation of the lectures—bound in white, as was the custom—was presented to the Holy Father in Rome, who was well pleased with them. But the opinion of the Curia in general was one of disapproval, and the lectures were even threatened with referral to the Holy Office. There was another difficulty. Manning's political outlook inclined him to the cause of popular sovereignty, so he defended the States of the Church not on the grounds of legitimacy— the grounds used by the Austrians, and by the English and

---

[51] English College Archives, Talbot Papers, 572, Patterson to Talbot, 20 May [1860].
[52] Reynolds, 127.
[53] Purcell, II. 152.

Irish Catholics—but on the contention that the Pope needed a territorial basis to preserve his independence. Early in the 1880s he dropped even that view, regarding the matter as having been, in effect, settled by the turn of events.

As a defender of Ultramontane doctrines and disciplines Manning was both orthodox and consistent. His defence of the *Syllabus of Errors* in 1864, and of the Definition of Infallibility in 1870, gave him an international reputation as a champion of the 'Roman' view of the Church. To opponents of Ultramontanism, he became something of a symbol of the new dogmatism of the Vatican. Ferdinand Gregorovius encountered him at a party in Rome during the Vatican Council and recorded his impression. 'Closely observed the fanatic', he noted in his diary; 'a little grey man, looking as if encompassed by cobwebs.'[54] Manning's strict adherence to Ultramontanist teachings, in fact, is a further indication of the discontinuities of his life. As an Anglican he had been noted for moderation, for compromise on disputed ecclesiastical issues, for accommodation. As a Catholic he was sure of the ground he had occupied, and his Catholic life was dedicated to its preservation and enhancement—against the potentially corrupting influence of English 'Gallicanism'. He believed the English Catholics had absorbed far too much of the practice of a 'national' Church from their Protestant fellow countrymen, and that the sort of liberal ecclesiastical or theological attitudes represented by Newman, or the English 'Inopportunist' bishops on the Infallibility question, like Errington and Clifford, were liable to separate the English from the centre of unity—from the very authority by which all truth was known. In 1859 he told Talbot that the Old Catholics were 'one of the greatest evils in England'.[55] He was opposed to the APUC as an embodiment of the wrong attitudes, and his Pastoral Letter on the issue, in 1866, was regarded as something of a manifesto for the Ultramontanist position—'the best thing he has written,' as his supporter Morris reported to Rome.[56]

[54] *The Roman Journals of Ferdinand Gregorovius, 1852–1874*, ed. Friedrich Althaus, London 1911, 354.

[55] Purcell, II. 99.

[56] English College Archives, Talbot Papers, 521, Morris to Talbot, 26 Feb. 1866.

Manning tended to an apocalyptic view of society; he was impressed with the sense of some impending cataclysm in which the fight for the survival of Christian truth would require its clear definition, that men might behold the light and the dark in dramatic contrast. In England, the conflict was against the seemingly respectable countenance of liberalism and progressive enlightenment. 'The tendency of both metaphysics and science in England', he said in 1867, 'is to eliminate the supernatural and to limit the basis of philosophy to the span of sense and experiment.'[57] In an Address to the Young Men's Catholic Association in 1871 he said: 'Individuals are becoming more anarchical, the intellect more licentious, the wills of men more stubborn; and this self-will expresses itself in their actions, so that it is true to say that the principles upon which the Christian world was founded, and by which it has hitherto been preserved, have been rejected and are being violated on every side.' The world, he argued, was not progressing; it was 'going back'. This was the purpose of the *Syllabus*, he continued, with its rejection of the notion 'that the Roman Pontiff can and ought to reconcile and adjust himself to Progress, Liberalism, and Modern Civilization'.[58] With such an apostasized world the Church could have only 'partial' relations—sufficient to secure the benefits for society of 'the natural order of mankind'.[59] The strife of the nineteenth century was only, for him, a version of the normal conditions of things, however. 'In one sense the conflict of the Church and the World is always the same,' he wrote in *Caesarism and Ultramontanism* (1873); 'The enmity of the world is one, and the truth is one; nevertheless the forms of that enmity are endless and always changing.'[60] In the same paper, Manning gave his clearest definition of Ultramontanism—'the essence of which is that the Church being a Divine institution, and by Divine assistance infallible, is, within its own sphere, independent of all civil powers; and, as the guardian and interpreter of the Divine law, it is the proper judge of men and of nations in all things touching that

[57] Manning, 'French Infidelity' (1867), in *Miscellanies*, I. 205.
[58] Manning, 'On Progress' (1871), ibid. I. 322-3.
[59] Manning, *The Catholic Church and Modern Society*, 15.
[60] Manning, *Caesarism and Ultramontanism* (1873), in *Miscellanies*, II. 129.

law in faith or morals.'[61] Caesarism, by contrast, 'is in human nature'; it has 'always been striving to reassert itself'.[62] Modern Caesarism was evident in the German Falk Laws of 1873, but it was everywhere a threat to spiritual independence. It claimed 'not only that the State has supreme power over the Church in all persons and causes, but supreme right to determine the limits of the rights of the Church, its liberties, offices, and duties.'[63] There were implicit objections here to aspects of the growth of the modern State—which were incompatible with some of Manning's contentions, made in reference to social reform in England, about the widening of the action of the State. He did not himself sense any inconsistency. His concern was to emphasize the sacerdotal aspects of religious authority, not to sort out a coherent scheme for Christian involvement with social change. The claims he made for the priesthood were high and personally demanding. 'They are ambassadors from God,' he wrote, 'having, therefore, commission to treat and conclude in His name.'[64] The priest's responsibility was ultimate: 'He is called to the nearest approach to our Divine Redeemer, and to be a fellow-worker with Him in gathering out the elect from this evil world.'[65]

Since Manning regarded the battle for Ultramontanism as involving the highest considerations of ecclesiastical autonomy and Christian doctrinal purity, it was hardly surprising that he should seek to contain the influence of 'worldly Catholics' like the Old Catholics of England (as he believed them to be), and of 'liberal' Catholics like Newman. Purcell has written of Manning's 'persistent opposition to Newman', and there is a good deal of truth in the assessment. Newman, for his part, felt 'a distressing mistrust' of Manning.[66] Their relations were important from the start, because of the coincidence that Newman's *Apologia* and Manning's elevation to the Archbishopric had projected both men into the forefront of English Catholicism at about the same time. From the obscurity of the Birmingham Oratory Newman was in 1864 suddenly received into public discussion and, in general, a very sympathetic appraisal resulted. But the *Apologia* disclosed

[61] Ibid. II. 140. [62] Ibid. II. 148.
[63] Ibid. II. 153. [64] *The Eternal Priesthood*, 20.
[65] Ibid. 108. [66] Purcell, II. 305.

a Catholicism which was not Ultramontane in tone, and
Manning sensed the damage its success might do to the
'Roman' influence his appointment was intended to foster.
The two men were later to differ over the question of the
Temporal Power, over the establishment of an Oxford Cath-
olic College, and over Infallibility. In each disagreement,
Manning saw Newman as providing an intellectual cover for
the anti-Papal party in England—for 'worldly Catholicism'.
The matter was urgent. 'I see much danger of an English
Catholicism, of which Newman is the highest type', Manning
wrote to Talbot in 1866; 'It is the old Anglican, patristic,
literary, Oxford tone translated into the Church.'[67] The
observation is a revealing one. Newman, he was saying, had
not undergone the discontinuities necessary for an authentic
acceptance of the Catholic faith. His life was a single development. The genuinely Catholic content of his religious
understanding must therefore be questioned. Newman was a
'minimizer' of Catholic doctrine. Hence Manning's hostility
to Newman's plans for a hall or college in Oxford, and to the
suggestion, made by the Duke of Norfolk and Lord Ripon in
1878, that Newman should receive a cardinal's hat. He forwarded the request to Rome, though avoiding personal endorsement, and then allowed Newman's own self-effacing
language about not wishing to accept the honour if it meant
residence in Rome to be interpreted, publicly as well, as a
refusal to accept it: Leo XIII was more open to Newman's
friends than Pius IX had been, however, and in 1879 the
cardinal's hat was duly conferred. It was an extraordinary
illustration of the extent to which Manning was prepared to
go in order to preserve the English Church from tendencies
whose influence he lamented.

Many have regarded the Vatican Council as the highest
point of Manning's life. There he was recognized as one of
the leading exponents of Infallibility, as an ecclesiastical figure
of international dimension. He needed to be: the English
bishops elected Grant, not Manning, as their representative on
the most important of the four Deputations of the Council—
De Fide. Manning got on to the Deputation because the Italian

bishops elected him.[68] He worked as a diplomatist rather than as a theologian, both in securing support for the Infallibility cause and in explaining the Council to the outside world. 'The true motive of the Vatican Council is transparent to all calm and just minds,' he later wrote. 'For three hundred years no General Council had been held, for three hundred years the greatest change that has ever come upon the world since its conversion to Christianity had steadily passed upon it.'[69] The hostile and often extremely uninformed reporting of the Council in the press had created a climate of opinion in which a Bavarian plan to intervene and protect the liberties of Catholics had achieved some weighty support—including that of Gladstone, the English Prime Minister. Manning was released by the Pope from the oath of secrecy in order to provide the British representative in Rome, Odo Russell, with a more accurate account of the purpose of the proceedings. He particularly sought to discredit the opinions of Lord Acton, who was in Rome at the time on his own behalf, and whose opposition to the Infallibility cause was regarded by many as influential. But whatever Manning's diplomatic success with securing bishops for the Infallibilist side, with Odo Russell he achieved nothing. Purcell actually supposed that Russell, whose mother was a Catholic, had some sympathy for Infallibility, and was persuaded by Manning, during their walks along the Pincio, that the British Government should discountenance an intervention by the Powers.[70] In reality, however, Russell got his opinions from Acton. In February 1870, Russell was telling the Foreign Office that Acton 'inspires me with so much respect and confidence, that I should like to be always of his opinion';[71] and in March he wrote, 'all Lord Acton's views appear to me to be admirable'.[72] Gladstone dropped the idea of intervention in the Council because he was defeated on the question in his own Cabinet.

[68] But see Dom Cuthbert Butler's alternative account: it was not 'the Italian bishops who put him on their list, but that he was on the list circulated by his own committee', Cuthbert Butler, *The Vatican Council, 1869–1870*, London 1962, 148.

[69] H. E. Manning, *The True Story of the Vatican Council*, London 1877, 31.

[70] Purcell, II. 433–6.

[71] Noel Blakiston (ed.), *The Roman Question. Extracts from the despatches of Odo Russell for Rome, 1858–1870*, London 1962, 397.

[72] Ibid. 411.

Manning's failure to persuade him was rather publicly manifested in the controversy produced by Gladstone's pamphlet against the Vatican Decrees, published in 1874–to which he wrote a reply early in 1875. Over the Definition of Infallibility he had performed an extremely effective service at the Council itself, and afterwards his authority in the English Church was enhanced by the reputation he acquired among the bishops of the world gathered in Rome. Manning himself saw this as the centre of his life's work. The Definition had just the triumphalist qualities that most suited his sense that a battle with the world needed exclusive and clear understandings of religious authority. The circumstances of the Definition, also, caught his imagination: as the bishops voted a storm broke over Rome, and lightning flickered around the dome of St. Peter's. 'Critics saw in this thunderstorm an articulate voice of divine indignation against the definition,' he later wrote: 'They forgot Sinai and the Ten Commandments.'[73]

In his administrative work in the diocese of Westminster, and in his general leadership of the English Church, Manning's achievements were uneven. In 1863, two years before his appointment, he had written an article for the *Dublin Review* outlining the priorities of the Church as he then saw them. First came the provision of 'proper diocesan seminaries, according to the decrees of the Council of Trent'.[74] Second was education for the poor.[75] There was also a need for a more efficient use of the laity and for training for foreign missions. His great priority was the spiritual oversight of his own clergy, and on this he expended most of his energies in a largely unseen (because personal and localized) ministry which was valued and successful. Canon Morris, a year after Manning's appointment, hoped he would 'not kill himself' with the effort he put into it. 'The amount of good he does is wonderful', Morris observed; 'I have never yet seen a sign of the least weariness about him, and however pressed he may be, his readiness to listen to everyone and to help everyone,

---

[73] *The True Story of the Vatican Council*, 145.

[74] 'The Work and Wants of the Catholic Church in England' (1863), in *Miscellanies*, I. 43.

[75] Ibid. I. 45.

and to take part in every good work, I never saw in any one in my life.'[76] He retained personal control of diocesan affairs —unlike his predecessor. Indeed, it was during Wiseman's tenure of the archbishopric that Manning had, of course, really begun the administrative work which he continued in his own name after 1865. Right up to the end of his life Manning saw to every detail. He consulted with the Hierarchy about large general issues—the University question, the parochial school maintenance grants from the government, and so forth—but in his own diocese he sought advice rarely, concentrating virtually all decisions in his own hands. Wiseman had entrusted him with administrative work from the start of his Catholic ministry: in 1855 he had communicated with the War Department, along with Bishop Grant, about Catholic army chaplains, and in the same year Wiseman had made him Diocesan Inspector of schools. It was over the establishment of the Oblates of St. Charles, in 1857, that Manning showed his skill in approaches to the Curia. In 1856, he had gone to Milan and drawn up a Rule for the Oblates based on the original of St. Charles Borromeo. He had also managed to procure, from the Archbishop of Milan, two relics of the saint's blood—'there was no portion of the body to be obtained', as Manning wrote to Wiseman at the time.[77] The Archbishop, in return, received a copy of Wiseman's novel *Fabiola*. In January 1857, the Pope and Cardinal Barnabò approved the Oblates, but in circumstances which turned Manning's joy into sorrow: for Robert Wilberforce, his close friend, who was in Rome studying for the priesthood, died of gastric fever during the visit. Each sentence of the Rule, as Manning later wrote to Talbot, was settled 'after long and repeated consideration, and much advice in Rome'.[78] In December Wiseman, pleased with the thoroughness of the work he had entrusted to Manning, sent the final version to Rome for Papal sanction.[79] The experience had also earned Manning the lasting confidence of

[76] English College Archives, Talbot Papers, 521, Morris to Talbot, 26 Feb. 1866.
[77] Purcell, II. 60.
[78] English College Archives, Talbot Papers, 477, Manning to Talbot, 3 Sept. 1858.
[79] Ibid. 1138, Wiseman to the Holy Father, 25 Dec. 1858.

Roman officials, so that a decade later Cardinal Antonelli could assure the British government that Manning's opinions were those of the Papacy.[80] The success over the foundation of the Oblates, and the dedication with which, as Superior, Manning established their work in Bayswater, was unhappily tarnished by the dispute with the Westminster Chapter about the work of the Oblates in St. Edmund's College. Wiseman and Manning were obliged to withdraw the Oblates, due to the opposition of the bishops. It was, as Manning realistically reported to Propaganda, 'a matter of peace and charity'.[81] Barnabò, at Propaganda, was 'not pleased' to hear of the withdrawal; and Manning himself admitted, in reporting this opinion to Wiseman, that it was, for the Roman cause in England, 'a step backward'.[82] In 1869 Manning sought to reverse the situation—confirmed in the Decree of 1863—by setting up a proper diocesan seminary, on the Tridentine basis, in the convent at Hammersmith. Students were transferred from St. Edmund's. But the venture failed. Manning discovered, as Wiseman had done, that on controversial issues he had no real support among the bishops. This became clear with his other great educational venture: the Catholic University College in Kensington, founded in 1874. This also failed. The blame here lay partly with Newman, whom Manning invited to participate in the establishment but who declined: Newman's instincts were probably correct over this, for his idea of a University was radically different from Manning's hope of a middle-class, technical, and scientific institute. The College also failed because of the choice of Rector—the unfortunate Mgr. Thomas Capel: the choice was made by Manning himself. It failed also because the laity wanted to send their sons to Oxford and Cambridge, and not to Kensington. Manning had continued Wiseman's policy of prohibiting the attendance of Catholics at the Universities. With the repeal of University Tests in 1871, Clifford petitioned Rome for the removal of the ban. Propaganda replied by urging the creation

---

[80] See Norman, *The Catholic Church and Ireland in the Age of Rebellion*, 358.

[81] Propaganda, *Scritture* 16 (1861-3), 206; Manning to Barnabò, 1 July 1861 [in Italian].

[82] Westminster Dioc. Archives. Wiseman Papers, Bishops' Letters R79/5, Manning to Wiseman, 25 Sept. 1861.

of a Catholic University in England. It failed too, because the Jesuits were opposed: their own plan for a College had been rejected. But above all, it failed because the bishops took no real interest after the initial foundation, and made no financial contributions towards its maintenance. Manning was left with a sad legacy which included the long proceedings at Rome consequent upon Capel's suspension in the Westminster diocese, in 1883, for what Purcell called 'grave moral offences'.[83] There was an unhappy background of personal disagreements between Capel and Manning, with the usual appeals to Rome by both parties—Manning feeling 'that in Rome I was being undermined' by Capel's friends.[84] He withdrew priestly faculties from Capel, telling him that he 'must absent himself from England'—to Australia—but 'he refused to go away'.[85] Manning believed that he had 'every day fresh evidence and new proofs of great scandal', and was oppressed with the conviction that 'if he stays here the facts of his case will become public and his ruin irreparable'.[86] Capel, for his part, complained that Manning had taken away all possible alternatives, since he had told him that 'whatever diocese I went to he would have to inform the Bishop of the accusations.' He complained of how terribly he was 'crushed by the jealousy and envy of others.'[87] It was a cause of great anxiety to Manning also; but in the end Capel departed to America.

In another area, Manning's administrative and diplomatic accomplishments were more successful. In 1867 he acted as intermediary between the Irish Catholic bishops and Gladstone, at the time when Gladstone was formulating his new Irish policy of Disestablishment and Disendowment of the Protestant Church. In 1868 he continued these contacts—this time with Disraeli, who was seeking to conciliate Irish opinion by granting a Royal Charter to an Irish Catholic University. In 1873 he mediated over the University Bill proposed for

[83] Purcell, II. 581.
[84] Bristol Record Office 35721, Clifford Papers, Manning to Clifford, 31 May 1879.
[85] Ibid. Manning to Clifford, 10 June 1879.
[86] Ibid. Manning to Clifford, 22 June 1879.
[87] Ibid. Capel to Clifford, 26 June 1879.

Ireland by Gladstone. Again, in 1881, it was Manning who tried to persuade the Irish bishops to accept the Land Act, acting closely with Gladstone; and in 1885 he advised the Irish Viceroy, Lord Carnarvon. In 1885–6 he followed Gladstone's conversion to Home Rule. In 1887 he counselled Mgr. Persico, who was sent on a special mission to Ireland by the Papacy in order to ascertain the realities of the agrarian agitation—and whose report led to the condemnation of the Plan of Campaign by the Holy See in 1888. Manning actually believed this last act imprudent: 'Pontiffs have no infallibility in the world of facts . . .'.[88] Yet these essays in mediation were not in themselves particularly fruitful: the Irish policies whose acceptance he urged were not always adopted. Manning gave assurances to the parties concerned when he should not have done so, because they had no foundation in the opinions of others; and he led men to suppose that he had the entire confidence of others when he did not.[89] Such errors of judgement are easily made by those caught up in the close exchanges of semi-confidential negotiations. But Manning's Irish ventures *were* successful in another sense. His real objective was to re-establish a union of sentiment and action between the English and the Irish Catholic Churches. For this purpose he maintained close links with Cardinal Cullen and with his successor in Dublin, Archbishop Walsh. The motive was there from the beginning. In 1865 Manning had written to Cullen with the assurance that they had 'such an identity of principles that we need only a fuller and more personal knowledge of each other to renew the union which once partially existed'.[90] An alliance of the two Ultramontanes would strengthen the 'Roman' influence generally in the Church, and cancel out the remembered legacy of differences between English and Irish Catholics over the Veto question, early in the century, and over Irish political demands subsequently. Heavy Irish immigration to the English cities had, in the mid-century, reinforced the need for an understanding with the Irish Hierarchy. In 1866, Manning began inviting Irish Catholic

[88] Leslie, 429.

[89] Norman, *The Catholic Church and Ireland in the Age of Rebellion*, 245.

[90] Shane Leslie, 'Irish Pages from the Postbags of Manning, Cullen and Gladstone', in *Dublin Review*, Oct. 1919, 163.

Members of Parliament to his Tuesday evening receptions at Archbishop's House. To Manning belongs the credit of having achieved the working union he sought with the Irish. Few others could have managed it.

In another area of old conflict he was successful. It was Manning who contrived to secure a Roman definition of the place of the religious orders in the work of the English Church which brought stability to an area that had, throughout the century, been rich in the fruits of discord. Manning had, anyway, become a critic of the regulars: their involvement in parochial and educational work in England he seemed to find too worldly. He complained about Franciscans who wore gold watches. The Orders, for their part, disliked the encroachment of the bishops upon their schools—a feature which became more common as the dioceses responded to Manning's calls for more educational expansion. It was a dispute with the Jesuits which provided the immediate cause of confrontation. Despite his early connections with Farm Street, Manning had become markedly cold towards the Society over the years, and never allowed them to establish any secondary schools or colleges in the diocese of Westminster. At the Provincial Synod of 1873—Manning's only Provincial Synod—matters were discussed fully but without a solution. Manning objected to the privileges of the regulars; they objected to the attempt to restrict their educational work. In 1875 the dispute with the Jesuits over Fr. Gallwey's establishment of a school in Vaughan's diocese of Salford, without his permission, extended into a full-scale debate about the relations of the regulars and the seculars in England. Manning took the issue to Rome, where the ultimate solution was decided in 1881: the Bull *Romanos Pontifices*. His claims that the educational work of the Orders should come under episcopal control were upheld. As a result the work of the bishops was helped by the elimination of some unnecessary internal friction. The Orders, for their part, were not in the end unhappy with the new definition of their position. A settled relationship with the bishops was to their advantage. The Bull was one of Manning's most notable and enduring achievements.

Politics was the one area of his life in which Manning traced an uninterrupted development from early years. His youthful liberalism was conventional enough—rather like Pusey's—and had something of 'Tory Radicalism' about it. He supported the Reform Bill in 1832, but had opposed Catholic Emancipation in 1829 because it appeared to undermine the position of the Church of England. He became an advocate of Free Trade, and supported Peel. His responses, both then and throughout his life, were very similar to Gladstone's. Like Gladstone, he wanted a political career. He, too, moved over to the Liberal side, and then to a sort of populist radicalism whose rhetorical externals, when adjusted to real political action, were not unlike the Gladstonian style of the Midlothian Campaign. In 1889 Manning declared 'I am a Mosaic Radical. My watchword is, For God and the People.' The sentiment was Gladstonian; the reality was an adhesion to traditional institutions, suitably adapted to the circumstances of the times. In political outlook therefore, though not really in questions of social reform, Manning was a Gladstonian Liberal. The dislocated friendship of the two men was a major thread in his life. After the close correspondence of views on ecclesiastical matters following their first acquaintance at Oxford, Manning passed out of contact with Gladstone for ten years after his conversion. Then, from 1861 to 1873, their meetings and letters resumed; only to be interrupted again in 1875 by the public controversy over the Vatican Decrees. In 1887, following Manning's conversion to Home Rule for Ireland, by then Gladstone's adopted policy, their communications were resumed. Despite the blank years, the development of the two men disclosed many common features. Manning's association with radical groups was sometimes more overt than Gladstone allowed himself. Thus his support for the United Kingdom Alliance, which began in 1867, was very public: he spoke on their platforms at Manchester and elsewhere and became a Vice-President. When he died, members of the Alliance carried banners in his funeral procession. Manning was initially attracted to the Alliance because its central purpose was Temperance; but the Alliance was also a radical political movement whose integration with similar pressure-groups helped to give a popular basis to Gladstonian Liberalism. Manning must have known that by supporting the Alliance he was making a political statement. His support of Trade Unionism, however, and especially of rural Unionism, was an exception to his Gladstonianism: Gladstone himself tended to regard Unions as impediments to free contractual relationships in industry, they offended his sense of *laissez-faire* orthodoxy. Manning saw them as a matter of social reform. In 1878 and 1879 he made donations in support of agricultural labourers' unions, and spoke publicly in favour of Joseph Arch, the Dissenting and Radical leader of rural Unionism. By these years, his earlier 'Tory' characteristics had gone, buried forever by his antipathy to the traditional Catholic families in England whose Tory politics he found almost as unsympathetic as their 'worldly' religion. 'The old Catholic Toryism is the Toryism of Laud and Strafford's instincts, feelings, and tradition,' he wrote: 'without reason, principle, or foundation in the law of England.'[91] The Catholic Church should side with the people, he believed. The Anglicans had shown themselves unable to create a popular Church: but the example of Ireland, he argued, was of a union of sentiment between people and religion. The future of English Catholicism should lie in that, too, and not in the country estates of the Old Catholics.

The law of England was important to his political vision. He venerated the Constitution, which he regarded as a Catholic instrument: 'The Constitution of England is a Catholic structure inherited from our fathers.' But this sort of attitude did not result in traditionalism. Like many popular radicals, Whig historians, and Tory reformers, in the first half of the nineteenth century, Manning adhered to a belief that free institutions had existed in Saxon England—'it was the Norman and Angevin Kings that brought in Absolutism'—and that political society should move towards a restoration of the popular government which was then supposed to have existed. 'I believe', Manning wrote in 1890, 'the extension of the franchise and the admission of nearly two-thirds of the grown men of the people in the parliamentary suffrage to be a real return to the spirit of our old Saxon monarchy'.[92] Trade Unionism, too, he traced back to this event. 'If you go back to the earliest period of our Saxon history,' he said in 1874, 'you will find that there always were associations distinct

[91] Purcell, II. 631.   [92] Ibid. 636.

from the life of the family on the one side and from the State on the other.'[93] There was, at this juncture of Manning's political thinking, a faint and unconscious affinity with guild socialism and even with later doctrines of the corporate state. Between the state and the family, he contended, there was an area of 'the free action of men . . . which must be regulated by a law of its own'. Associations protected and expressed the life of that area—'as soon as we begin to trace anything in our Saxon history, we begin to trace the rise of guilds'.[94] Thereafter he developed the idea in support of labour organization, but not in order to unfold a political scheme for society in general. Combined with his belief in popular politics and universal suffrage, however, a certain similarity to guild socialism emerged. In 1864, he had written: 'If I have any politics they are popular, learned in the school which teaches that princes are for the people, not the people for princes.' It was a principle he accepted 'with all its consequences and corollaries'.[95] In 1890 he wrote, 'The rich can take care of themselves, and their underlings can help them. . . . My politics are social politics.'[96] Yet he was not a socialist. He added a measure of collectivism to the duties of the state —in an uneasy coexistence with the free-contract idealism of classical Liberalism—but socialism he regarded as the enemy of individual spiritual integrity. He was acquainted with the philosophical content of the European socialism condemned in the *Syllabus of Errors*. 'Socialism seems to me to denote an abnormal treatment of social needs and of society itself,' he observed in 1891; 'Socialism is to society what rationalism is to reason.'[97] He had no vision of social transformation by political or economic change: his was an advocacy of reforms for the people, an extention of the old 'Tory Radical' ideal, into the circumstances of the collectivist state. '*Salus populi suprema lex*', he quoted, in 1880; '"Class legislation" is treason against a commonwealth—legislation that does not reach and benefit the whole people is a political injustice.'[98]

[93] Manning, 'The Dignity and Rights of Labour' (1874), in *Miscellanies*, II. 86.
[94] Ibid. 87.
[95] Manning, 'The Visit of Garibaldi to England' (1864), ibid. I. 126.
[96] Purcell, II. 635.　　　　[97] Leslie, *Manning*, 378.
[98] Purcell, II. 630.

Manning disapproved of party political allegiances among the clergy, as he did for himself. This was in some degree because he disapproved of the parties: 'A desire for the welfare of the people in the largest sense, which eliminates the party politics of classes and of sectional interests, and above all, the dictates of a higher order of truths, would incline me to view with sympathy whatsoever is for the welfare of the people.'[99] There is again, here, a whiff of corporatism. He said, 'I have no faith in either Party.'[100] Yet he did believe that it was right for the clergy to have political opinions, provided they were not involved with party allegiances. 'I do not recognize any incompatibility between the sacred office I bear and the public treatment of these topics', he wrote in his *Letter to Earl Grey* (1868), in preparation for unfolding a scheme of reforms for Ireland. 'It is not our belief that ecclesiastics cease to be citizens or that anything affecting the common weal of our country is remote from our duty.'[101] In 1884 he directed the Catholic voters, in the anticipated general election, to support only those candidates favourable to increasing the grants to the Voluntary Schools. But that was a singular occurrence. He *did* believe that political life and institutional religion should be linked. Although he advocated Irish Disestablishment he was in favour of a union of church and state in England, even though the Protestant Establishment was, to him, a very imperfect representation of the Christianity which should inhabit the centre of national life. He was not concerned with the political claims of the Protestant Dissenters, whose secular and atomistic view of the state he found very deeply antipathetic. He was opposed to the atheist Charles Bradlaugh being allowed to take his parliamentary seat in 1881. His view of the state, in ideal terms, corresponded with the Christian confessional structure whose moral purposes were described by negative deduction in the *Syllabus of Errors*. That his own, English, belief in popular sovereignty was incompatible with the scheme there laid out does not seem to have troubled him.

It was for his social ideas and works that Manning was

[99] Manning, 'The Visit of Garibaldi to England', in *Miscellanies*, I. 126.
[100] Purcell, II. 608.
[101] Manning, 'Ireland, A Letter to Earl Grey' (1868), in *Miscellanies*, I. 214-5.

perhaps best remembered. He has generally been represented as a pioneer of Christian involvement in social reform and working-class causes, as being 'in the vanguard of the working class movement'.[102] His beliefs and actions in this area were not, however, particularly unusual. Manning reflected the social service idealism which was actually spread rather thickly across the Church leadership of England in the second half of the nineteenth century. Reference to the speeches made by Anglican bishops and divines at the Church congresses, held annually from 1861, will show how preoccupied they had become with discussion of the need for collectivist social reforms in such matters as working-class housing or sanitation, and with employment and industrial questions; statements issued by the Anglican Lambeth Conferences of 1888 and 1897 on social issues were progressive in tone.[103] Manning is remembered for his mediation in the Dock Strike of 1889, as a member of the Committee of Conciliation set up at the Mansion House—and for his patient endurance when the Anglican Bishop of London, Frederick Temple, having alienated the strikers' leader Ben Tillett, left the negotiations in order to go on holiday in Wales. The end of the strike was popularly called 'the Cardinal's Peace'. Afterwards Manning wrote to Lord Buxton, 'the more I think, the more I am on the side of Labour'.[104] But other Anglican prelates mediated in strikes: Bishop James Fraser of Manchester in 1878, Bishop Brooke Foss Westcott of Durham in 1892, and Bishop Mandell Creighton of Peterborough in 1895. Indeed, it was Manning's social interests which showed how close parts of his thinking remained to the developing attitudes of the English intelligentsia, however much his Ultramontanism was offended by the rationalism and infidelity of contemporary learning. Most of his Catholic contemporaries were shut out from all this; they lacked his acquaintance with the social service idealism of the Protestant universities and the Protestant intellectuals. Vaughan attributed his support of labour causes

[102] Gordon Wheeler, 'The Archdiocese of Westminster', in *The English Catholics, 1850–1950*, ed. Beck, 162.

[103] See Norman, *Church and Society in England, 1770–1970*, 123–67.

[104] V. A. McClelland, *Cardinal Manning. His Public Life and Influence, 1865–1892*, London 1962, 147.

to senility.[105] What appeared singular and, in the perspective of later developments, pioneering in Manning was, however, a view only from within English Catholicism. In the wider context of the English Churches his interests looked quite normal, and abreast of the times. That Manning was often more *successful* in his work for social causes did indeed put him in a separate category, but that is another matter from regarding his vision as a novel one.

Manning's social attitudes closely paralleled the general shifts of thought and practice within the established classes. As an Anglican he shared the paternalism and charitable instincts which were then regarded as the proper duty of a parson. He took an interest in the social issues of the times—education, the poor law, factory reform, the penal code, the housing of agricultural labourers—and his *Charges* as Archdeacon of Chichester urged attention to them. He shared, too, the prevalent adhesion to the principles of Political Economy, and to the limited view of state action required for their free operation. When, in the mid-century, the leaders of opinion began to criticize *laissez-faire* practices, and to move towards an acceptance of state intervention in areas where social reform was too urgent or too protected by vested interests to occur by individual initiative, Manning moved along with the tide. Whilst retaining a general belief in the principle of Political Economy, he contended for exceptions in cases of pressing need. The adjustment is seen most clearly in his most celebrated social statement: *The Dignity and Rights of Labour*, a lecture delivered to the Leeds Mechanics' Institute in 1874. First came the—by then conventional—critique of capitalism; it was necessary to realize that skill as well as capital was the cause of wealth, he argued: 'I claim for labour the rights of property.'[106] He went on to defend the organization of labour to protect its own freedom. Yet he also declared that contractual relationships 'cannot be meddled with by the public authority of the State;—I mean the whole order of commerce'. He added, 'Clearly, therefore, there is a certain field which must be regulated by a law of its own.'[107] This

---

[105] Snead-Cox, *The Life of Cardinal Vaughan*, I. 477.
[106] Manning, 'The Dignity and Rights of Labour' (1874), in *Miscellanies*, II. 81.
[107] Ibid. II. 87.

was classical *laissez-faire*. Next, he produced what he called 'a politico-economical heresy'. Declaring his 'great respect' for Political Economy, he said: 'I entirely believe—as you may have seen—in the law of supply and demand and free exchange and safety of capital, which are the first conditions of industry'; but he could not go along with those who denounced all state intervention. 'The principle of free-trade is not applicable to everything'; this was because 'it is met and checked by a moral condition'.[108] It was, of course, just such a consciousness of this 'moral condition' which had made the factory reformers in the 1830s and 1840s violate the principles of Political Economy by state intervention in contractual relationships. Manning's was not an original or even an unusual position. He was rather more open to the idea of state intervention in land contracts than was usual, however: this was an area which even quite advanced critics of *laissez-faire* in England were inclined to leave alone. In discussing the Irish land question, indeed, in 1868, he laid down some natural law principles which should govern landed relationships. There was, he wrote in his *Letter to Earl Grey*, 'a natural and divine law' by which 'every people has a right to live of the fruits of the soil on which they are born'. This was 'a right older and higher than any personal right'.[109] In the actual conditions of Ireland, he argued, this required legislation to secure to the tenants a just return for their labour. 'There is no right of private property which is not modified, not only by those higher laws, but also by a multitude of positive enactments, based only on public utility.[110] There could be quite radical implications from this, and Henry George, who was also, of course, interested in the Irish land problem, visited Manning in 1886 and came away with the impression that the Cardinal shared his views—on the single tax and agrarian socialism.[111] Manning did not, however; he believed, also as a natural and divine law, in the legitimacy of private property. George, who in the year of his visit, received support from the Catholic clergy in his campaign for Mayor of New York City, probably supposed that

[108] Ibid. II. 93.
[109] Manning, 'Ireland. A Letter to Earl Grey' (1868), in *Miscellanies*, II. 239.
[110] Ibid. II. 240.   [111] Purcell, II. 649; Leslie, 353.

Manning's social involvement was like theirs. Believing as he did in social justice applied in landed relationships it was not surprising, given his disposition to defend the rights of labour to protect itself, that Manning should have supported rural Trades Unionism. Thus in 1872, the year of the great agricultural workers' strike organized by Joseph Arch, Manning not only gave his support to the cause but also attended a public demonstration on behalf of the Unionists. Arch said, 'The testimony at such a time and in such a place of a man so respected was of the greatest value to the Union.'[112]

Most of the progressive causes of the day which were outside the area of industrial relations or social reform did not attract Manning, perhaps because they were promoted by interests or parties which were secular. He refused to receive feminists at Archbishop's House, regarding the place of women as in the home. He rejected progressive educational schemes because of their frank secularity. Though an advocate of working-class recreations he was actually opposed to most of the recreations they enjoyed. His reputation as a social reformer, which is amply justified, rests on his championing of the cause of the poor, and his perception that society had somehow to adjust so that their condition might be improved by justice rather than by charity. 'The accumulation of wealth in the land, the piling up of wealth like mountains, in the possession of classes or of individuals, cannot go on,' he declared; 'No commonwealth can rest on such foundations.'[113] It would be an error to exaggerate Manning's international influence as a social reformer, however. Cardinal Gibbons of Baltimore acknowledged the inspiration his own campaign on behalf of organized labour—his defence of the Knights of Labor against potential censure at the Vatican—had received from Manning's example. But the supposition that Leo XIII's great 'social' encyclicals, and especially *Rerum Novarum* (1891), were in some large measure inspired by Manning cannot be substantiated and is in itself unlikely.[114] The European Catholic world in the second half of the nineteenth century,

---

[112] Leslie, 350.
[113] 'The Dignity and Rights of Labour', in *Miscellanies*, II. 97.
[114] For accounts of Manning's supposed influence on the Encyclicals see Leslie, 378–80; McClelland, 158; Holmes, 184.

like the English sceptics of *laissez-faire* orthodoxy, had furnished its own social critiques. Manning was not an original social thinker.

It was his *action* in social reform that made him most impressive—the more so since the notion of a Catholic Cardinal taking a prominent part in English public life was an unusual one for Protestant and Catholic observers alike. In 1870 he was invited to become a member of the Mansion House Relief Fund for those who suffered in the Paris Commune; and thereafter, throughout his life, he served on numerous Mansion House Committees for charitable and social purposes. Manning was also appointed, in 1884, to the Royal Commission on the housing of the working classes, which sat under Sir Charles Dilke and reported in 1885. Like many churchmen and philanthropists in the nineteenth century, he was impressed by the connection between moral behaviour and environmental circumstance. Between 1887 and 1888 he was a member of the Committee on Distress in London. He was also particularly concerned to promote medical care, and was among those who encouraged Florence Nightingale. His love of animals converted him into an anti-vivisectionist: he was Vice-President of the Victoria Street Society from its foundation in 1876. In 1886 he became concerned with systematic emigration, as another way of helping the poor to a better life. He joined the National Association for Promoting State-Directed Colonization. The most important of his philanthropic enterprises, however, was undoubtedly Temperance. Here, the influence of environment upon the moral behaviour and prospects of the poor was especially dramatic, and in 1867 Manning was persuaded by the arguments of the United Kingdom Alliance in favour of more restrictive liquor licensing to help reduce the social evil of drunkenness. In 1872 he managed to get 170 of the Catholic clergy in his diocese to petition Parliament in support of Bruce's Licensing Bill.[115] In that year also, and fired by the example of the Salvation Army, Manning established the League of the Cross, a Catholic campaign for Temperance, with the help of

---

[115] Brian Harrison, *Drink and the Victorians. The Temperance Question in England, 1815–1872*, London 1971, 268.

Fr. Nugent. It was to be his most important philanthropic undertaking—it was also his most controversial, attracting the hostility of many Catholics unpersuaded by his arguments and example. Manning signed the pledge himself.

Manning's most important social work was unquestionably education. It was his own priority: the values which children acquired in the classroom affected their eternal salvation and furnished the spiritual climate of family and national life. Education had to be distinctly Christian, and in the circumstances of England that meant denominational, since it was a society of plural religious allegiance. Secular education promoted Indifferentism and Scepticism. The teaching of a common formula of Christianity (as in the Irish National Schools after 1831 and the English Board Schools after 1870) was not really Christian but secular, because it divided real education—the acquisition of values and not just of knowledge—from the area of Revealed Truth, as represented by the Churches. 'The national character was chiefly formed in its Christian schools', Manning wrote in 1886, as he surveyed the preceding centuries of educational endeavour; 'What character will be formed in schools without Christianity?'[116] The Board Schools set up by the state, and the Voluntary Schools of the Churches, were 'mutually exclusive'. Every year the Board Schools, 'fraught with antagonistic principles', were 'penetrating the legislation and structure of the commonwealth, and tainting the brain and blood of the governing classes'.[117] Religious understanding in England was the first victim—'Dr. Colenso is a fair sample of the actual and dominant tendency of religious belief among us'.[118]

A concern with education, and particularly (because the most urgent), with primary education, had preoccupied Manning from his earliest years. As Rector of Lavington, and as Archdeacon of Chichester, he had worked to promote the denominational ideals of the National Society, and had even then endeavoured to separate the question of the schools from political entanglement. The Education issue, he wrote

[116] H. E. Manning, *The Future of the Primary Schools*, London 1886, 4.
[117] Ibid. 7.
[118] Manning, 'The Work and Wants of the Catholic Church in England', (1863), in *Miscellanies*, I. 70.

in 1838, 'wears only by accident a political, or civil aspect; its real character is moral and spiritual: and its importance not temporal alone, but eternal; involving the everlasting welfare of souls for whom Christ died'.[119] As a Catholic his educational priorities remained intact. His first three Pastoral Letters, as Archbishop of Westminster, were taken up with educational questions—with the need for more Catholic schools for poor children. He laid aside plans to build a cathedral in London, as a memorial to his predecessor, in order to promote fund-raising for education. In 1866 he established the Westminster Diocesan Education Fund and had, within a year, set up twenty schools. Yet despite his opposition to non-denominational education, and a scepticism about the wisdom of accepting state grants towards the maintenance of Church schools which dated from his Anglican years, Manning believed in co-operating with the government over education. This was, in part, because he believed, as many Catholics and Anglicans did not, that the state had a right to involve itself with education—both because the educational needs of an expanding society were outstripping the resources of the Churches and because of the nature of civil government itself. The state, he wrote in 1886, 'has a right to protect itself from the dangers arising from ignorance and vice, which breed crime and turbulence'. It had 'a duty also to protect children from the neglect and sin of parents, and to guard their rights to receive an education that shall fit them for human society and for civil life'.[120] In 1870 he committed the Catholic Church to co-operation with the new 'Dual System', of Voluntary and Board schools, created by Forster's Education Act. Most of the bishops were sceptical; some were hostile. They were in Rome at the time, for the Vatican Council. But before departing from London, Manning had already proposed a compromise to the government: Catholic inspectors would be given up in return for the advantage of increased maintenance grants, and a guaranteed statutory basis for denominational education. Despite Professor McClelland's contention that Manning did not even

---

[119] *National Education*, 10.
[120] H. E. Manning, *Is the Education Act of 1870 a Just Law?* London 1886, 4.

consult the bishops in Rome on the matter,[121] he did in fact call a meeting at the English College. An account of it exists in a letter of Ullathorne's, now in the Birmingham Diocesan Archives. It was not, from the bishops' point of view, a very satisfactory occasion. Ullathorne, according to his account of the meeting, questioned Manning closely about his actual knowledge of Forster's Bill. 'He said he knew nothing', Ullathorne recorded; 'This surprised everyone.'[122] Manning himself subsequently began to have some doubts about the wisdom of co-operating with the new system,[123] and his later years were filled with attempts to get the level of support from taxation for the denominational schools put on the same basis as the Board Schools. But he retained a belief in the practical importance of co-operation with the state: it gave the Catholics a share 'in the treatment of questions which may affect us', as he told Ullathorne.[124] 'To propose the repeal of the Education Act of 1870 would be like proposing the repeal of the Gregorian Calendar', he observed in 1886: 'The principles embodied in the Act of 1870 cannot be rescinded; they ought rather to be carried out to their full and complete application'.[125] The Education rate should be extended to the Voluntary Schools; it was a matter of ordinary justice that those who paid tax should benefit equally by it.[126] Manning's preparedness to co-operate with the state over the education question placed him in a position somewhat at odds with the other bishops. This had become evident in 1869, when he had approved the principle of state intervention to modernize the legal trusts of the endowed schools; the differences of 1870 widened the divergences. But there was never a disruption over the schools question. Manning pursued a moderate and conciliatory course with the bishops, carrying them along as the years proceeded. In no other field was his skill as a diplomatist so exhaustively tested. The Voluntary Schools Association, founded in 1884 as part of the

[121] McClelland, 80.
[122] Birmingham Dioc. Archives, B.4796, Ullathorne to the Vicar General, 23 Feb. 1870.
[123] Purcell, II. 494.
[124] McClelland, 70.
[125] *Is the Education Act of 1870 a Just Law?*, 3.
[126] Ibid. 11.

campaign to get a Catholic share of the education rate, was intended to stimulate a public scrutiny of the 1870 Act and to oblige Parliament to reconsider, not its principles, but its terms. In 1885 there was some success: Salisbury's administration set up the Cross Commission to enquire into the working of the 1870 Act, and Manning was himself appointed to serve on it. 'The Denominationalists are in large majority', Manning wrote to Clifford, on his appointment to the Commission; but they were not 'united in our needs'.[127] The majority report of 1888 endorsed the policy of extending the rate to the Voluntary Schools. It was not, however implemented. Manning had, during all these years, also been concerned to foster secondary education. By the time of his death in 1892, he had founded twelve secondary schools in London, often with the help of the Marist Brothers. It was an impressive achievement; an enduring and visible sign of his social service. Manning is rightly remembered for his love of the poor.

[127] Bristol Record Office, 35721, Clifford Papers, Manning to Clifford, 28 Dec. 1885.

7
Catholic Learning

The mid-century conversions of Anglicans to the Catholic faith made an enormous difference to the intellectual culture of the English Catholics. However much university reformers and liberals of the time may have complained about the condition of the ancient universities, the infusion of Oxford standards of academic endeavour raised the entire level of Catholic higher studies—especially since the leading converts, like Newman and Ward, were by any evaluation men of quite outstanding intellectual distinction. The contrast, between the new Catholics and the old, was not lost on contemporaries: it was the occasion of much ill-feeling following the *Rambler* articles dismissive of Catholic education; for the *Rambler* was the vehicle of the converts' continuing pursuit of the sort of academic enquiry they had been accustomed to at Oxford and elsewhere. The article on 'Catholic and Protestant Collegiate Education' in 1848, written by the editor, John Moore Capes, was based upon his knowledge of the standards and methods of Prior Park, where he had been Professor of Mathematics.[1] It caused great offence to Ullathorne and others. So did a similar article in 1856, which was explicit in its contention that the English Catholics were ignorant of intellectual culture. Wiseman was particularly incensed by it.[2] In fact, although the contrast between the academic sophistication of the converts and the Old Catholic scholars—as well as those recently educated in Rome—was in general a real one, it did a considerable injustice both to the extent and the quality of existing scholarship within the English Catholic Church. At the time of the large-scale conversions, the state of Catholic higher studies in England was in transition. It had been dominated at the start of the century by the returning regular

[1] Joseph Altholz, *The Liberal Catholic Movement in England*, Montreal 1962, 16.
[2] Wilfrid Ward, *The Life and Times of Cardinal Wiseman*, II. 207, 229.

orders, at Ushaw and Downside, and by the higher studies section at Stonyhurst. The regulars' control of higher education was, indeed, an important element in the controversies between the Vicars-Apostolic and the orders, and lay behind some of the disputes over diocesan seminaries. But just as in the Anglican Church the reforms of the century witnessed the transfer of the control of the ancient universities from the clergy to the laity, so within Catholicism, too, there was a movement from the regulars to the seculars in higher education, and then from the seculars to the conciliation of increasing demands for lay participation. The arrival of the converts accelerated the existing impulses. The regulars did not relinquish their position without misgivings: Kensington University College, set up by the bishops in 1873, was met with reservations by the Benedictines and with hostility from the Jesuits. Though under a clerical Rector, it had a largely lay teaching staff. The lay and Liberal Catholic campaigns for the relaxation of the episcopal prohibition of attendance at the national universities was a further impulsion towards the 'secularization' of Catholic higher education.

Though broadly correct in their assessment, the converts tended to exaggerate the humble attainments of existing Catholic learning. They probably expected poor standards of those to whom the formal outlets of professional life had been denied by the penal laws; but what shocked both the converts and the Old Catholic 'Liberal' scholars, like Acton, however, was the style of learning characteristic of those who had spent years at the prestigious pontifical institutions of education. Roman intellectual discipline appeared to reside in an ordered representation of scholastic thinking and in categorizations of the later canonists, rather than in critical analysis. It is fundamental to an understanding of the scorn some liberal Catholics felt for the Ultramontanists in England —most of whom were educated in Rome—that they held this view of Roman scholarship. Newman, when he studied at Propaganda in 1846–7, was shocked by the condition of theological education in the city.[3] Acton held Wiseman's scholarship in low esteem—and Wiseman was regarded as one

---

[3] Meriol Trevor, *Newman. The Pillar of the Cloud*, London 1962, 402.

of the best of the Roman scholars in England. Of his *Recollections of the Last Four Popes* (1858), Acton remarked: 'There is absolutely nothing new to be learned from it.'[4] Yet there were some fine scholars among the English Catholics in the first half of the nineteenth century. Men like Thomas Eyre, Bishop William Gibson, John Gillow, and Charles Newsham, belonged to a style of learning which still reflected the English Colleges on the continent and was characterized by accuracy of knowledge and detail rather than by critical thought; but they could stand comparison with the typical Anglican divines of Oxford or Cambridge of the period—rather than with leading Anglican scholars like Paley or Whately.

It was a feature of nineteenth-century intellectual life that it thrived through periodical literature: and of that the Catholics, too, had developed an interesting range before the arrival of the Oxford converts. The polemical sharpness, characteristic of the times, was also much evidenced in it. But as a stimulant to Catholic intellectual awareness these papers and journals were important. The *Catholic Magazine*, begun in 1801, had a short existence, as did the *Conciliator* of 1813. The *Orthodox Journal*—which its opponents called the 'Pseudodox'—was the first successful publication. It was founded by a Norwich journalist of extreme views (used against the Catholic Board) called William Eusebius Andrews. The first numbers appeared after his move to London in 1813, and publication continued until 1820. A brief revival in the 1840s was unsuccessful. 'My sole motive', Andrews wrote, 'was to aid the cause of the Catholic Church, and to caution my Catholic brethren against the workings of a party, who have entailed more disgrace upon the Catholic name by their casuistical policy, than all the calumnies raised against it by our enemies since the Reformation.'[5] Bishop Milner used the columns of the *Orthodox* in order to attack Bishop Poynter. In 1815 the *Publicist* appeared (known after 1816 as *Catholicon*); and in 1818 Charles Butler founded the *Catholic Gentleman's Magazine*. That so many of these publications

---

[4] Altholz, 67.
[5] Bernard Ward, *The Eve of Catholic Emancipation*, II. 174.

were ephemeral was not an indication of the absence of a receptive readership. Protestant journalism of the time was just the same. Papers tended to be founded to combat or promote particular issues—phases of the Catholic Emancipation question, for example—and their steam ran out with the passing of the selected issue. *The Tablet*, founded by Frederick Lucas in 1840, at the suggestion of Father Lythgoe, Provincial of the Jesuits,[6] was the most famous, as well perhaps as the most forthright, of the Catholic journals of the pre-convert era. Lucas promoted his Whig principles by describing his opponents, in its pages, as 'scoundrels', 'plunderers', and 'rogues'. He frequently compared the acts of Tory adversaries with those of 'common pickpockets'.[7] In 1850 *The Tablet* moved to Dublin—a reflection of Lucas's increasing preoccupation with Irish politics. It returned to London with Lucas's successor as editor, John Edward Wallis, who changed the whole tone of the paper: he was a Tory. In 1868 it was sold to Vaughan. In 1860 the *Universe* was founded—Wiseman's attempt to produce an English equivalent of Veuillot's *L'Univers*. It was run by the Society of St. Vincent de Paul. The *Month* began in 1864, with considerable support from the Jesuits, as a Catholic literary journal. In 1882 Gasquet established the *Downside Review* as an academic periodical. The Catholic Truth Society, founded by Vaughan in 1884, was conducted by James Britten, a convert who worked in the British Museum. It was to have an enduring importance in the dissemination of information about Catholic doctrines, especially in its output of pamphlets and its publication in English of Papal documents.

The great exception to the belief that little authentic learning was to be found among the English Catholics in the first half of the century was John Lingard, author of a successful and widely acclaimed *History of England*. He was born in Winchester in 1771, the son of a carpenter, and educated, from the age of eleven, at Douai. When the forces of the French Revolution occupied the College in 1793 he escaped to England, and joined Lord Stourton's household as a tutor.

---

[6] Edward Lucas, *The Life of Frederick Lucas, M.P.*, London 1886, I. 31.
[7] Bernard Ward, *The Sequel to Catholic Emancipation*, II. 33.

It was there that he made his first acquaintance with leading Catholic figures. In 1794 he moved to Crook Hall in order to join up with part of the reassembled Douai. He was ordained a deacon there in 1794, and was raised to the priesthood by Bishop Gibson at York in the following year. Thereafter he taught at Ushaw—and in 1821 was awarded a DD by the Pope for his work there—but in 1811 he left the College, having failed to succeed Eyre as President in the preceding year. He lived the rest of the forty years of his life at Hornby, near Lancaster, devoting himself to his historical writing. He retained a great affection for the College, visiting often, and leaving it his library and his railway stocks in his will. A measure of his distinction was the widespread supposition— shared by Lingard himself—that at the consistory of 1826 Leo XII had created him a cardinal *in petto*. Wiseman later claimed it was Lamennais, and not Lingard, who was elevated in 1826.[8] There is no doubt about the offer of a bishopric in 1817, however. Lingard declined it in order to continue his historical studies. His first book, *Antiquities of the Anglo-Saxon Church*, was published in 1806. It was thorough but unremarkable. Research over the years for his great *History of England* proceeded at the State Paper Office in the Tower of London. The work was initially rejected by two Catholic publishers, and accepted by a Protestant one—Joseph Mawman, who brought out the first three volumes in 1819. They were attacked by Milner in the *Orthodox Journal*—for not being *Catholic* history at all. They were, that is to say, the fruit of genuine historical research, and not polemical or partisan writing. The volumes, Milner wrote, were 'only calculated to confirm Protestants in their errors'.[9] By later standards of historical scholarship, Lingard's *History* appears, despite that judgement, rather uncritical; but it was a landmark in English historical writing for its use of original sources. He was, indeed, dismissive of Macaulay's *History*, published in 1848, precisely because, in his judgement, it lacked objectivity. 'Macaulay does not write history', he contended; 'His work abounds in claptrap of every description.'[10] Phrases used by

[8] Martin Haile and Edwin Bonney, *Life and Times of John Lingard, 1771–1851*, London 1912, 220–2.
[9] Ibid. 171.   [10] Ibid. 343.

Macaulay, like 'Popish idolatry and superstition', were cited to illustrate his point. The book, he concluded, was 'factless'.[11] The last of Lingard's own eight volumes appeared in 1830, and the entire work went through seven English editions up to 1883. The success of Lingard's study led to translations into Italian, French, and German. In 1821 the agent of the English bishops in Rome testified to the esteem in which the work was held at the Vatican.[12] As well as these labours of authorship, Lingard took an active part in Catholic issues of the day, especially Catholic Emancipation—on which question he showed markedly Cisalpine tendencies[13]—and in the affairs of the Northern District. He also wrote many pamphlets, championing the seculars against the regulars. In later life 'his advice was asked on every conceivable subject'.[14] He died at Hornby in 1851 and was buried in the cloister at Ushaw.

Just as intellectual life in general was not so negligible as the converts alleged, so the Catholic Colleges, too, were capable of better learning than was sometimes supposed. Nor were they particularly good, however: a balance of view is needed. Thus Wilfrid Ward's judgement of St. Edmund's College, Ware, on the eve of W. G. Ward's arrival in the 1840s —'There was not much intellectual culture . . . Theology was not a welcome subject of discussion'[15]—conveys more of the author's desire to heighten the impact of his father's beneficial influence than it relates about the actual condition of the College. The higher studies at Stonyhurst and Oscott achieved very respectable standards—but they were not a satisfactory substitute for a proper university course with a recognized degree. There could be no real entry of English Catholics into the professions until they could get degrees. The fruits of Emancipation still waited on the bough. A few Catholics did reside at colleges of the ancient universities in the first half of the century, but they could not proceed to

---

[11] Ibid. 345.

[12] Westminster Dioc. Archives, Gradwell Papers, Letter Books B3(22 March 1821).

[13] See Joseph P. Chinnici, *The English Catholic Enlightenment: John Lingard and the Cisalpine Movement, 1780–1850*, Shepherdstown (West Virginia), 1980.

[14] Haile and Bonney, 359.

[15] Wilfrid Ward, *William George Ward and the Catholic Revival*, 7.

degrees until the reforms of the 1850s: from 1854 Catholics, along with other Dissenters, could proceed to the BA degree, and from 1856 they could proceed to the MA degree at Cambridge—which had always been more liberal in this respect. English Catholics had attended Trinity College, Dublin since 1793. London University acquired its charter in 1835, and this proved beneficial to Catholics in a limited way. It was a secular institution, to which colleges could apply for affiliation and then prepare and present students for degrees. Ushaw, Stonyhurst, Prior Park, Downside, Oscott, and St. Edmund's all affiliated, and this resulted in considerable internal changes in their curricula, in order to make them coincide with the new degree courses. To some Catholics, however, the secular nature of London University was as distasteful as the secular Queen's Colleges were to prove to the Irish Catholic hierarchy in 1845. W. G. Ward assailed the London arrangements as not really being university *education* at all: there was no association of religion and learning.[16] The Irish, prompted by Propaganda, were to solve their problem by the creation of a Catholic University. The English bishops, while aware of the small numbers and the more limited financial resources of English Catholicism, began to consider this possibility quite early. Baines had originally intended to found a Catholic University at Prior Park in 1834, but ran into the opposition of Wiseman. As President of Oscott in 1840, Wiseman himself had hoped it might evolve into a university.[17] It is not true, as some have imagined, that it was the arrival of the Oxford converts in the Church which first awakened the English Catholics to the need for proper higher learning. In 1861 Wiseman set up his 'Academy of the Catholic Religion' in London, in an attempt to cultivate a sense that Catholicism and scientific learning were naturally united. Liberal Catholics suspected it of being window-dressing for Ultramontanism.[18] By 1863 Wiseman and Manning were again considering the possibility of a Catholic University—and perhaps, also, of a new Catholic academy for English students in

---

[16] V. A. McClelland, *English Roman Catholics and Higher Education, 1830–1903*, Oxford 1973, 65.
[17] Ibid. 17.
[18] Holmes, *More Roman than Rome*, 121.

Rome. It was such aspirations which provided the background to the Oxford Oratory schemes of the 1860s.

The first steps towards the foundation of a Catholic Hall in Oxford seem to have been taken in the second half of 1863, by Edmund Ffoulkes, a convert who had formerly been a fellow of Jesus College. He proposed a committee for the purpose, mostly of the Catholic aristocracy, and to include Newman. His attempt to secure the support of Bishop Grant merely had the effect of bringing the plans to the attention of the hierarchy.[19] Wiseman had before this shown himself enthusiastic for a Catholic College at Oxford: it was 'the very fulfillment of the desire of his heart'.[20] But recent evidences of the condition of thought at Oxford—now controlled by liberal dons and seemingly heterodox theologians—together with Manning's opposition, had swung him round. The publication of *Essays and Reviews* in 1860 had seemed to indicate how hazardous the English universities were to faith. The undisciplined life of the undergraduates had already established that there were dangers to morals. After receiving warning signals from London, Propaganda instructed the hierarchy to consider the matter at the Low Week Meeting of 1864. There the bishops rejected the Oxford Hall project and decided in principle to instruct the clergy to dissuade Catholic parents from sending their sons to the national universities. They also decided against a Catholic university. No public pronouncement of the policy was made.

Ullathorne, meanwhile, though he fully endorsed the line taken by the hierarchy (and especially the decision to make no formal prohibition of attendance at the universities) was worried about the pastoral condition of Catholics in Oxford, which was in his diocese. So he invited Newman to set up an Oratorian house in the city. From Newman's point of view the advantages were enormous. He had just completed the *Apologia* and had every expectation of emerging from the shadows; boys were already evidently being prepared for university entrance in the courses at the Oratory School in Birmingham; in Oxford he could resume something of his old

[19] McClelland, *English Roman Catholics*, 193.
[20] Purcell, *Life and Letters of Ambrose Phillipps de Lisle*, II. 2.

influence. In August 1864, he purchased land in Oxford for the Oratory, which, he hoped, would take in student lodgers —though having no other link with the University as such— and so could well evolve into a Hall or College in due time. At an episcopal meeting in December 1864, however, the hierarchy drew up a letter to Propaganda offering explicit objections to a Catholic presence at Oxford, and spelling out the policy agreed at the Low Week gathering. Two of the bishops actually favoured an outright ban on attendance at the Universities. No actual mention was made of Newman or the Oratory plans. In February 1865, Propaganda confirmed these decisions and generally condemned 'mixed education' —the education of Catholics and Protestants in the same institution—since this, in the course of things, tended to separate sacred and secular learning, and so fostered Indifferentism. By a *Rescript* of August 1867, Propaganda formally declared that Catholics sending their sons to the universities would be guilty of their exposure to the occasions of sin. There was still no formal prohibition, which might be enforced by ecclesiastical penalties. The bishops were instructed to declare these judgements to the laity, which they did through their individual pastoral letters in 1867.

In 1866, however, Ullathorne again invited Newman to set up an Oratory in Oxford. In the light of the episcopal discussion and the instructions of Propaganda he doubtless felt he could do so in the knowledge that neither Newman nor anyone else could mistake the move for an attempt to create a Catholic presence in the University. Ullathorne was still concerned about the pastoral care of the city. Newman, who had abandoned the earlier scheme and sold the land he had purchased, now prepared once again to return to Oxford. Propaganda sanctioned the new proposal—but with the proviso, which Ullathorne withheld from Newman, because he hoped to be able to get it rescinded, that Newman himself should not reside in Oxford. The Pope himself had supposed that Newman's presence in Oxford would attract Catholic youths to the University[21] and so nullify the *Rescript* of 1865. Newman must have realized how critical the question

[21] McClelland, *English Roman Catholics*, 222.

of students would become and how impossible, in the nature of a university like Oxford, whose colleges are distributed throughout the city, would be any attempt to separate the pastoral and academic work of the proposed Oratory. In November 1864, when the first scheme had run into episcopal opposition, he had written to Ullathorne to say that he made his 'going to Oxford dependent upon a great existing need, the fact of Catholics being in the University'. He added: 'If they are not there, an Oratory is unnecessary.'[22] The circumstances had not changed. Hence the fears at Rome. But Newman had other episcopal support apart from Ullathorne's. Clifford wrote to express his delight that Newman was to return to Oxford (and to enclose a personal donation of £20 for the proposed Oratory): 'I bless and thank God for thus allowing you, after so many strange events, to gather in with your own hand in gladness some portion of the harvest which long ago was sown by you in sorrow.'[23] But the reaper remained in Birmingham. Unable to act as the superior of the Oxford house himself, Newman could see no purpose in pressing the scheme further, and it lapsed. Vaughan reported him to Talbot as saying 'that nothing could now induce him to go to Oxford'.[24] No further Oratories were established in England, and the Birmingham and London houses alone represented the rule of St. Philip Neri in English Catholicism.

Catholic opposition to the Oxford schemes did not rest entirely on the foundation provided by the theological liberalism of the Protestant divines. But it was an important motive—combined with the suspicion, entertained by Ultramontanes, that Newman himself participated in some of the errors. W. G. Ward regarded the Oxford of the period as the seed-bed of Indifferentism, and attacked the plans for a Catholic presence in the University in the *Dublin Review*. Catholic higher education, he contended, must be in institutions where the students acquire 'the instinctive habit of

[22] *The Letters and Diaries of John Henry Newman*, ed. C. S. Dessain, London 1971, xxi, 319.
[23] Bristol Record Office 35721, Clifton Diocesan Archives, Clifford Papers, Clifford to Newman, 5 Feb. 1867.
[24] English College Archives, Talbot Papers, 715, Vaughan to Talbot, 6 May, n.d.

obedience to ecclesiastical authority'.[25] Newman had a rather different view of university education. Opponents of the Oxford schemes could also turn to the condemnation made by Rome of the Queen's Colleges in Ireland, set up explicitly to provide 'mixed education' and rejected by the Irish Catholic hierarchy precisely for that reason. Oxford, like Cambridge, was also the chief place of training for the clergy of the State Church: Anglican theological colleges were only just beginning to be founded at this time. Some Catholic bishops disapproved of Catholic youths being educated at Oxford just for that reason. 'The Universities are the stronghold of the National Establishment, where the clergymen are trained to continue its worship and where statesmen are found who must be its defenders in the senate of the kingdom', Grant wrote in his *Pastoral* of 1867; 'the atmosphere is pervaded by Protestant opinion.'[26] Furthermore, the reforms of the 1850s, which had admitted non-Anglicans to the degrees of ancient universities, were themselves inspired by the very liberalism and latitudinarianism which the Catholics most dreaded.[27] Petitions organized by the laity in support of the attendance of Catholics at the universities, in 1865 and 1867, indicated to some Church leaders, as to Talbot in Rome—who regarded them as an insult to the bishops—that Catholics were already showing signs of picking up some unsound critical attitudes from their Protestant neighbours. Propaganda still pressed the English hierarchy to consider a Catholic university of their own, and they discussed the matter at episcopal meetings in 1868 and 1869.[28] While this plan had priority at Rome, there was little chance of any substantial concessions which would allow Catholics to secure degrees in the national universities. Nor should it be forgotten that these were also the years when Ambrose Phillipps de Lisle was urging his Reunion initiatives upon the Church. His support for the Oxford Hall proposals, and for Catholic attendance at the Universities,[29] was actually

[25] Wilfrid Ward, *William George Ward*, 192.

[26] O'Meara, *Thomas Grant. First Bishop of Southwark*, 233.

[27] H. O. Evennett, 'Catholics and the Universities', in *The English Catholics 1850–1950*, ed. Beck, 293.

[28] Westminster Dioc. Archives, ACTA, *Meeting of the Bishops in Low Week, 1869* (6 April), 3 (repeats the resolutions of ACTA, 1868, 22).

[29] Purcell, *Ambrose Phillipps de Lisle*, II. 2.

intended by him to help the general reconciliation of Anglicanism and Catholicism—and induced fresh fears among the bishops accordingly. Wiseman, particularly, was sensitive to the dangers here, just before his death in 1865. Finally, there was Newman's position. He was still the subject of great suspicion in Ultramontane circles, and was not rehabilitated from the taint of heresy at Rome until 1867. His successful return to the esteem of English Protestants by the appearance of the *Apologia* in 1864 did nothing to assist his reputation with those whose fears about Oxford derived from its apparently indelible Protestantism. The *Apologia*, in the eyes of many Ultramontanes, seemed far too sympathetic to certain features of Anglicanism, even if it spelled out reasons for the falsity of its historical claims.

The practical ban on the attendance of Catholics at the national universities was repeated by Propaganda in 1885 and remained in force until after Manning's death. The position of Catholics remained unaltered by the University Test Act in 1871. Intended by Gladstone primarily as a concession to the Protestant Dissenters, who had been demanding the removal of religious qualifications for offices at the ancient universities for forty years, the reform actually lessened the prospects for Catholics. For Cardinal Barnabò, as to the English bishops, its effect would be to make the universities even less religious, and so even more hazardous to the faith of Catholics.[30] But the problem of how to provide Catholics with higher education remained, and in 1871, at a joint meeting of the heads of Catholic Colleges and the bishops, attended by superiors of the religious orders, a sub-commission was set up to canvass the prospects. Its findings indicated considerable support for a Catholic hall at Oxford or Cambridge.[31] As this was unacceptable to Manning and to a majority of the other bishops, the provision of a Catholic substitute institution began to become a serious possibility—Rome had been urging the establishment of a full Catholic university in England all along. The hierarchy appealed to Propaganda for guidance in 1872, and in return was instructed to debate the whole matter

[30] Evennett, in Beck, 302.
[31] Ibid. 300; McClelland, *English Roman Catholics*, 247.

at the Fourth Provincial Synod of Westminster, in 1873. The result was the decision to create a senate—an examining body, with two-thirds of its members laymen, on the model of the University of London; and there was to be a Catholic College, to train the laity for the professions, in existing buildings at Kensington.

The Catholic University College at Kensington, opened in January 1875, was not successful. Mgr. Thomas Capel, Manning's own choice as Rector, soon began to demonstrate an independence of episcopal policy and a degree of administrative incompetence.[32] He continued to raise funds for his projected Catholic Public School in London, although he had undertaken not to do so, in defiance of the bishops. There were allegations of moral improprieties among the students, and in 1877 Lord Petre complained that his younger son had been exposed to them. Among the results was an inquiry into the conduct of the College by an episcopal committee in 1878 and the discovery that no financial books had been kept. There were very heavy debts. Yet the professors had been well chosen, almost entirely from distinguished laymen, and the recruitment of students had reached fifty in the first three years—a large number in view of the size of the Catholic upper and middle classes. Indeed, the vision shown in at least one of the appointments—of Mivart to the chair of Biology— was to prove a further ground of discord. In 1877 the Bishop of Nottingham (Bagshawe) demanded his resignation, claiming that his opinions, as published, were not in accordance with Catholic teaching. Manning stepped in to prevent the boat being rocked, but it proved to be an early pointer to the later difficulties in Mivart's Catholic life. It was Capel's resignation which was obtained, by the 1878 Committee; and in the following year the College was reorganized and moved to Cromwell Place. It survived until 1882, when it was merged with St. Charles' College, Bayswater. Those closest to higher education had failed to give their support. The Jesuits were hostile, regarding the Kensington College as a rival to their own influence in higher education. Newman declined to cooperate with it as well: he did not believe the laity would be

[32] See chapter 6.

given any really effective control, and he doubted if the level of intellectual freedom to be tolerated would be adequate. The failure of the Kensington venture revived interest in an Oxford hall or college. In 1871 the Jesuits had opened their Oxford mission and within a few years, as Newman had always foreseen in his schemes, their priests were unavoidably involved in student life. An Oxford University Catholic Club came into existence in the 1880s, and towards the end of the decade there were about fifty Catholic students at the Universities.[33] At Cambridge, early in the 1890s, Anatole von Hügel was urging the hierarchy to alter its policy on the attendance of Catholics. In 1893 he succeeded in offending Vaughan by presenting an address to the Pope, attired in the gown and hood of a Cambridge MA. In 1894 the laity drew up a further address in favour of a change of policy, inspired by the Duke of Norfolk and Anatole von Hügel: 80 of the 436 signatures were of priests. The pressures were becoming inexorable, but the real reason for the abandonment of the policy of exclusion by the hierarchy, in January 1895, was the realization that the national universities had themselves changed sufficiently to make Catholic residence, with careful safeguards, morally acceptable. There had been an increase in liberalism and secularism, it was true: but the moral condition had improved and the Anglican monopoly had been broken. Three bishops dissented from the new policy—which Vaughan claimed had anyway been in Manning's mind for some years. His death had cleared the way.[34] Rome was successfully petitioned, though Propaganda still made it clear that it preferred a proper Catholic University, and the bishops drew up their safeguards. At the Low Week meeting, in April 1895, the hierarchy resolved 'that great prudence should be used in communicating the matter to the public, both in order to avoid arousing anti-Catholic animosity, and to obviate any appearance of inviting or encouraging Catholics to go to Oxford or Cambridge'. A Board was set up 'to collect the necessary means, and to propose arrangements to be made for Lectures, and whatever might appear desirable for the

---

[33] Evennett, in Beck, 304.
[34] For an account of the change of policy, see chapter 8.

Catholic training and instruction of the Catholics attending the universities'.[35] Chaplains for the two ancient universities were sanctioned by Propaganda in June 1896. A number of minor points had also to be cleared up—Vaughan addressed Propaganda on the question of whether priests and ecclesiastics could read for degrees at the Universities.[36] He had also to report that the three bishops who had declined to agree to the new policy were also refusing to sign the Instructions for priests to convey to parents.[37] There were some practical difficulties. The priest named by the Board as Catholic chaplain at Cambridge had been received by the Bishop of Northampton only as an assistant to the parish—who seemed, as Vaughan told Propaganda, 'unwilling to recognize him in any other position'.[38] But the policy worked well despite these early complications. Campion Hall was founded at Oxford by the Jesuits, and St. Benet's Hall by the Benedictines. At Cambridge Benet House was established by the Downside Benedictines, and St. Edmund's House was founded with the co-operation of St. Edmund's College, Ware. Complications about the status of this last, set up in 1896, were raised by opposition within the university itself. In May 1898, the Senate of the University, in a mood of anti-Catholic feeling got up by the non-resident MAs, declined to recognize St. Edmund's House as a public hall of the University. In a report to Propaganda on the state of Catholic education in general in England, which Vaughan made in January 1903, the sections on higher education show a satisfactory outcome of the new policy: 'Catholics have done themselves credit in both universities.' He also urged action on the provision of Catholic higher education for women. Oxford and Cambridge, he judged, were not suitable places for them—there was 'not a Catholic atmosphere' there. But women students could well attend at London, Liverpool, or Birmingham, where they could reside in convents.[39]

[35] Westminster Dioc. Archives, ACTA, *Low Week Meeting of the Bishops, 1895* (23 April) V, 1–2.
[36] Ibid. Vaughan Papers, 34/2, 'Draft for Propaganda', 29 Feb. 1896.
[37] Ibid. 341, 'Draft to the Cardinal Prefect', 28 Feb. 1896.
[38] Ibid. 402, Vaughan to the Cardinal Prefect, 19 May 1896.
[39] Ibid. 230 a, 'Draft to the Cardinal Prefect of Propaganda', Jan. 1903.

Whatever the strength of the pressures brought against the old policy of a practical prohibition of Catholic attendance at the Universities, it remained something of a tribute to the bishops that they were able to change course just at a time when the intellectual waters were becoming disturbed. For by the 1890s the crisis of Modernism was already upon them: conditions for the reception of Catholics at the universities may have improved from a moral point of view, but the intellectual hazards were increasing and were now well represented within English Catholicism itself. Comparable problems had always existed for the hierarchy. But in at least some of its leading features, the liberal Catholicism of Lamennais, Montalembert, and Döllinger, in the mid-century, had seemed less threatening because they were already part of the received outlook of the English Catholic leaders. Lamennais' ideas in the *Avenir*, founded in 1830, were easily recognizable as a version of the sort of political radicalism espoused by those in England who sought reforms of the constitution in the same period. Lamennais preached a free press and freedom of thought and religion; he sought an independence of the Church from the State. That, too, was the burden of Montalembert's famous address at the Malines Congress in 1863: a free Church in a free state—the slogan of the Italian *Risorgimento*. Hence the attack on Montalembert by Ward,[40] precisely because the union of Church and State had always been Catholic teaching, and because its disruption lay at the heart of the Italian liberals' assault upon the States of the Church in Italy. But those principles were just the ones that the Irish Catholic hierarchy were opposing, in their campaign for the disestablishment of the Protestant Church in Ireland, and which, during the Catholic Emancipation movement in England, the Vicars Apostolic had absorbed from the surrounding pool of English liberalism and radicalism. It was only after Lamennais's death that English Catholics really seem to have been conscious that his difficulties with the Church were ones about the nature of religious ideas themselves and not just matters of ecclesiastical obedience.[41]

---

[40] Wilfrid Ward, *William George Ward*, 158.

[41] W. G. Roe, *Lamennais in England. The Reception of Lamennais's Religious Ideas in England in the Nineteenth Century*, Oxford 1966, 125.

Dominic Barberi had detected heretical influences in his writings before then, but Lamennais's Ultramontanism, for many English Catholics—who were very much aware of his opinions —seemed to guarantee respectability. Lamennais himself did not apply critical techniques or the atmosphere of scientific inquiry to his view of Biblical authority (as the later Modernists were to do) and so his liberalism, expressed in terms of political reform, was easily compatible with English Catholicism, Ultramontane and 'Old Catholic' alike. Although they did not seem aware of it, the condemnation of Lamennais's political doctrines by Gregory XVI in *Mirari Vos* (1832) was in effect a censure of the political ideas which those English employed who sought the political reforms of the first half of the nineteenth century. Liberal Catholicism was a complicated and uneven phenomenon, however, and by the later 1840s it was clear that not all Liberal Catholics were liberal in politics. As a view of the relationship between ecclesiastical authority and the pursuit of intellectual culture, Liberal Catholicism could and did attract conservatives. To the extent that Newman was a 'Liberal Catholic' he fell into this category. The publication of the *Syllabus of Errors* in 1864 was an interesting test of Liberal Catholicism, helping, in its effect upon opinion, to separate out the Ultramontanes. Döllinger interpreted the *Syllabus* and *Quanta Cura* as an attack upon modern society and government, and, impelled also by his opposition to the Temporal Power, gave up his Ultramontanism. Newman, who was not in most senses an Ultramontane, was not opposed to the *Syllabus* precisely for the reasons which Döllinger gave. The censured propositions were just things which had appeared, in the guise of the English political liberalism of the 1830s, to threaten Oxford and the Church. 'I see little which would not be condemned', he wrote, 'by Keble or the great body of the Anglican Church thirty years ago.'[42] By the 1860s Liberal Catholicism in England had anyway lost political clarity and was, in the hands of some of the most distinguished converts, and of Sir John Acton, already probing the defences of ecclesiastical

---

[42] Hugh A. MacDougall, *The Acton-Newman Relations. The Dilemma of Christian Liberalism*, New York 1962, 97.

authority on questions of education and theological liberty. They were concerned above all with raising the level of intellectual life among Catholics. The difference of view with the hierarchy over the Oxford hall schemes was one indication of the determination of the bishops not to allow intellectual life to escape their regulation. The controversy over the *Rambler* was another.

From its beginning, the *Rambler* showed an interest in French and German Liberal Catholicism.[43] The journal started as a weekly in 1848 with John Moore Capes, the proprietor, as editor. He was a converted Anglican clergyman. During his period in sole control, the journal concerned itself with social issues and the conditions of the poor; it was also sympathetic to Ultramontane positions—supporting the new devotions and Faber's *Lives of the Modern Saints*, for example. In 1856 Richard Simpson (another Anglican convert—he had been Vicar of Mitcham in Surrey until 1845—) became sub-editor, and in 1857 he became editor in the reorganization resulting from Sir John Acton's becoming part-proprietor. Simpson was a very effective journalist and polemical writer. 'He had the gift—the fatal gift it may be called in the circumstances— of catching the comical side of serious matters, which made him not always a respecter of those persons in authority who were accustomed to look for reverence and obedience.'[44] The *Rambler*, despite Acton's position in its management, was also pretty clearly the organ of converts: it did not express a coherent, comprehensive view of the converts, for they were divided themselves between 'Liberal' Catholics and Ultramontanes, but it represented the views of those approximating to 'Liberal' opinions. Newman's influence over the contributors was, as Gasquet observed, 'very considerable at all times'.[45] It was, indeed, his association with, and brief editorship of the journal, which helped create the impression—certainly within the Ultramontane wing of the hierarchy—that he was himself a 'Liberal Catholic'. The *Rambler* caused early offence to the bishops by articles critical of the educational attainments of the English Catholics; and then went on to opinions and

[43] Altholz, 12.
[44] Ibid. xlv.
[45] Abbot Gasquet (ed.), *Lord Acton and his Circle*, London 1906, xxii.

attitudes which, to Wiseman and the Ultramontanes, were much more serious. The whole tone of editorial policy—and this was the core of the row over the journal—expressed a belief that literary, political, and intellectual positions should be adopted without direct reference to ecclesiastical authority. Though stated moderately, the ideas of the *Rambler* contributors were clearly a challenge, not to Catholic teachings as conventionally understood in England, but to the Ultramontane leadership. By 1856 Wiseman was already complaining of its independence,[46] and in 1858 he got Ward and Oakeley to use the *Dublin Review* as an antidote. In a report to Propaganda of 1861, he gave examples of this in order to demonstrate what he called 'the numerous hellish sentiments of the *Rambler*'.[47] Even Ullathorne, normally a defender of moderate 'English' Catholicism against extreme 'Roman' influences, was offended by the journal. 'It is doing great mischief', he wrote in 1859; and added—'I am happy to say that though there is a restless party who hold with the *Rambler*, the large majority are on the side of orthodoxy.'[48] He wrote in January of that year; in February Wiseman, Grant, and Ullathorne met to discuss the journal, and approached Newman to use his influence with Simpson to moderate the tone of the articles. In the event, Newman himself became editor in April and produced two issues in 1859—one of which contained his controversial essay 'On Consulting the Faithful in matters of Doctrine'. He found the duties of editorship clearly very onerous, and, as Acton recorded, 'he bitterly complains of his old age'.[49] (He had thirty more years to live.) The editorship returned to Acton and Simpson, who were joined by T. F. Wetherell. In July 1862, the journal changed its name to the *Home and Foreign Review*. Its tone and purpose remained unchanged; in the following year Vaughan was complaining to Talbot in Rome that it was undermining faith. It had already, he wrote, caused a monk

[46] Wilfrid Ward, *Wiseman*, II. 228.

[47] Propaganda, *Scritture Riferite nei Congressi, Anglia* 16 (1861-3), 303 (25 Nov. 1861) [in Italian].

[48] *Letters of Archbishop Ullathorne*, ed. by the nuns of St. Dominic's Convent, Stone, London 1892, 100.

[49] Gasquet (ed.), *Lord Acton*, 71.

to apostasize; and believed 'many young men think it *intellectual* to support the Home & Foreign.'[50] Propaganda had already asked the bishops to warn the faithful about the journal. The pressures, in the end, were too great. After the Papal Brief of December 1862, condemning the liberal ideas of the Munich Congress (September 1863), Acton and the managers decided to end the *Home and Foreign* rather than face the possibility of action against them by the ecclesiastical authorities. The journal ceased in April 1864.

The issues of higher education and journalism had thus provided two occasions of confrontation between Catholic ecclesiastical authority and lay and 'liberal' thought. There was a third before the Modernist 'crisis' of the end of the century—the most well known: the question of Papal Infallibility at the Vatican Council of 1869–70. To some, it appeared to raise the questions of intellectual freedom, and of the relationship of the Church to modern knowledge, in a particularly stark fashion. It was the circumstances of the definition of Infallibility, rather than the doctrine itself, which caused alarm to traditional English Catholics and to those liberals who were opposed to Ultramontanism. For the doctrine had been implicit in the Church through the centuries, representing the centralization of the infallibility of those protected in all truth by the promise of Christ himself. It had been expressed in a systematic theological form by Bellarmine. As a symbol of the 'Roman' influence of the nineteenth-century Ultramontanes, however, the issue of Infallibility only too easily came to appear as a weapon of neo-triumphalism in a Papacy anxious to exercise a spiritual autocracy over a world which had stood aside while the temporal patrimony of the Church was stripped away. Most English Protestants completely failed to understand what the doctrine was actually about; and some Catholics, perhaps offended by extreme opinions like those of Louis Veuillot or W. G. Ward—who appeared to attribute Infallibility even to the Pope's private conversations and letters—showed little comprehension of what was a technical matter relating to the *magisterium* of

[50] English College Archives, Talbot Papers, 703, Vaughan to Talbot, 20 June 1863.

the Church. Thus Ambrose Phillipps de Lisle, addressing Bishop Clifford in 1866 about Infallibility, denied that 'any Pope, or any Bishop, or any single man on earth could ever possess that attribute which belongs alone to the Church Herself in her *Collective Action* and not in her individual Pastors, or even the highest of them'.[51] He also supposed that a definition of Infallibility would wreck his Reunion schemes.[52] The immediate stimulus to the cause of definition came not from the fate of the Temporal Power but from the definition of the Immaculate Conception in 1854. This expression of the will of the Church, as Manning noticed, 'powerfully awakened in the minds of both clergy and laity the thought of infallibility'.[53] In the 'keen and bitter controversy', as Dom Cuthbert Butler called it,[54] preceding the Council, some theologicial objections to a definition were raised by liberal Catholics. There were also the more common expressions of those who subscribed to Infallibility but thought the moment to declare it an article of faith inopportune. Among the English bishops both views were to be found among the opponents— Clifford and Errington tended towards actual theological objection, but never pressed the matter on those grounds, while Vaughan (of Plymouth, uncle of Herbert Vaughan), Amherst (of Northampton), and Turner (of Salford), though not formally Inopportunists when it came to the voting, were inclined to regard the matter as best not raised. Manning, of course, was the leader of those English bishops in favour of the definition—indeed he was one of the leading members of the Council[55]—and Ullathorne, Grant, and Cornthwaite (of Beverley), supported him. Only four of the English bishops actually spoke in the Council sessions: Manning, Vaughan, Errington, and Clifford. Only Brown (of Newport) and Goss (of Liverpool) were absent from the Council; the first stayed in England to keep a watching-brief on the affairs of the Church, the second was ill. Escaping the dominance of

[51] Bristol Record Office, 35721, Clifford Papers, Phillips de Lisle to Clifford, 7 April 1866.
[52] Purcell, *Ambrose Phillipps de Lisle*, II. 32.
[53] Manning, *The True Story of the Vatican Council*, 43.
[54] Cuthbert Butler, *The Vatican Council, 1869–1870*, 85.
[55] See chapter 6.

Manning, Clifford and Errington co-operated with Moriarty (of Kerry in Ireland), who was an Inopportunist, and with the American Bishops, among whom there was a sizeable Inopportunist group. The Americans, in fact, who had regarded themselves as thoroughly Roman in spirit, discovered that the Romans of Rome actually condemned 'hundreds of opinions hitherto held or tolerated' by American Catholics.[56] Bishop Martin Spalding of Baltimore wanted the English-speaking prelates 'to act as a body', and proposed this to Ullathorne through the mediation of Moriarty.[57] Ullathorne's views on the Council have become especially familiar, because Dom Cuthbert Butler used his letters from the Council as the basis of his study. They have survived among Ullathorne's papers at St. Dominic's Convent, Stone.[58] Although the Council was not, for Ullathorne, as it was for Manning, 'the great time of his life', he was 'among the bishops that counted'.[59] He was enthusiastic for a definition of Infallibility, but wanted to balance it by some statement on the divine origin of the episcopate in order to ensure that *ex-cathedra* utterances rested upon a broad foundation of universal assent.

The first session of the Council was held in December 1869. News of it in England came mostly from the *Times* reports, which were astonishing for their inaccuracy. The newspaper had sent, as its special correspondent, Thomas Mozley, an Anglican parson (who was also Newman's brother-in-law). He could speak neither Italian nor French, and, like other correspondents in Rome, supposed that the official secrecy imposed upon the debates and upon the participants was a cover for sinister attempts to curtail the freedom of Catholics in the various countries. 'The lies with which people have deluded the poor correspondent are so huge, so ludicrous, so utterly antagonistic to the facts', Ullathorne

[56] Robert D. Cross, *The Emergence of Liberal Catholicism in America*, Cambridge, Mass. 1958, 20.

[57] Ullathorne Papers, St. Dominic's Convent, Stone, Box X(3), Ullathorne to Estcourt, 14 Dec. 1869.

[58] There are 15 letters to his secretary, Canon Edgar Estcourt, and to Dr J. S. Northcote, the President of Oscott; 36 to Mother Imelda Poole, Superioress of St. Dominic's Convent, (Nov. 1869–Apr. 1870), and 14 to Mother Imelda Poole or to Mother F. R. Drane (May–July 1870).

[59] Cuthbert Butler, *Ullathorne*, II. 40.

recorded, 'that we read them at our table as they arrive from London with roars of laughter.'[60] But the irresponsibility of *The Times* had a more serious consequence. As Ullathorne noticed prophetically, 'I suppose England will believe all this, and it will become part of the Protestant tradition.'[61] The *Times* reports, together with hostile commentary supplied by Acton, who was in Rome as a freelance observer, provided Gladstone with the incentive to consider the intervention of the European powers, and later, in 1874, with materials for his pamphlet assault upon the Vatican Decrees.

The discussion of Infallibility began in May: it had not originally been on the Council's agenda at all, but there was an accepted inevitability about its eventual inclusion by the *De Fide* deputation. Manning was a leading figure in urging the matter forward. On the 25 May he made his great speech on Infallibility. 'The Pope's infallibility *is* Catholic doctrine of divine faith, and all are already obliged to hold it,' he declared, 'to question it is at least material heresy, for it is not an an open theological opinion, but a doctrine contained in the divine revelation.'[62] This was a clear statement of Ultramontanism. The definition, Manning believed, would have a good effect in England—it would 'more than anything else promote conversions and the return of the country to the Faith'.[63] He was later to be rigorous in its enforcement. His *Pastoral* of 1874 declared that any Catholic who could not assent to Infallibility 'does by that very fact cease to be a Catholic'.[64] On the day that Manning made his speech in the Council, Ullathorne observed, 'after human means and wits have exhausted themselves, the Holy Ghost will settle the matter'.[65] And so, on 18 July, as the thunderstorm descended upon Rome, the Decree was passed: 533 *placet*, 2 *non placet*. The next day war was declared between France and Prussia. The disappointed minority—whose numbers were of course much larger than the formal *non placets* indicated—awaited

[60] Butler, *Ullathorne*, II. 54.
[61] Butler, *Vatican Council*, 151.
[62] Ibid. 308.
[63] Ibid. 309.
[64] Downside Archives, VII.A.3.a, Abbots' Papers (File marked '1871–1880'), letter of Manning 'to be read in churches', 22 Nov. 1874.
[65] Butler, *Vatican Council*, 326.

events. 'It is evident that any active measure taken at present by members of the minority', Clifford wrote to Newman in August, 'would at once provoke action on the part of the violent party, and then schism would be the only alternative which of course is evidently wrong.'[66] One by one the bishops of the minority made their formal adhesions to the Decree—Clifford himself on 3 December. The Ultramontanists had won. Pius IX, who had all along hoped for this outcome, was modest in his personal claims. At least, he told Cesare Cantù, 'I am not infallible in choosing my snuff.'[67]

Manning's large hopes of a stimulus to Catholic growth in England, as a result of the successful passing of the Infallibility Decree, were radically diminished by Gladstone. In the elections of February 1874 his government was defeated. Gladstone was resentful of the Irish Catholic bishops, who had directed the Irish Members of Parliament to vote against the Irish University Bill and so precipitated the demise of the administration. Released from office, Gladstone composed a pamphlet on the Vatican Decrees which was a classic of traditional English anti-Catholicism—*The Vatican Decrees in their bearing on Civil Allegiance. A Political Expostulation.* Now that he no longer had to worry about the Irish vote, he really let himself go.[68] He set out to show—mostly by copious reference to the *Syllabus* of 1864—that Rome 'has refurbished and paraded anew every rusty tool she was fondly thought to have disused'; that 'no one can now become her convert without renouncing his moral and mental freedom, and placing his civil loyalty and duty at the mercy of another'; that Rome 'has equally repudiated modern thought and ancient history'.[69] Again: 'The modern Church of Rome has abandoned nothing, retracted nothing.'[70] The triumph of Ultramontanism, at the Vatican Council, was a sinister assault upon

[66] Bristol Record Office, 35721, Clifford Papers, Clifford to Newman, 15 Aug. 1870.

[67] Edmund Campion (ed.), *Lord Acton and the First Vatican Council: A Journal*, Sydney 1975, 62 (22 Dec. 1869).

[68] For a summary of the pamphlet, see Norman, *Anti-Catholicism in Victorian England*, 92–5, 212–22.

[69] W. E. Gladstone, *The Vatican Decrees in their bearing on Civil Allegiance*, London 1874, 12.

[70] Ibid. 11.

liberty—'individual servitude, however abject, will not satisfy the party now dominant in the Latin Church: the State must also be a slave'.[71] It was an extraordinary outburst, and acquired huge publicity; in its first month, between November and December 1874, it sold 145,000 copies.[72] Leading Catholics produced replies. Manning's, in 1875, denied that the Council's decrees had any effect on civil allegiance, which was 'as full, perfect and complete since the Council as it was before'.[73] Ullathorne's made the same point.[74] Acton's, in a letter to *The Times*, purported to defend the Vatican Decrees by showing that English Catholics had in the past always ignored extreme pronouncements from Rome, and would do so again.[75] On reading the letter Newman said he was 'shocked beyond what I can easily say'.[76] Similar in tone to Acton's letter was a pamphlet by Phillipps de Lisle; and in correspondence with Gladstone he distanced himself from 'Vaticanism' as representing only 'an element' in Catholicism—an element against which Gladstone's essay had been 'the most powerful indictment'.[77] Of the *Syllabus*, he wrote: 'The idea of the modern civilized world accepting it as a rule of conduct, if it ever entered into the narrow and prejudiced conception of some besotted theologian in the obscure corner of a darkened cell, it is too ridiculous to be entertained by any serious thinker who knows what is passing in the outer world.'[78] Newman received many letters urging him to make a public reply to Gladstone, and when he did he produced a work of lasting value.[79] Among those writing to him was the Duke of Norfolk, the first layman of the English Church; and it was to

[71] Ibid. 29.
[72] Norman, *The Catholic Church and Ireland in the Age of Rebellion, 1859–1873*, 458.
[73] H. E. Manning, *Vatican Decrees in their bearing on Civil Allegiance*, London 1875, 18.
[74] W. B. Ullathorne, *The Döllingerites, Mr. Gladstone, and Apostates from the Faith*, London 1875.
[75] *The Times*, 9 Nov. 1874.
[76] MacDougall, 132.
[77] Purcell, *Ambrose Phillipps de Lisle*, II. 44.
[78] Ibid. II. 46.
[79] For an analysis, see J. D. Bastable, 'Gladstone's *Expostulation* and Newman', in J. D. Bastable (ed.), *Newman and Gladstone. Centennial Essays*, Dublin 1978, 15.

him, therefore, that Newman chose to address his essay. *A
Letter Addressed to His Grace the Duke of Norfolk* dismissed
the notion of a divided allegiance: 'so little does the Pope
come into the whole system of moral theology by which (as
by our conscience) our lives are regulated, that the weight of
his hand upon us, as private men, is absolutely unappreci-
able'.[80] There was no interference in civil society: 'The Pope,
who comes of Revelation, has no jurisdiction over Nature.'[81]
These sentiments were hardly calculated to flatter Ultramontane sensibilities, but they were correct in point of Catholic
teaching. What offended the Vatican about Newman's pamphlet were implied criticisms of the Curia, and references to
the culpability of certain former pontiffs. The centre of the
essay was about conscience—which was seen 'not as a fancy
or an opinion, but as a dutiful obedience to what claims to
be a divine voice, speaking within us'.[82] The defence of conscience, exercised within the knowledge of the divine supplied by the Catholic *magisterium*, elevated the whole debate
about Catholic civil allegiance above the knock-about anti-
Catholicism of Gladstone's pamphlet. It was characteristic
of Newman to have seen enduring and eternal principles in
the issues from which others had derived only surface judgements.

In turning now to the contributions of the two leading
intellectual converts from Anglicanism—Newman and Ward—
something must first be said about their place in this study.
Since Newman was the most outstanding and well-known
English Catholic of the nineteenth century, whose writings
have permanent importance in Christian thinking, it may at
first seem strange that he has not been made the subject of a
separate chapter.[83] There are two reasons for this, and both

[80] John Henry Newman, *A Letter Addressed to His Grace the Duke of Norfolk*,
London 1875, 47.

[81] Ibid. 68.

[82] Ibid. 69.

[83] Newman's early life and career are surely too well known to be reproduced
here. For further details, see Meriol Trevor's two volumes, *Pillar of the Cloud* and
Light in Winter (London 1962) which have, in most particulars, superseded the
older, standard life by Wilfrid Ward, *The Life of John Henry, Cardinal Newman*,
London 1912 (2 vols). There is also *John Henry Newman* (London 1966) by
C. S. Dessain, the editor of Newman's letters; and numerous smaller biographical
studies.

have to do with the balance to be maintained in a general historical survey of this sort. There was an occasion towards the end of his life when Ullathorne visited the Oratory and Newman insisted, against his protestations, in kneeling to receive his blessing. 'I have been indoors all my life, whilst you have battled for the Church in the world,' Newman said.[84] It was a modest and a true remark. Newman's learning was generally put to active use—he wrote to help prove the Christian causes he espoused; but in the general perspective of the growth, administration, and external relations of the English Catholic Church he was not a leading figure. His Catholic life was passed almost exclusively in the Birmingham Oratory—the only exception being his visits to Dublin to conduct the affairs of the Catholic University in the 1850s. Men looked to him for learning and guidance on Catholic issues of the day, yet Newman held no office in the Church until he was made a cardinal in 1879, by Leo XIII (he was, by then, seventy-eight years old, and said the honour was 'a strange turn-up'[85]). He was an isolated figure, always at the centre of men's perception of English Catholicism, but at the periphery of the institutional Church. His learning is itself the second reason why this sketch of Newman is integrated with this chapter rather than laid out in a separate one. This is a study of the Church; it is not a history of ideas or of Catholic thought. In what follows, therefore, Newman's contribution is assessed as it touched others or affected the institutional Church in England. It is not an attempt—inappropriate in a study of this dimension—to summarize Newman's thought.

His life spanned the century, from 1801 to 1890, yet his intellectual development has a considerable measure of consistency about it. There has been so much emphasis on Newman's conversion in 1845—especially by himself, in the *Apologia*—that it is easy to assume that it marked an enormous break in his intellectual life. In fact it scarcely did so. What changed were the externals: loyalties, old friendships, his residence in Oxford. Hence the desolation of his letters at the time. 'All that is dear to me is being taken from me,' he

[84] Ullathorne, *From Cabin-Boy to Archbishop*, Introduction (by Shane Leslie), xxiii.

[85] Meriol Trevor, *Newman. Light in Winter*, London 1962, 563.

wrote; 'My days are gone like a shadow, and I am withered like grass.'[86] A closer look even at the *Apologia*, however, will show that Newman steadily developed a view of the Church as a universal institution, of divine origin, with a structure of authority, and that by a series of stages he substituted, as its contemporary embodiment in England, the Catholic for the Anglican tradition. Catholicism most seemed to him to correspond to the Church of Antiquity, just as Anglicanism was the modern version of the sort of ecclesiastical irregularities seen in the early heresies. His study of the primitive Church had begun in 1828; in 1832 he published his *Arians of the Fourth Century*. It was in 1839, while working on the Monophysites, that his position suddenly clarified: 'My stronghold was Antiquity; now here, in the middle of the fifth century, I found, as it seemed to me, Christendom of the sixteenth and the nineteenth centuries reflected. I saw my face in that mirror, and I was a Monophysite.' The conclusion: 'The Church of the *Via Media* was in the position of the Oriental communion. Rome was, where she now is.'[87] Furthermore, 'The drama of religion, and the combat of truth and error, were ever one and the same.'[88] As Newman put it in his *Letter to the Duke of Norfolk* in 1875, 'I say then the Pope is the heir of the Ecumenical Hierarchy of the fourth century;' and, in contrast—'Does any Anglican Bishop for the last 300 years recall to our minds the image of St. Basil?'[89] A *national* Church seemed to him a contradiction in terms, for the Church had of its nature to be common to all men, with the same doctrines and discipline.

Newman belonged to no particular theological school of thought; he was indebted to no dominant writer for his ideas. But there were influences at each stage. As a young man in Oxford he had got from Edward Hawkins, Provost of Oriel, the notion that the Bible needed to be interpreted within the body of the tradition in which it was written, that, as in the doctrine of Baptismal Regeneration, religious truth had an

---

[86] *Letters and Correspondence of John Henry Newman during his Life in the English Church*, ed. Anne Mozley, London 1898, II. 415 (April 1845).
[87] Newman, *Apologia Pro Vita Sua*, 217.
[88] Ibid. 218.
[89] Newman, *Letter to the Duke of Norfolk*, 28.

objective basis and did not depend upon subjective experience. From Richard Whateley, who became Archbishop of Dublin—and especially from his (anonymous) *Letters on the Church by an Episcopalian*—of 1826, he came to respect the spiritual autonomy of the Church, and to suspect the facts of English erastian practice as incompatible with the divine authority of the Church. From Richard Hurrell Froude, a Fellow of Oriel from 1826 and the closest friend of Newman's Oxford days, he gained an insight into Catholic devotional life. Froude himself was a High Church Anglican whose spiritual practices, apparently almost entirely Catholic in style, were to shock Protestant opinion when they were first revealed with the publication, by Newman, of his *Remains* in 1838, two years after his death. The two men were quite different. Froude was 'daring, high-spirited, strong-willed and gay'.[90] Newman shared none of these characteristics—not even the last one. He also lacked Froud's association between Gothic taste and right principles of religious faith[91]—a quality shared with Pugin —and Froude's interest in politics. Newman was introspective, philosophical, theoretical. Theirs was an attraction of opposites. It was from Wiseman that Newman derived the final incentive to apply his studies of Antiquity to the world of the nineteenth century. In September 1839 he read the article on the Donatist heresy in the *Dublin Review*, and was transfixed by the words of St. Augustine quoted by Wiseman. They were a test of ecclesiastical authenticity and orthodoxy which seemed chillingly to apply to the isolated condition of the Anglican Church: *securus judicat orbis terrarum*. 'By these great words of the ancient Father,' he wrote, 'the theory of the *Via Media* was absolutely pulverized.'[92] He had seen 'the shadow of a hand upon the wall'.[93] The defence of Anglicanism in his *Lectures on the Prophetical Office of the Church* (1837) seemed to have fallen to pieces. In persuading Newman that his doctrine of the Church was incompatible with Anglicanism, because Anglicanism lacked the authority to define and preserve authentic religious truth, Wiseman had

[90] Trevor, *The Pillar of the Cloud*, 78.
[91] Piers Brandon, *Hurrell Froude and the Oxford Movement*, London 1974, 54.
[92] *Apologia*, 219.
[93] Ibid. 220.

provided the last proof that Newman needed. As a Catholic his opinion did not change; he adopted no new ideas when he was finally received into the Church by Father Dominic Barberi in 1845. His knowledge of the actual Catholic Church, indeed, both in England and in Rome, was fairly sketchy, even at the time of his conversion.[94] He had arrived at his position quite independently. It was a matter of logic applied to a belief in dogma. Newman was certainly not drawn to Rome, as so many of his Protestant contemporaries appeared to suppose, by a taste for ritual. He was unmoved by it, and, as it happens, frequently made mistakes in the services he conducted as a Catholic.[95]

This independence of Newman's mind is important in understanding his continuing isolation as a Catholic. It did not prevent others from seeking to categorize him; to label him with the less subtle party distinctions which for so many appeared necessary. Newman had been anxious to keep clear of parties even in the Oxford movement: that, he said, had been 'but a floating opinion, it was not a power'.[96] As a Catholic he was claimed both by the 'Old Catholics' and the 'Liberal Catholics', but he was close to neither. His social conservatism and his belief that educational endeavour should be suited to the needs of gentlemen—a feature which was to cause difficulties with the Irish bishops in the conduct of the Catholic University—were accidents of his background and his lack of interest in political change. They were not the reflection of any personal sympathy for the styles of the English gentry and certainly not of the lingering 'Gallican' element in 'Old Catholic' views of the Church. That was too much like the national church ideology of Anglicanism, from which he had just escaped. His political conservatism was not really important either, simply because, despite attempts to identify a 'corpus of political ideas' in the writings (even if not systematically expressed),[97] Newman was distrustful of political idealism. It substituted impersonal categories for the

[94] Trevor, *The Pillar of the Cloud*, 120.
[95] Ibid. 197.
[96] *Apologia*, 172.
[97] Terence Kenny, *The Political Thought of John Henry Newman*, London 1957, 2.

real personal duties which religion taught in men. In 1883 he wrote, 'It has never been my line to take up political or social questions, unless they came close to me as matters of personal duty.'[98] There is no reason to suppose that he had ever departed from that position. His youthful Toryism at Oxford, which he imbibed with his learning from the Anglican atmosphere of the University—a bulwark against reform—was without a theoretical basis. It was unlike Coleridge's, or the young Gladstone's, and burned away with the years, as he became more or less apolitical. Unlike Coleridge he had no conception of the state as a mystical or organic entity. His empiricism was thoroughly English, and he came to prefer a neutral state if that secured non-intervention in the affairs of the Churches. He retained his social conservatism, continuing, in that, to preserve the Tory paternalism of his background. He never showed much interest in the sort of social reform which made others, like Manning, advance towards a limited acceptance of collectivism. He regarded the evils of the age as residing in wrong intellectual attitudes towards faith and the means by which it is known; social conditions were a lesser matter.[99] Newman regarded the spiritual nature of men as being in much greater immediate hazard than their material situation. As a matter of ordinary Christian duty, of course, he offered succour to the afflicted if he could. It is recorded that he used to pay the medical bills of the poor in the district of Birmingham surrounding the Oratory.[100] His social paternalism was certainly comparable to the practices of the 'Old Catholics', but it is difficult to see many other similarities. But the 'Old Catholics' looked to him for his 'Englishness': it was in contrast to the Italianate religion of the Ultramontanes; and they may have sensed in him a moderation of view. His published opinions on the position of the laity must also have been conducive.

It is difficult to see that Newman was much nearer the Liberal Catholics' various positions—except in a highly qualified sense—despite the fact that the Papacy seems periodically

[98] Dessain, 70. See also *Apologia*, 154.

[99] J. Derek Holmes, 'Factors in the development of Newman's political attitudes', in Bastable (ed.), *Newman and Gladstone*, 78.

[100] Joyce Sugg, *A Saint for Birmingham?*, London (CTS), n.d., 5.

to have identified him as a liberal. He had a deeply pessimistic
view of human nature and of the capability of men to make
moral progress. He emphasized Original Sin and recognized
that corruption is the normal lot of mankind and of human
institutions. This was very far from the social progressivism
of the earlier Liberal Catholics, and of the liberal rationality
of Acton and the later Modernists, with their conviction that
enlightened political principles were inseparable from the
establishment of Christianity. He shared none of the political
radicalism of the Lamennais tradition, and none of the distrust of ecclesiastical authority of Acton's position, or of
Döllinger and Montalembert. When Ullathorne condemned
the *Home and Foreign Review* in 1862, Newman wrote to
Acton to say that Ullathorne's was 'the voice of the Church'.
Acton said that Ullathorne's letter was 'singularly absurd'.[101]
And Newman endeavoured to keep the *Rambler* contributors
from offending the ecclesiastical authorities. In 1859 he tried
to dissuade Acton from writing theological articles in order
to avoid controversy.[102] That he often fell foul of the authorities was due to rejection or misunderstanding of his ideas,
both as an Anglican and as a Catholic. In both periods of his
life—it was a central paradox—he upheld the very exercise of
ecclesiastical authority which was used against him. His opposition to the Temporal Power of the Papacy in Italy, and
his 'minimalistic' interpretation of the Vatican Decrees, were
certainly in sympathy with Liberal Catholic positions.

He was not opposed to Infallibility as such however—
merely to the circumstances of the definition. He applied,
indeed, the logic of the Augustinian formula that had brought
him into the Catholic Church in the first place—*securus judicat orbis terrarum*: how could God 'allow 530 bishops to go
wrong?'[103] 'As to myself personally, please God, I do not
expect any trial at all,' he wrote to Ullathorne about Infallibility, early in 1870. But he feared for those who did, and
'at the prospect of having to defend decisions, which may

[101] Altholz, 195.
[102] *Letters and Diaries*, XIX (London 1969), 167 (July 1859); Gasquet (ed.),
Lord Acton and his Circle, xxiii.
[103] Brian Martin, *John Henry Newman. His Life and Work*, London 1982,
123.

not be difficult to my private judgement, but may be most difficult to maintain logically in the face of historical facts'. He referred to 'the store of Pontifical scandals in the history of eighteen centuries'.[104] In another place he said he was 'not bound to defend the policy or the acts of particular popes'.[105] Such sentiments did not endear him to the Rome of Pius IX, but they were neither unorthodox nor particularly 'Liberal'. If they had to be categorized at all, they were probably, indeed, 'Old Catholic'—nearer to the Cisalpine tradition. Newman's belief in ecclesiastical miracles was certainly very far from the later Liberal Catholic outlook, which sought to reconcile Catholicism and modern knowledge. Despite his developed view of the importance of conscience in the acceptance of religious ideas, furthermore, Newman's thought was deeply wedded to the dogmatic principle as the basis of faith. Its absence in Anglicanism induced the beginnings of his dissatisfaction with that Church as an authentic embodiment of Christian truth. His complete rejection of liberalism in religion, as an Anglican in Oxford, and in opposition to the leading tenets of the Liberal Catholics, was a constant characteristic of his religious sense. For liberalism was 'the anti-dogmatic principle'.[106] It pervaded the Anglicans of his day: there is a brilliant passage in *Loss and Gain*, Newman's novel of 1848 about a young man converted to Catholicism at Oxford, in which one of the characters (Bateman) surveys the attitudes of the bishops to the Articles of Religion of the Church of England and concludes that their various interpretations indicated that they 'have no sense at all', the Articles could be made to mean anything.[107] In such a Church, as Newman remarked in the *Apologia*, there could be no defence against the inroads of alien ideas; Anglicanism appeared able to absorb anything.[108] In a famous attack upon Sir Robert Peel, in a series of letters to *The Times* in 1841—the unfortunate Peel, in opening a Reading Room at Tamworth,

[104] *The Letters and Diaries of John Henry Newman*, ed. Dessain, Oxford 1973, XXV 18–19 (Jan. 1870).
[105] *Letter to the Duke of Norfolk*, 37.
[106] *Apologia*, 163.
[107] J. H. Newman, *Loss and Gain. The Story of a Convert* [1848], London, 1962 edn., 76.
[108] *Apologia*, 149.

had spoken of his hope that 'controversial divinity' and 'party differences' in religion could be avoided—Newman spelled out the basics of his lifelong conviction. 'Christianity is faith, faith implies a doctrine, a doctrine propositions, propositions yes or no, yes or no differences,' he wrote. 'Differences, then, are the natural attendants on Christianity, and you cannot have Christianity, and not have differences.'[109]

In Rome to receive the red hat, in 1879, Newman confirmed his continued resistance to liberalism, 'the doctrine that there is no positive truth in religion, but that one creed is as good as another'.[110] Now that, as a definition of liberalism in religion, may not prove satisfactory to some; but it establishes Newman's belief that he was still far from willing to be identified with 'liberalism'. His real war was with Indifferentism, as his remarks in Rome made clear. To the extent that Liberal Catholicism fostered or even encouraged it, he was clearly an opponent. It is arguable, however, that most Liberal Catholicism in the second half of the century did not. Its enemy was ecclesiastical authority over intellectual enquiry, and here Newman's ideas did have some affinity. He was found on the Liberal Catholic side during most of the disputes of the 1860s precisely because he favoured a view of academic freedom which differed from the Ultramontanes. Newman contended for authority, but also for authority to be exercised upon Christian truth as agreed by the general sense of the Church, and not just by *fiat* of the Curia. His view veered towards collegiality. The whole atmosphere of his *Grammar of Assent*, published in 1870, with its affirmation of religious certainty established upon the 'illative' faculty applied through reason, suggested a religious polity in which the individual believer was active in arriving at the truth which authority then declared. Similarly, the famous article on the laity in the *Rambler* of July 1859 saw authority as resting upon a wide base, necessary 'because the body of the faithful is one of the witnesses to the fact of the tradition of revealed doctrine, and because their *consensus* through Christendom is the voice of the Infallible

[109] J. H. Newman, *Discussions and Arguments on Various Subjects*, London 1872, IV, 'The Tamworth Reading Room', [1841], 284.
[110] Reynolds, *Three Cardinals*, 249.

Church'.[111] Gillow had already denounced this view as heretical, and Bishop Brown now brought the article before the authorities in Rome. Newman had caused particular outrage to the Ultramontanes by showing that in the Arian controversy of the fourth century the bishops had defected from orthodoxy while the laity remained faithful. Almost ten years later, Talbot was still citing the article as having encouraged the laity in a wish 'to govern the Church in England by public opinion'. He concluded: 'Dr Newman is the most dangerous man in England.'[112] It was not surprising that Newman should have become associated with the Liberal Catholics in the eyes of those who desired to allocate the entire definition of Christian truth to the episcopacy—or perhaps even only to the Papacy. The section on intellectual freedom in the last part of the *Apologia* was similarly disliked in Ultramontane circles. In reply to such objections to his ideas about ideas, Newman pointed to the narrowing of Catholic experience. Thus to Ward, in 1867, he wrote to say 'You are making a Church within a Church', just like the Evangelicals within Anglicanism. 'As they talk of "vital religion" and "vital doctrines", and will not allow that their brethren "know the Gospel", or are Gospel preachers, unless they profess the small shibboleths of their own sect, so you are doing your best to make a party in the Catholic Church.'[113] Yet, with characteristic balance, Newman was opposed to unbridled intellectual enquiry: ideas had to be explored within the community of believers. In his Dublin lectures of 1852, *The Idea of a University*, he warned of the dangers of 'intellectualism' —of elevating philosophical theories above Revelation. 'Revealed Religion furnishes facts to the other sciences, which those sciences, left to themselves, would never reach.'[114] In 1870 he observed: 'The Church moves as a whole; it is not a mere philosophy, it is a communion.'[115] To his mind, the Ultramontanes were just as likely to convert the faith into a

[111] [J. H. Newman] 'On Consulting the Faithful in matters of Doctrine', *The Rambler*, I (new series), July 1859, 205.

[112] Purcell, *Manning*, II. 318 (April 1867).

[113] Wilfrid Ward, *William George Ward*, 267 (9 May 1867).

[114] J. H. Newman, *The Idea of a University. Defined and Illustrated*, London, 1907 edn., 73.

[115] Trevor, *Light in Winter*, 482.

series of theoretical propositions as were, for very different reasons, the Liberal Catholics.

It will be appreciated, from these evidences, that there is no satisfactory way of identifying Newman's thinking with 'Liberal' Catholicism, the more so since the Liberal Catholic position was not stable, and changed enormously during his lifetime. But there was one area in which Newman was able to put some of his ideas into action, and the result helps an understanding of his general position on a number of the matters which concerned the Liberal Catholics. In 1851 Archbishop Cullen visited Birmingham and invited Newman to be the Rector of the Catholic University which the Irish Hierarchy were about to establish in Dublin. Newman accepted, though he retained his office as Superior of the Oratory, and in the seven years which followed he made some sixty crossings of the Irish Sea to administer the new venture. The Irish University was the direct result of the condemnation of the Queen's Colleges, and of the 'mixed education' they embodied, both by the Irish bishops and by Propaganda in 1847 —a condemnation repeated at the Synod of Thurles in 1850. Propaganda suggested that the needs of Catholic higher education should be met by the creation of a Catholic University on the model of the successful one set up by the Belgian bishops in 1834 at Louvain. The Catholic University in Dublin had a difficult start: there were differences of view over fundamental matters of policy between Newman and the Irish bishops. Much subsequent commentary has emphasized Newman's attempt to reproduce Oxford education in Dublin. In some measure he did, indeed, try to do so. Newman originally intended a collegiate structure, until Cullen prevailed against him; and there can be little doubt that the college he envisaged would have been like Oxford ones. Yet Louvain, too, was collegiate in structure. Newman also projected an education for 'gentlemen', and although the Irish bishops had intended a university for Irishmen, he hoped to attract English Catholics in quite large numbers. The bishops sought training for their youth in the professions; Newman had a vision of general liberal education. 'Whether or no a Catholic University should put before it, as its great object, to make its students "gentlemen",' he wrote, 'still to make them something or

other *is* its great object, and not simply to promote the interests and advance the dominion of science.'[116] The purpose of
a university was 'in one word the culture of the intellect'.[117]
He added, however, 'and I do not deny that the characteristic
excellencies of a gentleman are included in it'.[118] There are
some indications of this in the Dublin college. Newman had a
billiards room built and a cricket field laid out; undergraduates were allowed to hunt; and as a rather scandalized Cullen
noted—fearing the corruption of Irish youth by alien English
ways—'the young men are allowed to go out at all hours, to
smoke etc.'[119] Serious though such considerations may have
been for some, however, the more interesting consequences
of Newman's attempt to give his religious and educational
ideas a physical reality lay in the clarity with which the ideas
themselves appeared. At Oxford, he had had to fight against
secularizing liberal tendencies; in Dublin the reverse was the
case. There the battle with the bishops over various issues of
control was essentially .concerned with avoiding too much
ecclesiastical interference. Newman clearly intended the University to be largely a lay institution; the bishops envisaged it
as a sort of lay seminary. This central issue was a key issue in
the controversies between the Ultramontanes and the Liberal
Catholics in England: the balance between free intellectual
enquiry and religious authority. Newman was concerned with
knowledge for its own sake. That was the educational purpose
of a university: 'If its objects were scientific and philosophical
discovery, I do not see why a university should have students;
if religious training, I do not see how it can be the seat of
literature and science.'[120] All knowledge, on the other hand,
had to be related to religious Revelation: once again it was a
matter of establishing a balance. 'If the Catholic Faith is true,
a university cannot exist externally to the Catholic pale, for
it cannot teach universal knowledge if it does not teach Catholic theology.'[121] The appointments which Newman made to

[116] *The Idea of a University*, xiv.
[117] Ibid. xv.
[118] .Ibid. xvi.
[119] John Coulson, 'Newman's Idea of an Open University and its consequences
today', in Bastable, *Newman and Gladstone*, 223.
[120] *The Idea of a University*, ix.
[121] Ibid. 214 ('Duties of the Church Towards Knowledge').

teaching posts at Dublin caused some disquiet because they included many Englishmen—including the son of Dr Arnold of Rugby, a curious turn of fate—but much more disquiet was caused by their liberal attitude to knowledge, and because of the thirty-two professors only five were priests. When six Young Irelanders were given posts matters looked serious to the bishops: the Young Ireland party had been identified by the hierarchy as 'Mazzinians', enemies of Catholic faith and morals. Newman was concerned with intellectual excellence. He was innocent of affairs in Ireland and had, in fact, never been there before arriving to start the University.[122] Difficulties with the main body of the bishops—'those wild Paddies', as Ambrose St. John called them[123]—got worse. 'Every individual who helps me will be grudged,' Newman exclaimed to J. D. Dalgairns in 1854.[124] The irritations at that level were not really the cause of division: that remained the difference between Newman's liberal view of education and the bishop's insistence on a circumscribed religious framework for all knowledge. As the bishops, so it seemed to Newman, increased their obstruction, he came to depend more and more on Dr David Moriarty, President of All Hallows College, Drumcondra (and later Bishop of Kerry).[125] Now Moriarty was a noted Liberal Catholic, who was later to be an Inopportunist at the Vatican Council. Newman's reliance on him heightened the impression that he was moving towards a 'Liberal' position. The matter should not be exaggerated, however, and Cullen, who was the doyen of the Irish Ultramontanes, later actually testified at Rome to Newman's doctrinal orthodoxy at a time (1867) when he was still suspected of heretical tendencies. That Cullen worked in 1854 to prevent the bishopric being conferred on Newman which Wiseman had procured for him (and which had already been made public) was probably an indication, not of his doubts about Newman's soundness of doctrine, but of his wish to retain control of the management of the University. When Newman determined to resign the

---

[122] Fergal McGrath, *Newman's University. Idea and Reality*, Dublin 1951, 125.
[123] Trevor, *Light in Winter*, 63.
[124] *Letters and Diaries of John Henry Newman*, ed. Dessain, XVI (London 1964), 168 (June 1854).
[125] McGrath, 153.

Rectorship in 1858, Cullen tried to persuade him to stay. Yet Cullen's opposition to his vision of education was unquestionably among the considerations which determined Newman's decision to relinquish the office. The more important reason, however, was probably his desire to attend to the affairs of the Birmingham Oratory. 'I left the University literally because the Oratory *demanded* it,' he wrote to Robert Ornsby.[126] His hopes of English support had not materialized, either financially or through the supply of large numbers of students. He had failed to get financial control of the University away from the bishops, and into lay hands. The University had not received a Charter from the Crown, and so could not confer legally-recognized degrees—although as Newman pointed out to his successor, Dr Bartholomew Woodlock, Louvain had no charter either and yet flourished.[127] Irish secondary education, furthermore, had not adequately—again from Newman's point of view—prepared youths for a university education. The Dublin University survived until 1882 when it was integrated with the Royal University of Ireland.

There was another intellectual area in which Newman was suspected in his own day of 'liberal' tendencies: his view of the relationship between historical evidence and Revealed truth. Here his thought achieved lasting insights. Yet Döllinger appears to have been impressed by Newman's ignorance of history. 'I am amazed at the naive confidence with which Newman presents the most obvious untruths without any semblance of proof', he observed, 'I can defend his character only at the expense of his learning.'[128] Certainly Newman's detailed knowledge of the history of the Church in all but the Early and Reformation periods was thin,[129] and the works he admired, like Fleury's *Church History* (of which he published a translation in 1838) were scarcely critical. But Newman did have an extraordinary grasp of the subtlety of the relationship between ideas, material events, and the formulation of

---

[126] *Letters and Diaries*, ed. Dessain, XIX (London 1969), 455 (Jan. 1861).

[127] Ibid. XXIV (Oxford 1973), 40 (Feb. 1868).

[128] Victor Conzemius, 'Acton, Döllinger and Gladstone: A Strange Variety of Infallibilists', in Bastable, *Newman and Gladstone*, 43.

[129] Nicholas Lash, *Newman and Development. The Search for an Explanation in History*, London [1975], 1979 edn., 44.

doctrine. It was, again, a balanced and moderate approach: 'For myself, I would simply confess that no doctrine of the Church can be rigorously proved by historical evidence; but at the same time that no doctrine can be simply disproved by it.'[130] His *Essay on the Development of Christian Doctrine*, written while he was still an Anglican and published after his conversion in 1845, was Newman's greatest work. Its essential thesis is that religious development is according to the same sort of cultural and historical influences as define the process of change in all things, that Revealed truth is transmitted through human agency in the historical Church and that, however guided by mysterious forces, the intellectual patterns and real events of each successive age will mould and transform men's perceptions of the original deposit of faith. It was an expression of Newman's observation that all life is change; and that men cannot stand outside their own history.[131] Development, Newman remarked, was 'discernible from the first years of Catholic teaching up to the present day, and gave to that teaching a unity and individuality'.[132] It accounted for the authenticity of Catholic teachings—on the Papacy and on Marian devotions, for example—which were not evident in Antiquity. In his article of 1859 'On Consulting the Faithful in Matters of Doctrine'—which was itself actually about Development—he suggested that the definition of the dogma of the Immaculate Conception in 1854 was an example of the process at work.[133] Development valued the place of tradition, yet set it upon a dynamic rather than a static calculus. In this it differed from the theory of Development in Cardinal Franzelin's *De Divina Traditione et Scriptura*, conceived in opposition to certain aspects of German dialectical philosophy, and which regarded Development as a process of logical deduction. Newman was within the English empirical tradition, and wrote in order to provide a correct interpretation of an aspect of Catholic history which Protestants had always highlighted in their anti-Catholic polemicism—the claim that true doctrine could issue from institutions in which there were

---

[130] Newman, *Letter to the Duke of Norfolk*, 118.
[131] Lash, 134.
[132] *Apologia*, 287.
[133] *Rambler*, I (new series), July 1859, 209.

evidences of corruption. Some have believed that Newman's theory had affinities with nineteenth-century evolutionary thought,[134] but this is unlikely, and the organic images in the *Essay* more probably derive from Biblical language.[135] If the *Essay* can be compared with any nineteenth-century secular thinking, it is to the accumulation of historical relativism. Whately saw this; he said the work was more likely to turn men into sceptics than into Romanists.[136] This assessment was quite common at the time. 'Were I an Infidel, and did I possess the species of intellect which Mr. Newman possesses', wrote the Revd. George Faber, Prebendary of Salisbury, of the *Essay*, 'the mode, which, in the present day, I should select for the most effectual propagation of Infidelity, would be the precise mode adopted by that gentleman in his recent Work.'[137] The *Essay* was denounced by the most famous theologian in Rome, Perrone.

Twentieth-century admirers of·Newman have tended to attribute all their own favoured ideas to him; in the nineteenth century his detractors represented him as the repository of all dangerous ones. It is a measure of the true independence of his mind, and of his lack of indebtedness to any party or men, that he was such an isolated and suspected figure. It gave him, in his own day, a very limited influence inside the Catholic Church. His influence, indeed, as the Duke of Norfolk noticed in 1878, was much greater with the non-Catholic public.[138] It had not always been so. At the time of his conversion, when he was widely believed to have been a secret 'Romanist' for some years (largely because of the adverse reception of Tract XC in 1841) and in his Catholic life until the publication of the *Apologia* in 1864, he was a despised and misunderstood figure. All kinds of extraordinary rumours about him were accorded credence—'The report grows stronger', he wrote to Faber in 1850, 'that I am married, and have shut up my wife in a convent.'[139] The Achilli

---

[134] Trevor, *The Pillar of the Gloud*, 282.
[135] Nicholas Lash, 'Literature and Theory: Did Newman have a "Theory" of Development?' in Bastable, *Newman and Gladstone*, 165.
[136] Trevor, *The Pillar of the Cloud*, 370.
[137] G. S. Faber, *Letters on Tractarian Secession to Popery*, London 1846, 75.
[138] Reynolds, 246.
[139] *Letters and Diaries*, ed. Dessain, XIV (London 1963), 163 (Dec. 1850).

case added to the hostility. In the course of his *Lectures on the Present Position of Catholics in England* in 1851, Newman had depended on allegations made by Wiseman to accuse Giacinto Achilli (an ex-Dominican priest who had become a popular anti-Catholic lecturer in England) of moral improprieties. The result was that Achilli, who was sponsored by the Evangelical Alliance, brought an action against him for libel. Wiseman, unhappily, was unable to find his evidence and after delayed court hearings, in 1853—which even *The Times* judged prejudicial—Judge Coleridge had deplored Newman's moral deterioration since his conversion. Newman was found guilty. The fine of £100 and costs was fortunately light. But Newman had to endure a terrible sequence of events and his reputation sank to its lowest level in Protestant society. For him it was, as he had written to Talbot (in seeking evidence against Achilli from Rome), 'a most important crisis'. 'Indeed it is not my cause, but the cause of the Catholic Church,' he urged: 'Achilli is going about like a false spirit, telling lies, and since it is forced upon us, we must put him down, and not suffer him to triumph.'[140]

It was in Rome, however, that Newman came to have opponents, and it was in fact Talbot who denounced his article on the Laity as 'certainly detestable', in 1859.[141] On receiving Bishop Brown's delation of the article for heresy, Barnabò had asked Ullathorne, as Newman's bishop, to seek an explanation from Newman. Newman had been willing to provide this, but had asked for specification of particular alleged offences in the piece. Wiseman failed to pass this request on to Rome—another indication of his chaotic conduct of routine business[142]—and Propaganda concluded that Newman had refused to comply. Newman was, in consequence, suspected of unsound views at Rome until 1867. In 1860 a report even circulated in the city that he was sympathetic to Garibaldi.[143] The opposition of Manning and the Ultramontanes in England, some of whom suspected that Newman had

[140] Ibid. XIV 344 (Sept. 1851).

[141] Holmes, *More Roman than Rome*, 114.

[142] The matter occurred at the height of Wiseman's dispute with the Westminster Chapter and with Errington, and so may well have been overlooked.

[143] MacDougall, 64.

never really espoused truly Catholic principles and attitudes, was symptomized in the dispute between the Birmingham Oratory and the London one—which was the embodiment of Faber's Ultramontanism. Manning's suspicions of Newman eventually extended to a clumsy attempt to prevent his elevation to the dignity of a cardinal in 1879. At least, in all his isolation, Newman had the consolation of Ullathorne's support. 'You have ever been indulgent towards me', he wrote to Ullathorne in 1886, as he contemplated death; it encouraged him 'in the prospect of the awful journey which lies close before me'.[144] By even the mid-1860s, Newman was writing of having 'got hardened against the opposition made to me', particularly 'on the part of certain influential Catholics'.[145] The publication of the *Apologia* in 1864 had at least removed the hostility of many Protestants, who were moved by the fairness of its tone, its evident spirituality, and its logic; but it had enhanced the opposition of the Ultramontanes. Other Catholics were delighted: the Birmingham Diocesan Synod presented Newman with an address. He had, after all, taken on one of the most well-known Anglicans of the day and succeeded. Charles Kingsley, whose allegations about the moral honesty of the Catholic priesthood the *Apologia* was written to disprove, was at the time Professor of Modern History at Cambridge, a Chaplain to the Queen, tutor to the Prince of Wales, and a much-read novelist. A sign of Newman's rehabilitation came in 1869: he was invited to attend the Vatican Council as an advisory theologian by several bishops —including Brown of Newport, his detractor in 1859. He declined, both on grounds of age, and because he was working on the *Grammar of Assent*. Yet it was not really until the cardinalate that Newman felt that 'the cloud is lifted from me for ever'.[146] When he died in 1890 the transformation of his reputation was complete: all the newspapers carried generous tributes to his life and work.[147]

William George Ward's conversion to Catholicism had followed the condemnation of his book *The Ideal of a Christian*

[144] *Letters and Diaries*, ed. Dessain, XXXI (Oxford 1977), 160 (Sept. 1886).
[145] John Henry Newman, *Autobiographical Writings*, ed. Tristram, 260 (*Journal*, Feb. 1865).
[146] Trevor, *Light in Winter*, 600.   [147] Ibid. 646.

Church, because of its sympathy for 'Roman' doctrines, by the convocation of Oxford University in 1845. He was thereafter known as 'Ideal Ward'. He was the son of the proprietor of Lord's Cricket Ground in London, and inherited his uncle's wealth so that, as a Catholic layman, he lived the life of a rich and independent scholar and *savant*. Educated at Winchester and Christ Church, he had become a Fellow of Balliol and proceeded to Holy Orders in the Church of England. As the *Ideal* had made clear, he was a leading figure of the Oxford Movement. After conversion he lived a secluded existence for three years in a little house Pugin had built for him near to St. Edmund's College, Ware; and it was at the College that he became Professor of Dogmatic Theology from 1851 to 1858. Throughout the 1860s he edited the *Dublin Review*, finally transforming the journal into a vehicle of extreme Ultramontane opinions: assailing Liberal Catholicism, upholding the Temporal Power, and advocating a very advanced interpretation of Infallibility. It was these articles which first made him well known to the English Catholic public.[148] In 1858, after his temporary (as it turned out) removal to the Isle of Wight, local residents were 'astonished' by 'the large number of "popish ecclesiastics" who visited him'.[149] He found the sea air at Cowes detrimental to his health and returned to Hertfordshire, yet in 1871 again took up residence there. Ward enjoyed public controversy and was good at it. Although to most Protestant Englishmen of his day Ultramontanism was the least rational of attitudes, he was listened to with respect by some of the leading intellectuals—as, for example, in the Metaphysical Society, after its formation in 1869. He was a correspondent of John Stuart Mill's from 1865 up to Mill's death in 1873.[150] A critic once said that Ward was more a 'theopolitician' than a theologian,[151] and although that does the quality of his thought an injustice it has a flavour of truth about it. When Cashel Hoey became sub-editor of the *Dublin*, Ward told him: 'You will

    [146] Purcell, *Manning*, II. 386.
    [149] Wilfrid Ward, *William George Ward*, 214.
    [150] Though it is hard to escape the impression that Ward was more enthusiastic about the exchange of views than Mill.
    [151] Wilfrid Ward, *William George Ward*, 134.

find me narrow and strong—*very* narrow and *very* strong.'[152]
It was no exaggeration. He shared with Faber, who was a
friend, exclusivity of opinion; both were extreme in their different areas of expertise. Disagreements with Newman, for
this reason also, became more extensive with the years: Ward
projected an ideology of ecclesiastical authority which left
just the sort of individuality which Newman so treasured
with no room for cultivation or expression. From de Maistre,
Ward got the conviction that authentic religious truth could
only be preserved if the Papacy established the criteria by
which the fruits of modern knowledge were to be received.[153]
He saw that the intellectual culture of the age tended to secularism and rationalism, and spoke of a 'war of principles' as
the necessary condition between Catholicism and modern
learning as a consequence. Christianity was exclusive. 'It
could not logically deal with all phases of thought as on a
level; with all standards of moral judgement as equally valuable studies.'[154] Newman, of course, would have agreed with
that; the two men did not differ over the dogmatic principle
as such, but about the means by which actual dogma was
established and verified. Nor did they differ over the place of
political experience in the Christian life. Ward, like Newman,
had a considerable antipathy to political liberalism, especially
since the English Liberal Party was so sympathetic to the
Italian *Risorgimento*, and like at least the Catholic Newman
he distrusted traditional Toryism. Both men eschewed political affiliation, not from high-minded detachment from the
mere traffickings of politicians, but because both regarded
political values as having in themselves a low priority. Like
Newman, again, Ward was not greatly exercised over the
social issues of the day. His knowledge of social facts was
limited. When he felt the need to inform himself about the
living conditions of the working classes, for example, in
1848, he consulted Mill over the literature he could read up.
'I feel most painfully my total ignorance on this subject,
arising, partly, from an Oxford life, but more from an (in
one sense) *unpractical* turn of mind,' he told Mill. 'I mean,
I have no powers at all to go among the poor and judge for

---

[152] Ibid. 223.   [153] Ibid. 146.   [154] Ibid. 148.

myself; my faculty of observation is so deplorably inadequate.'[155]

It was Ward, of course, who was the most persistent critic of the Liberal Catholics in England, and who frequently savaged the articles which appeared in the *Rambler*. He regarded Montalembert's famous address on religious and civil liberty at the Malines Congress in 1863 as simply a demonstration of the principles of Indifferentism, and privately circulated a critique of it. Wiseman, who was at the Congress, disapproved of the separation of Church and State which Montalembert advocated, as a departure from Catholic practice, but did not regard the speech as courting heretical tendencies, as Ward did.[156] With that exception, Ward always had the support of Wiseman, and of Manning, for his opinions. With the latter he shared a near identity of views over the *Syllabus* and over Infallibility. He regarded the *Syllabus* as itself an infallible statement and used the *Dublin Review* to say so. Two years later, in 1866, he published *Authority of Doctrinal Decisions* which enlarged the area of Infallibility to embrace any religious guidance given by the Pope personally, whether in public declarations or private letters and utterances. It was an opinion which he confirmed in *De Infallibilitatis Extensione* (1869). Since this went considerably beyond orthodox attitudes to Infallibility it drew a lot of criticism—from Dupanloup, who rightly recognized an affinity to the views of Veuillot, and from Ullathorne, representing moderate 'English' Catholicism.[157] Newman, too, publicly opposed Ward's interpretation in 1868, drawing further opposition from Rome. Canon John Morris, of the Westminster Chapter, wrote to Talbot: 'Ward is publishing his articles as a book, and I think that if Roman theologians read it, they will endorse it absolutely.'[158] Infallibility as decreed by the Vatican Council, however, fell far short of Ward's definition.

Around the time of the Council, Ward began to become increasingly subject to ill-health. He interested himself more in

[155] Ibid. 24.
[156] Wilfrid Ward, *Wiseman*, II. 460.
[157] Butler, *Ullathorne*, II. 44.
[158] English College Archives, Talbot Papers, 521, Morris to Talbot, 26 Feb. 1866.

philosophical than in theological speculation, and did so for the remainder of his life. In his later years he admitted that some of his earlier theological opinions may have been too extreme, that he had 'pressed one or two' of his points 'much too far' in 'the heat of polemics'. This was due, he confessed —in a moment of great frankness to which few intellectuals are given—'to a certain hankering after premature logical completeness'.[159] His exposition of the Ultramontanist position had attained very great theoretical coherence, none the less, and Ward must be judged a major intellectual influence within the English Catholicism of the nineteenth century. He spent the last years of his life on the Isle of Wight, reading French plays. 'I sometimes get through six in an evening', he said.[160] He died in 1882.

In direct contrast to Ward were the Modernists. The Modernist 'crisis' as it is usually called—the controversy surrounding the condemnation of the opinions of these later Liberal Catholics by the Vatican—was at its height at the end of the nineteenth century, where this study ends, and some of the most important developments took place in the first decade of the present century. But the leading English figures of the movement belonged to the nineteenth century: Mivart, who died in 1900; Acton, who died in 1902; and Tyrrell, whose death did not occur until 1909, and von Hügel, who lived to 1925. These men produced their most seminal work before the start of the new century. Modernism was as difficult to define as Liberal Catholicism had been—and, like it, the movement underwent internal transformation. Yet it is perhaps not too crude to say that in essence it was the attempt by some Catholic scholars to apply historical and scientific knowledge to Biblical criticism, and to seek to claim for intellectual enquiry, and the methods by which it is conducted, a measure of autonomy from ecclesiastical authority. In political outlook the Modernists tended to a sort of progressive liberalism, élitist but enlightened; in learning they were opponents of scholasticism. They eschewed just those dogmatic principles of religious definition which lay at the

[159] Wilfrid Ward, *William George Ward*, 264. (He said this in 1881.)
[160] Ibid. 387.

heart of both Ward's and Newman's understanding of Christian truth. Their quarrel was with received notions about the *magisterium* of the Church, about the relationship between the Papacy, the episcopate, and the laity, in the construction of religious truth and the authority by which it is delineated. Since a measure of scepticism about authority has been a leading characteristic of later twentieth-century Christian intellectual endeavour, it is not surprising that the thought of the Modernists has attracted recent sympathetic attention. In 1893 Leo XIII's Encyclical, *Providentissimus Deus*, attempted to set limits to the sort of Biblical criticism that the Church could approve, and this seemed to open the counter-attack by authority upon the Modernists. Loisy rejected its contentions and von Hügel explained it away.[161] In 1900 Cardinal Vaughan and the English hierarchy issued 'A Joint Pastoral Letter on the Church and Liberal Catholicism', mostly directed against Mivart's ideas, which upheld traditional teachings about the authority of the *magisterium*. In July 1907 came the Encyclical *Lamentabili Sane* of St. Pius X, a syllabus of sixty-five 'errors of the Modernists', of which the last was that 'Modern Catholicism can be reconciled with true science only if it is transformed into a non-dogmatic Christianity.'[162] A second Encyclical, *Pascendi Dominici Gregis*, in September of the same year, defended scholastic theology against Modernism—'the synthesis of all heresies'—and warned of threats to the Church 'by arts entirely new and full of deceit'.[163] In these reactions, which, like the *Syllabus* of 1864, seemed to deny the religious validity of some of the basic concepts of modern intellectual culture, there was a fundamental concern by the Papacy and by the local hierarchies to protect the authority of the teaching office of the Church against academic individualism exercised without reference to it. What was the contribution of the English Modernists to the 'crisis'? In the analysis which follows, the thought of the Modernists is considered—as was the case in the preceding observations on Newman and Ward—more or less solely as it explains their

[161] Lawrence F. Barmann, *Baron von Hügel and the Modernist Crisis in England*, Cambridge 1972, 39.
[162] Anne Freemantle (ed.), *The Papal Encyclicals*, New York 1956, 207.
[163] Ibid. 197.

relationship to the institutional Church, rather than as an examination of their place in intellectual history.

Acton, though for good reasons not conventionally regarded as a Modernist, illustrated one feature of the Modernists which it is always important to realize: as Archbishop Mathew pointed out, his influence within English Catholicism was slight. It lay with Protestant academies and literary men. 'Gasquet raised a tomb to him: but the *Cambridge Modern History* is his true sepulchre.'[164] His rejection of so many aspects of ecclesiastical authority placed him outside identification with the institutional Church. He recognized this himself, and made a virtue of it. He belonged, he told the electors during the Bridgnorth election of 1865, 'rather to the soul than the body of the Catholic Church'.[165] His exuberant denunciations of past Popes as 'murderers', and his triumphalist pitting of historical evidence against received dogmas, conveyed a sense almost of satisfaction in discomfiting the bearers of religious authority. His passionate desire to disclose evidence of past persecutions carried out by Papal authority made undergraduates at Cambridge, when they heard his lectures, say 'that he had persecution on the brain'.[166] He would perhaps have agreed with Tevor-Roper's assessment that his endeavours to present a reasonable version of Catholicism were frustrated because the English Catholicism of his day 'had reached its narrowest point of bigotry and obscurantism'.[167]

It was in Naples, in 1834, that Sir John Acton was born (he succeeded to the baronetcy in 1837); his father was a diplomat, and the family, an old landed one from Shropshire, had been converted to Catholicism in the eighteenth century. He was educated in Paris, and at Oscott, and then, in 1848, for two years in Edinburgh before a six-year period of study in Münich under Döllinger—the most important influence of his life. From Döllinger he acquired his passion for historical

[164] Mathew, 223.
[165] Altholz, *The Liberal Catholic Movement in England*, 234.
[166] Owen Chadwick, *Catholicism and History. The Opening of the Vatican Archives*, Cambridge 1978, 57.
[167] Lord Acton, *Lectures on Modern History*, London (Fontana edn.) 1960, Introduction by Hugh Trevor-Roper, 9.

learning and his belief, which was itself dogmatic, that history
provided the keys to the explanation of knowledge. He had
a Whiggish reverence for the English Constitution, which
seemed to him to embody true 'Catholic' principles of free
government. Though not especially concerned with party
politics, he entered Parliament for an Irish seat, Carlow, in
1859. His campaign, organized for him by the local Catholic
priest, was marked by 'a considerable amount of mob violence, and at least the suspicion of bribery'.[168] He favoured
the ballot, and agrarian and other reforms, and supported the
Liberals in the House of Commons. Gladstone made him a
peer in 1869, the year in which he lost his seat. But his
interests and his preoccupations were historical, not political.
Indeed he had a very elliptical knowledge of current events
and almost all of his predictions—including his belief that the
Pope would leave Rome and settle in Bavaria—proved false.[169]
Yet it was a central theme in his thinking that a Christian
should be committed to the politics of liberty: hence his well-
known antipathy to absolutism in both religious and civil
government. It was a consequence of his emphasis on the
ethics of religious systems. The Church, properly understood,
should be 'the irreconcilable enemy of the despotism of the
State'.[170] It was because of these beliefs that he regarded the
Münich Congress in 1863, and Montalembert's declaration
for religious and civil freedom, as 'the dawn of a new era'[171]—
another of his predictions which, as the Vatican Council was
to show, was rather less than accurate. He also disliked the
Temporal Power as tending to involve the Church with exactly
the sort of politics of which he disapproved. In March 1860,
in an article in the *Rambler*, he was still willing to defend it
in the belief that the anti-religious inclinations of the Italian
radicals would lead to 'the extermination of the Catholic
Church'.[172] He declared, 'The secularization of the Roman
system is simply contrary to the notion of a state which exists

[168] Altholz, 105.

[169] Gasquet (ed.), *Lord Acton and his Circle*, lxxxvii.

[170] Altholz, 66 (*Rambler*, Jan. 1859).

[171] Lord Acton, *Essays on Church and State*, ed. Douglas Woodruff, London
1952, 199 (*Home and Foreign Review*, Jan. 1864).

[172] MacDougall, 68.

as the property and for the benefit of the whole Catholic Church.'[173] A subsequent article appeared 'offensive' at Rome, as Talbot explained to Manning,[174] because it declined to uphold the status of the Church on theoretical and theological grounds. They were grounds on which Acton would not defend the Temporal Power, and in the next few years he became its opponent.

The whole movement of the Church towards the acclamation of Ultramontanism in the 1860s was regrettable to Acton. Like other liberals, he saw the *Syllabus* of 1864 as a rejection of intellectual and political dispositions which were essential for the achievement of academic freedom and personal liberty.[175] His work behind the scenes at the Vatican Council[176] was a self-conscious attempt to save the Church from what he considered, in Gladstonian style, a terrible slide into medievalism; it was the last chance to salvage the Liberal Catholic position. His attempts to influence the British government against the proceedings were certainly successful, but did not bear the fruit he had sought: an international intervention, his last desperate card. 'A decree proclaiming the Pope infallible would be a confession that the authority of General Councils has been an illusion', he wrote in 1867. The promoters of Infallibility regarded 'the preservation of authority' as 'a higher object than the propagation of faith'.[177] It was his constant theme. Authority, as exercised by Rome, was incompatible with individual conscience. His view of conscience was crucially different from that of Newman, for whom conscience was exercised within the mystical community of faith—it was not a sort of individual criterion by which the adherent could judge the sense of the *magisterium*. Acton's relations with Newman illustrated the depth of their religious differences. Despite their early cooperation over the *Rambler*, there was no real sympathy between them. Acton recorded a meeting on New Year's Day 1859, at which the two men discussed the position of the

---

[173] Acton, *Essays on Church and State*, 121 (*Rambler*, March 1860).
[174] Purcell, *Manning*, II. 165 (May 1861).
[175] Altholz, 233.
[176] See chapter 6.
[177] MacDougall, 111–12.

journal. Newman, he recalled, 'moaned for a long time, rock-
ing himself backwards and forwards over the fire, like an old
woman with a toothache'.[178] He came to believe that Newman
was really an Ultramontane—'he was heart and soul, far more
than he ever suffered to appear, an advocate of Rome'.[179]
With time, his judgement became more extreme. In 1880 he
called Newman an 'evil' man, and in 1896 he referred to his
religious opinions as 'a school of Infidelity'.[180] He declared:
'Newman professed liberalism, when in fact he was in favour
of the Inquisition.'[181] By these years, Acton was immersed in
his historical studies; he had been appointed, through Lord
Rosebery's influence, to the Regius Chair of Modern History
at Cambridge, and was engaged in editing the *Cambridge
Modern History*. The results of his enormous historical eclecticism, however, were intended for a massive and systematic
'History of Liberty'. It was never written.

Baron Friedrich von Hügel, even more than Acton, was
earnest about the moral seriousness with which he undertook
intellectual enquiry. Like Acton, he was a dedicated supporter
of the belief that Catholic teachings had to be brought into
correspondence with the methods and conclusions of contemporary scientific and historical knowledge. Like Acton,
also, he appealed more to non-Catholics than to members of
his own Church.[182] It was Charles Gore, the Anglican Bishop
of Oxford, who said—an extraordinary exaggeration—that he
was 'the most learned man living'.[183] He was, indeed, characterized by an enormous breadth of knowledge and a Germanic
style of systematic thinking which Englishmen tended to
find deeply impressive—or, if not impressive, at least the most
obvious thing about him. Archbishop Mathew remarked that
his thought was 'almost monumentally Teutonic'.[184] Nearly
three-quarters of his reading was of German works of scholarship, and during the First World War there were those who
supposed he must be a German spy.[185] His intellectualism
drew him to W. G. Ward (his neighbour in Hampstead), but it

[178] Gasquet (ed.), 47.   [179] Altholz, 170.
[180] MacDougall, 140.   [181] Ibid. 144.
[182] John J. Heaney, *The Modernist Crisis: von Hügel*, 150.
[183] Michael de la Bedoyere, *The Life of Baron von Hügel*, London 1951, xi.
[184] Mathew, 223.   [185] Heaney, 13.

was an attraction of like *minds* rather than of similar intellectual contents. Von Hügel's intellectualism impelled him to assess people by their ideas and their cerebral cultivation rather than by their characters or capabilities: his friends all agreed about 'his defective judgement of human nature'.[186] He was the son of an Austrian diplomat, born in Florence in 1852. His mother was Scottish, a converted Presbyterian, and his biographer has emphasized her contribution to his moral seriousness.[187] He never attended a school, but was educated, in succession, by an Anglican governess, a Lutheran layman, and a Jewish Hebrew teacher: it is necessary to look no further for the springs of his intellectual eclecticism. As a boy, he was interested in geology and entomology, and later testified that 'they helped to develop in me, I think, a double consciousness of cumulative evidence as an instrument of knowledge, of successive stages of development as a subject of knowledge'.[188] That ought to have produced at least some common ground with Newman's views on Development—whose virtues he did indeed acknowledge—but von Hügel's loathing of dogmatič principles of religion served to distance him from Newman. He conceived a personal dislike for Newman, in fact. When von Hügel was twenty-four, he and his wife had called on Newman (who was then seventy-four) in Birmingham, and both then, and on a number of occasions, had 'interviewed Newman'.[189] During the controversy with Kingsley, which resulted in Newman's *Apologia*, von Hügel sided with Kingsley.[190] He found Newman 'not easy to talk with, because he was so sensitive and easily pained, like a very refined sensitive old lady'.[191] There were those who did not find von Hügel easy to talk with either: he delivered monologues rather than conversed, a feature which in some measure was involuntarily produced by his deafness. He was extremely conscious of race and national characteristics in the determination of cultural and moral qualities. He found it, in fact, necessary 'to understand the racial background of a person, in order to size up his ideas'.[192] He regarded the British Empire

---

[186] Ibid. 18.
[187] Ibid. 13.
[188] de la Bedoyere, 17.
[189] Barmann, 6.
[190] de la Bedoyere, 32.
[191] Heaney, 23.
[192] Ibid. 17.

as 'greatly to the advantage of its subject races'.[193] He spoke out publicly against Irish Home Rule in 1886—partly because of his disgust at the Catholics' involvement with politics in Ireland.[194] Despite his cosmopolitan background, von Hügel lived his life in England, adopting in a rather heavily self-conscious form what he supposed were English attitudes and customs. The family lived at various times in very English places—Malvern, Torquay, Hampstead, and Kensington. Holidays were spent at Bournemouth. He sang selections from Gilbert and Sullivan operas to his young children; one of whom, Hildegard, recalled that the examinations he set them, to ensure their progression in enlightened knowledge, were 'far more exacting than those of the Public Schools or even the Universities'.[195] He had, as Wilfrid Ward observed, 'a picturesque personality'.[196]

Von Hügel was not a straightforward Modernist—perhaps none of those to whom the label has been applied were. Von Hügel's central emphasis was on intellectual freedom. From the Abbé Henri Huvelin, his spiritual director from the age of thirty-two, he acquired the principle that conscience was more important than orthodoxy. Döllinger seems to have had little influence in the formation of his thought, and his critical theological writings appeared to have owed more to Loisy, Blondel, Duchesne, and Tyrrell, with all of whom he corresponded. His personal friendship with George Tyrrell began in 1897, though there was never an identification of views. Von Hügel disliked ecclesiastical authority when it inhibited intellectual endeavour, but he was not an opponent of the spiritual or historical claims of the Papacy—as most of the Modernists in the end were in some degree or other. It is true in 1901 he declined to join what became the Pontifical Biblical Commission, and that this was because he wished to avoid commitments to an official body;[197] but his decision was not intended to convey any general rejection of Papal authority. In von Hügel there was no sense, as there was in Acton, that authority was being ransacked through the unavoidable compulsion of a personal claim to superior knowledge. Von Hügel

[193] de la Bedoyere, 127.   [194] Ibid. 51.
[195] Ibid. 54.   [196] Ibid. 57.
[197] Barmann, 88.

sought a pre-Tridentine form of Catholicism; he sought a work of restoration, a return to the collegiality, as he supposed, of the past. That was the pivot of his criticism of ecclesiastical authority. In von Hügel's critical theological writings, which began in the 1890s, there emerged a vision of a mystical element in Christianity, an absorption with the nature of God and the means of discussing his presence in the physical world whose laws and cultural variations the contemporary sciences were revealing. He was less concerned with the institutional Church. This became particularly clear in his most important work, *The Mystical Element of Religion*, published in 1908—a book which the Protestant Archbishop William Temple judged 'the most important theological work written in the English language during the last half century'.[198]

Von Hügel's friend, George Tyrrell, was perhaps the most extreme of the Modernists in England. He was in fact Irish, born in Dublin in 1861 to a Protestant family, and educated at Trinity College, Dublin. In 1879 he became a Catholic and in 1880 joined the English Province of the Society of Jesus. In 1894 he lectured in Moral Theology at Stonyhurst, moving to London, to Farm Street, in 1896. There he began writing. He was, as his biographer has remarked, preoccupied with analysis and synthesis. 'He could not help it. It was in his nature; it was in his blood.'[199] He also had a degree of intellectual perversity, which allowed his ordinary perversity (which was inseparable from his character) to be represented, to himself, as principled objections to Catholic authority. Hence the difficulties which he encountered, first with the Jesuit order, and then with the Church. He was 'by temperament', in the view of another student of his works, 'disposed to attack'.[200] The movement away from orthodox Catholic doctrine was first noticeable in December 1899 when he published an article entitled 'A Perverted Devotion' in the *Weekly Register*, which attacked Catholic teachings on hell and eternal punishment—the very issue which had involved a number of Anglican

---

[198] de la Bedoyere, xi.

[199] J. Lewis May, *Father Tyrrell and the Modernist Movement*, London (2nd edn.), 1938, 9.

[200] Mary Jo Weaver (ed.), *Letters from a "Modernist". The Letters of George Tyrrell to Wilfrid Ward, 1893-1908*, London 1981, xviii.

theologians in controversy earlier in the century.[201] The article was delated to the Provincial of the Jesuits. In the ensuing controversy, von Hügel supported Tyrrell. In 1903 Tyrrell wrote and circulated (though he did not publish) a critical—indeed dismissive—reply to the *Pastoral Letter* of the hierarchy on Liberal Catholicism (1900) entitled *The Church and the Future*. Thereafter came a number of works, which were considered heterodox by the leaders of the Church—some on Catholic devotional life. By then, he was living at the Jesuit mission in Richmond, Yorkshire, having had to depart from Farm Street because of his refusal to moderate his opinions. His opposition to the Church was also, by then, well advanced. 'The Church first kills and then devours her foes, and digests as much of the constitutions as matter for her purpose,' he wrote to Wilfrid Ward in 1900; 'no other philosophy of life is to live but herself; and she must rise and slay before she can eat.'[202] It was not the sort of sentiment which accorded well with the general atmosphere of the Catholic Church under Cardinal Vaughan. Tyrrell was deprived of the sacraments in 1907, and when he died, two years later, he was, in consequence, denied a Catholic burial. The priest who actually said the Catholic rites over his grave, in the Anglican churchyard at Storrington— Henri Bremond, a former Jesuit and a friend—was himself suspended from priestly functions as a result of doing so.

Mivart's heterodoxy also followed him into the grave. He was denied the sacraments in 1900, and when he died later the same year he was buried, without Catholic rites, at Kensal Green Cemetery. Four years later he was re-buried, as a Catholic, by special dispensation. St. George Jackson Mivart had been born in London, the son of a hotelier. Like von Hügel, he had a schoolboy passion for science and for collecting reptiles. He was sent to Harrow, where, he recalled, he 'learnt nothing'[203]—but enough, apparently, to become a Catholic, at

[201] See Geoffrey Rowell, *Hell and the Victorians. A Study of the nineteenth-century theological controversies concerning eternal punishment and the after-life*, (Oxford 1974). The book does not discuss Tyrrell's work, however.

[202] Weaver, 32.

[203] Jacob W. Gruber, *A Conscience in Conflict. The Life of St. George Jackson Mivart*, New York 1960, 8.

the age of sixteen, in 1844. He had been influenced by reading the Tractarians. Conversion itself followed a study of Pugin's *Contrasts* and a tour of recently-built Catholic churches. After a brief stay at Oscott he studied for the law in London and was called to the Bar in 1851. His mind continued to return to science, however, and a friendship with Thomas Huxley, whom he first met in 1859, convinced him that he should dedicate himself to scientific work. This proved successful, and in 1862 he became Professor of Comparative Anatomy at St. Mary's Hospital Medical School in London, a post he filled for twenty-two years. His research and writings, which were more systematic than original, were mostly about the skeletal anatomy of primates. After initially accepting Darwinian theories he returned to pre-Darwinian natural history—and was then criticized by the Darwinians and by Huxley.[204] His scientific work was acceptable to the Church: Newman commended his *Genesis of Species* (published in 1871), and Pius IX awarded him the degree of Doctor of Philosophy in 1876. He was appointed to a Chair in the Kensington Catholic University. His purpose, he wrote, was to show the 'compatibility' which existed 'between the most advanced science and the most orthodox Christianity'.[205] But it was his failure to retain the second of these that led to his difficulties with religious authority. Like the other Modernists, he elevated the concept of intellectual autonomy to a point at which it only became compatible with the *magisterium* of the Church according to his own, individual definition. In his *Contemporary Evolution*, published in 1876, he appeared to identify human rationality with the soul, and contended for a complete freedom of the conscience from ecclesiastical tradition. The Church, be believed, had no sovereignty over the intellect, and could concern itself only with faith and morals. In the later 1880s, he endorsed advanced attitudes to Biblical criticism. Like Tyrrell, he also became involved in controversy over the questions of hell and eternal punishment, in articles he wrote for the *Nineteenth Century* in 1892 and 1893. These articles were condemned by the Holy Office. Mivart refused to retract: 'The

---

[204] Ibid. 35, 92.   [205] Ibid. 50.

Roman Congregations consist of men who have obtained more or less of what most men care for—influence, power, and some "ways and means".[206] It was not the most conciliatory of rejoinders. Mivart, in fact, was an unbending man. His biographer wrote, 'There is little real humility in any of his writing; on the contrary, they display an author pompous and positive.'[207] He had also supported some of the causes which were most offensive to the Ultramontanes—the *Rambler* and the *Home and Foreign Review*, and the admission of Catholics to the national universities. This was not a passive support, either, for in the 1880s he was a member of the governing council of the Catholic Union, the chief organization of the laity. But Mivart never lapsed entirely from some sort of religious faith, and towards the end of his life his position was theistic or universalist. He had retained, to his own satisfaction, intellectual integrity and an openness to the phenomena of faith.

[206] Ibid. 194.   [207] Ibid. 215.

8

Cardinal Vaughan: End of an Era

Like Manning's, Vaughan's reputation has rather suffered at the hands of subsequent assessors of his work; he has been, if not damned, at least deflated by faint praise. Whereas the description of Manning comprised a caricature of schemes and ambition, the one contrived for Vaughan represented a man who was coldly efficient, a nuts-and-bolts administrator, too distant to be likeable. In the press notices following his death, as his biographer Snead-Cox noticed, 'the general impression appeared to be that he was hard, and unsympathetic —an estimable but rather narrow-minded prelate whose career had been redeemed from mediocrity chiefly by the unusual energy which had directed it'.[1] The centenary history of the Diocese of Salford, which Vaughan served for twenty years, allocates only one page out of 255 to his achievements— the author regarding him as 'essentially a missionary bishop' who treated the diocese as 'a small mission field'.[2] He wrote only one book, and that was left unfinished at his death; so that those who might describe greatness in terms of literary accomplishment or polemical ascendancy were unsatisfied by Vaughan's performance there, too. His mind, as Archbishop Mathew observed, was 'neither complex nor original'.[3] Vaughan himself was certainly aware of his poverty of conventional attributes. 'I do not excel as a preacher, an author, a theologian, a philosopher, or even as a classical scholar,' he wrote to the Pope in 1892, in seeking to represent his inadequacy for the Archbishopric of Westminster; 'Whatever I may be in these matters, in none am I above a poor mediocrity.'[4] It was a view that has continued to find supporters. His

---

[1] Snead-Cox, *The Life of Cardinal Vaughan*, I. v.
[2] Charles A. Bolton, *Salford Diocese and its Catholic Past*, Manchester 1950, 131.
[3] Mathew, *Catholicism in England, 1535–1935*, 220.
[4] Snead-Cox, II. 3.

most recent historical interpreter has concluded that Vaughan 'was not a great man'.[5]

The earthly institutions which hold together the treasures of eternity still require effective stewardship and management, however, and a case for greatness may surely be made for one whose achievements in that work were by any standards quite extraordinarily impressive. Vaughan founded and endowed the first English Catholic Overseas Missions; as Bishop of Salford he inspired a national movement for the preservation of the faith against proselytism and indifference which activated the laity for generations to come; at Westminster, as a symbol of resurgence and renewal, he left a Cathedral. In his lifetime, for these various undertakings, he collected enormous sums of money from the public—begging among the rich and influential, as well as arranging regular church subscriptions from the poor. It was, in his own words, 'hateful work'; and it is a tribute to the nobility of his character that he gave his life to it—that the Church he served might be institutionally sound in its assault upon the faithlessness of the world.

As a spiritual leader, Vaughan was made less impressive by a failure to inspire his own clergy. Very many seem to have found him aloof. Ill-health and central administrative duties meant that, during his time at Westminster particularly, he was unable to know the clergy individually. Vaughan actually had a very poor memory for faces: this led to embarrassing successions of re-introductions, and heightened the public image of distance and detachment from personal relationships. But his interior spiritual life, imparting strength to his institutional work—which would have hardened or dessicated most men—was rich, simple, and developed. He had, like Manning, a high view of the secular priesthood, and urged his clergy on in the 'perpetual treadmill', as he called it, of house-visiting and attendance on the sick and poor. In *The Young Priest*, the book which lay unfinished on his desk when he died, Vaughan wrote, 'The characteristic of the Apostolic life consists not in triumphs, but in labours and sufferings undertaken out of love for Jesus Christ.'[6] He always required

[5] Holmes, *More Roman than Rome*, 241.
[6] Herbert Vaughan, *The Young Priest. Conferences on the Apostolic Life*, ed. J. S. Vaughan, London 1904, 179.

Catholic institutions and associations to 'work with the local clergy and not without them'.[7] The priestly vocation was one of dedication and worldly privation: vicarious suffering is a theme which runs through his thought, especially in later years. 'The school of suffering is the school of Christ', he wrote, 'and happy they who study in it.'[8] Even Manning at times regarded Vaughan's clerical austerity as a little too demanding: 'You could be holier and happier', he told him, if he would 'learn to laugh'.[9] The centre of the spiritual life for Vaughan, was the pursuit of humility: 'You will never really labour to become humble until you are intellectually and conscientiously convinced of the value of this virtue', he wrote.[10] It was a quality which, beneath the exterior detachment, characterized his own spiritual life. He was impressed with the immanence of unearthly mysteries, of the speed with which the present life slides into eternity. He respected ecclesiastical miracles, in a culture which, like the English one—both Protestant and 'Old Catholic'—found them distasteful. In 1881, after witnessing the liquefaction of the blood of St. Januarius in Naples, he said: 'it seems to me to require a greater effort to disbelieve than to believe'.[11] His life and prayers were directed by the guidance of St. Joseph in whose honour he dedicated the Missionary College at Mill Hill. Indeed, it was by concealing a small statue of the saint in the house he sought to purchase in order to establish the College, in 1865, that he believed he had procured the assent of the reluctant vendor: St. Joseph had already taken up residence. One of the two pictures presented to the College in 1869 by Lady Herbert of Lea, his friend and benefactress, was of St. Joseph. The second was of the Sacred Heart—the other centre of Vaughan's spiritual life. Wherever he went he encouraged devotions to the Sacred Heart—at a time when the cult was achieving enormous popularity throughout the

---

[7] Westminster Dioc. Archives, Vaughan Papers, 199n, Vaughan to the Secretary of the Catholic Association, 14 Dec. 1893.

[8] Snead-Cox, II. 277.

[9] Ibid. I. 458.

[10] *The Young Priest*, 277.

[11] Arthur McCormack, *Cardinal Vaughan. The Life of the Third Archbishop of Westminster. Founder of St. Joseph's Missionary Society, Mill Hill*, London 1966, 161.

Catholic world. Soon after his elevation to the bishopric of
Salford, he took part in a national pilgrimage, led by the Duke
of Norfolk, to Paray-le-Monial, the central shrine of devotion
to the Sacred Heart. When Lady Herbert dwelt upon the separation and illnesses of her children—who had become wards
of Chancery, to preserve their Protestantism when she had
become a Catholic—Vaughan consoled her in the way most
natural to him: 'I can only find the interpretation', he said
of her suffering, 'in that Sacred Heart which was sad and
sorrowful and bled in the Garden and on the Cross.'[12]

Vaughan's relationship with Lady Herbert of Lea was in
fact closely linked to his growth in spirituality. Its origin lay
in the death of his mother, Eliza, in 1853—when he was a
young seminarist in Rome. She was a Catholic convert whose
faith was extremely intense. She wanted all her children to
become priests and nuns, and spent an hour each day in
prayer before the Blessed Sacrament to bring her children to
a sense of their vocations. All five daughters duly entered
convents, and six of the eight sons became priests. Vaughan
was desolated by her death. 'The Blessed Virgin will now
more than ever be to us a mother', he wrote to his father on
hearing the sad news.[13] Indeed, he began to pray to his dead
mother as he did to the Virgin, and when he became a cardinal, in 1893, he rededicated his life by noting, in his private
journal, 'in future the love of Jesus Christ, the example of my
mother, must be the sole motive'.[14] The lives of some un-
married men who formed close youthful attachments to their
mothers later disclose certain unconventional proclivities.
Not Vaughan's life however; yet his close relationship to Lady
Herbert of Lea—moving and beautiful, entirely spiritual and
completely wholesome—followed naturally enough from the
devotion he felt for his mother. Lady Herbert actually re-
sembled her physically. 'You seem to have come into my path
to change and modify me as no woman before', Vaughan
wrote to her in 1867; 'I never met anyone else so many ways
like my mother'.[15] She was the widow of Sidney Herbert, War

---

[12] *Letters of Herbert Cardinal Vaughan to Lady Herbert of Lea, 1867 to 1903*,
ed. Shane Leslie, 60 (Jan. 1868).
[13] Snead-Cox, I. 40.
[14] Ibid. II. 27.   [15] *Letters*, 21 (Aug. 1867).

Minister in Aberdeen's coalition administration, and her con-version to the Catholic faith followed his death. Vaughan first met her in 1866, and there followed a friendship and a correspondence which lasted all his life—his letters, revealing their spiritual and personal affinity over a period of thirty-five years, were later published by Shane Leslie. 'Lady Herbert of Lea was as deeply knit to the Cardinal's life and life's purposes', Leslie himself concluded, 'as St. Paula to St. Jerome'.[16] She died in 1911, and was buried near to Vaughan's grave at Mill Hill.

One of Vaughan's most well-known religious character-istics was his adhesion to Ultramontanism—to the 'Roman' influences in the English Church. He stood squarely in the tradition of Wiseman and Manning. His Ultramontane view of ecclesiastical authority was as uncomplicated as his spiritu-ality, and he used *The Tablet*, which he had purchased in 1868, as the vehicle of an exclusivist attitude to that issue which almost at once became the central loyalty test for Ultramontanes—Papal Infallibility. The opinions of the In-opportunists, and of Newman, were given no space at all in the paper; those doubtful about Infallibility were represented as the enemies of Catholic truth. He saw always a need 'to strengthen our attachment to the great principle of authority upon which our Saviour built up His divine plan for the sal-vation of souls'—the words were spoken in 1893, as he re-dedicated Catholic England to St. Peter—'The Author of Christianity made the acceptance of this principle the first condition of divine faith.'[17] Like Manning, he saw the dangers of error and apostasy on every side. 'The disloyal Catholic intellect is growing with a luxuriance and the strength of a weed', he said in 1865.[18] From Merry del Val in Rome—whose advisory relationship to Vaughan was not dissimilar to that between Talbot and Manning—he acquired a strengthened resolve to combat religious liberalism, the source of Indiffer-entism. He discerned a slide into national irreligion in England generally, affecting all the Churches and all of society. The

[16] *Letters*, Introduction, vii.
[17] *Address on the Re-dedication of Catholic England to Blessed Peter, by Herbert Cardinal Vaughan* (29 June 1893), London 1893, 23.
[18] Mathew, 220.

secularists, he wrote in 1868, were already large in number 'and rapidly increasing'.[19] By the last decade of the century the situation seemed to have fulfilled this prognosis. 'To some it appears as though the instinct of the Soul to thirst after God had been extinguished in this huge mass of English population, as though their spiritual appetite had been destroyed,' he wrote. Yet still there were 'reasons of hope', even if the evidences were rather secularized: 'Witness the way they listen for a while to anyone pretending to bring them a message.'[20] Such considerations confirmed his sense of ecclesiastical authority. The unity and permanence centred in Rome, if institutionally strong, would be ready when the time came to gather the harvest—if that unity was strictly maintained. Hence Vaughan's complete opposition to schemes for 're-union' with Anglicans on what he regarded as unsound principles, and hence, also, his sense that the education of the clergy was the first priority of the hierarchy. 'At present our Education is inferior', he reported to Propaganda in 1896; 'our Professors are not trained professors; our poverty has crippled us in many ways.'[21] At the time the Education question was being brought towards legislation in 1868 he was against compromise, believing it impossible to take an honest middle ground between the secular and the denominational position. 'Men who compromise their principles infallibly end by losing them, because they begin by losing their own firm grasp of them', he wrote.[22] Gladstone, he thought, demonstrated this, as his Vatican Decrees pamphlet finally revealed in 1874—the compromise by which he had stayed outside the Catholic Church while Manning followed the logic of things and entered had shown his true stamp. 'God cannot be served by compromise and very rarely his church can, either.'[23] As Archbishop of Westminster, however, and faced with actual legislative proposals in which some compromises were inevitable, he was realistically resigned to making them—provided,

---

[19] Herbert Vaughan, *Popular Education in England. The Conscience Clause, the Rating Clause, and the Secular Current,* London 1868, 53.

[20] *Address on the Re-dedication of Catholic England,* 26–7.

[21] Westminster Dioc. Archives, Vaughan Papers, 34/2, Draft Letter to Propaganda, 29 Feb. 1896.

[22] *Popular Education,* 8.

[23] *Letters,* 245 (Feb. 1874).

as he wrote to the bishops, on the advice of Propaganda, 'no scandal would be given to our people'.[24]

Once the essentials of the Catholic position were seen to be inviolable, therefore, he was quite prepared to consider timely adaptations to circumstance. He sponsored services in the vernacular, for example, and in 1874 composed a popular service of psalms and hymns in English—earning the criticism of Latin purists—so that when Cardinal Franchi, Prefect of Propaganda, visited Manchester in 1875, the hymns he heard in the cathedral were in English. Nor was his Ultramontanism 'sectarian'. Unlike Manning, whose public sense of the Catholic contribution was personal and social, Vaughan believed the Church should address itself to the entire nation, and see its ministry and office as directed to the whole people and not just, pastorally, to the Catholics. The building of Westminster Cathedral was a symbol of this; so was the call, made by the bishops at their Low Week meeting in 1902, for the Accession Oath of the Sovereign to be relieved of its anti-Catholic clauses.[25]

Vaughan was personally austere. He ate heartily but plainly, and, when need required it—as in the early poverty of the Mill Hill Missionary College—he was willing and glad to endure months of real privation. As a boy he had been keen on sports, and used, apparently, to say his rosary beneath hedgerows on summer evenings, with his gun in his other hand, waiting for the rabbits to come out. His health was unreliable, however, and with the years it got worse. Several times he believed he was near to death—once, in Rome as a student, this conviction secured a Papal dispensation allowing his ordination eighteen months before the canonical time. It was these illnesses which also prevented him becoming closely acquainted with the clergy, but which also made him acutely conscious of the poor health of the inhabitants of the crowded slums of Salford. He was socially awkward in the actual presence of the poor, however, and regarded the duty of visiting their homes as occasions of real suffering, to be offered up in the pursuit of sanctity. 'I must, it is my plain

---

[24] Westminster Dioc. Archives, Vaughan Papers, 48, 26 Dec. 1895.
[25] Ibid. ACTA, Low Week Meeting of the Bishops, 1902 (8 April), XVI.

duty,' he confessed about visiting the poor: 'the way to their souls is often through their temporal concerns.'[26] He expected the same of his clergy. 'We have ourselves, perhaps, offended God more grievously and against greater light than these poor people who do not attract us', he wrote in *The Young Priest*; 'Their faults, perhaps, are on the surface, while ours are in the substance of the Soul.'[27] He never managed to lose the common social assumptions of the old landed classes from which he came, and however earnest his desire to seek out the poor and befriend them the vocabulary and style of his background obtruded. Of the working class, of the 'gangs of navvies, broad-backed powerful animals', and of 'the brickies, the most universally debased on the scale of morality of all our workmen', he once observed: 'They are flesh and blood, and they think and speak of nothing else'. Their very language comprised 'words of the coarsest, foulest, and most degrading meaning'. But they were, he realized, only express-ing in one way a materialism and a practice of 'earthly satis-faction' which was to be found in the middle and upper classes in abundance. 'Their faith is in the present', he said of those last, 'and the present has absorbed them.'[28] He attacked the racial discrimination practised against blacks in the South-ern States. In 1897 he told the Sheffield Social Union Club that after attending Church on Sundays 'each member of the class or coterie goes his own way taking no interest in the life struggle of his neighbours'.[29] His sense of popular politics looked to the future. 'If the people are going to rule', he ob-served in 1867, at the time of the Reform Bill discussions—when Bright and others had spoken of a working-class 're-siduum' of hopeless dependence, and Lowe had spoken of working-class moral deficiencies in much the same way as he had done—'it is vital that we should not be strangers to them or bear a hostile name.'[30] Vaughan was a conservative in politics, and his sense of social compassion was a species of Tory paternalism. His opposition to Liberalism reflected a Roman perspective; and he employed *The Tablet* to express

[26] Snead-Cox, II. 11.
[27] *The Young Priest*, 294.
[28] *Popular Education* (1868), 56-7.
[29] McCormack, 277.
[30] *Letters*, 39 (Oct. 1867).

it: 'opposed by every instinct and principle to the spurious Liberalism and irreligious revolution of the Continent, we shall denounce it in all its forms—especially when it manifests its influence among ourselves'.[31] The question of denominational education guaranteed his Conservative sympathies. Yet he was not 'political'. Apart from advising Catholics to support parliamentary candidates who supported the Voluntary Schools in the 1885 general election, his life was unmarked by any political action. His social concern was pastoral rather than political in flavour; a quality in which it was rather different from Manning's. It was expressed, accordingly, within Catholic institutions under the control of the Church rather than, as Manning's had often been, in general philanthropic and public bodies. His support for state old-age pensions and graduated income tax were the two possible occasions of his offering a public voice on public issues: on both, he took no action. Over sanitary and housing reforms, and on the urgent need to abolish the evils of the cellar-dwellings of the poor, he urged Catholics to action first, as a yeast to produce a social ferment for change. His night-time wanderings through the slums of Manchester gave him a first-hand acquaintance with the conditions he condemned. He also began to show a marked preoccupation with mortality statistics during his years in Manchester, correctly linking the 'disgrace' of the slums to shortened life. 'In Salford there was an enormous procession of hearses throughout the year, and many of those hearses had no right to be there', he said.[32] Although less concerned about Temperance than Manning, he came to take the matter up as he became more familiar with the effect of drink on the domestic economies of the working classes. He proposed more controlled licensing rather than prohibition; and he dropped his earlier contention, made in the presence and to the great scandal of Manning, that drink was actually a food from which the poor could obtain some nourishment. The memorial to Vaughan's social concern was the network of Social Union Clubs, which he first started in the Mile End Road in London. By 1894 there were five of them, and then they spread throughout the

[31] Snead-Cox, I. 197.   [32] Ibid. I. 433.

Catholic parishes of the land. They were youth clubs for the recreation of the working classes, and within them there soon grew up the same atmosphere of social reformism which occurred in the Protestant Social Unions of the same decade.

The relationship of Vaughan and Manning was both interesting and important—Vaughan owed his advancement in the Church exclusively to Manning's friendship and approval. Yet they were of quite different backgrounds and temperaments. Vaughan was brought up in the isolated world of the Catholic gentry and was educated in Catholic Colleges; Manning belonged to the world of the establishment, to Harrow and Oxford. Vaughan was retiring by nature, whereas Manning became so only after his wife's death. Vaughan was unintellectual and naturally activist, while Manning was a thinker and a pietist. What they had most obviously in common was a developed interior life. They had got to know each other well in Rome, early in the 1850s, when both, despite the great difference in their ages, were students at the Accademia Ecclesiastica. It was Manning who later recruited Vaughan for the Oblates, sent him to St. Edmund's College, and eventually secured his appointment as Bishop of Salford. Between 1879 and 1881 it was Vaughan who did most of the spadework in Rome, preparing Manning's case against the Religious Orders in preparation for what became the Bull *Romanos Pontifices*. He was away from his diocese for a year and a half for this; but it was an invaluable experience of Roman procedures, completing the administrative accomplishments he had already displayed over the creation of the St. Joseph's Missionary Society. During the Salford years differences between the two men opened up. They were not fundamental: Vaughan's 'Roman' allegiance was never at issue; differences related to variations of practical policy. Vaughan was opposed to the creation of Tridentine seminaries in the English dioceses—but not for ideological reasons. He, like Manning, favoured the Roman discipline; he just did not believe that the resources available to the English Church were adequate for the provision of well-financed or educationally respectable seminaries. Vaughan supported the idea of formal diplomatic relations between England and the Holy See, which he supposed would help to impart that 'national' Catholic presence in the country which he so much wanted to encourage. Manning believed that diplomatic relations would be used by the government to interfere with the Church and with Irish policy: he saw the shadow of the old Veto controversy. Since the question did not become one of practical politics at this time it did not prove divisive. Vaughan assented for many years to Manning's continuation of Wiseman's policy of operating a practical ban on the attendance of Catholic students at the Universities. His adhesion was real enough here; since he had no personal knowledge of the Universities he was prepared to believe the accounts of the inherent Protestant and liberal tone given by Ward and Manning. When he later changed the policy, it was, as he thought, in accordance with a shift in Manning's own thinking on the question. Vaughan was unconcerned with public issues and political questions, and lacked the network of contacts in public life which Manning was at times able to activate. He had an English landowner's economy of sympathy for the Irish question. In this matter, the two prelates were at their farthest remove. Vaughan did not follow Manning's conversion to Home Rule in 1886. Ireland, indeed, despite the Catholic dimension in nationalist politics, 'was a question which was outside his life'.[33] His only political consideration over Home Rule appears to have been a reluctance to see the Irish MPs removed from the Westminster Parliament, since this would eliminate the Catholic members and destroy the political base the Church needed for the presentation of Catholic educational claims. His failure to appreciate the importance of the Irish question, at a time when a large section of the Church over which he was called to preside was in a state of extreme excitement about it, was a substantial contribution to his lack of popularity with the Catholics of the parishes.[34] There were also differences between Vaughan and Manning over vivisection and Temperance; and there was the accumulating distaste of Vaughan for Manning's social enterprises—not for the works in themselves, but for the diversion, as he saw it, of the functions of the Archbishop from proper administrative

---

[33] Snead-Cox, I. 470.
[34] Leslie, in the Introduction to the *Letters*, xiii.

concerns to rather ambiguous co-operation with Protestant philanthropy. Vaughan could never understand Manning's liking for the Salvation Army. But the friendship of the two men was undiminished by their growing dissimilarities, and Manning never doubted that Vaughan was the only person who should succeed him at Westminster. Vaughan's whole career had become a preparation for it, although he was the first to be appalled at the prospect.

Herbert Vaughan was a grand-nephew of Cardinal Weld. He was actually born in Gloucester when his parents were visiting relatives in the city in 1832; but the family home was at Courtfield in Herefordshire. His father, a Colonel in the local Militia, and a landowner, belonged to one of the oldest Catholic families in England. He intended his eldest son to pursue a military career, but Herbert disappointed him by realizing, under the influence of his mother, a priestly vocation. In 1841, when he was nine, he was sent to Stonyhurst. There his life was unremarkable enough—given to the intellectually undemanding studies and the sporting preoccupations of the Catholic gentry. In 1847 he went to Downside for a year, and then to the great Jesuit school at Brugelette in Belgium. There, in candid recognition of his English country style, he was known to the French-speaking boys as 'Milord Roast-beef'.[35] In 1851, when nineteen, he left for Rome accompanied by his cousin William Clifford—afterwards Bishop of Clifton—to begin his studies for the priesthood. His academic accomplishments in Rome were adequate and not in any way remarkable; but his time was intersected by poor health and frequent visits outside the city to recover. The death of his mother in 1853 added to his reduced condition. In October 1854, when he was twenty-two, and after a sojourn in Florence to improve his health, he was ordained. Despite his exceptional youth (and, it was supposed, at the suggestion of Manning) Wiseman at once offered him the Vice-Presidency of the Westminster diocesan seminary of St. Edmund's at Ware. He travelled around Europe in the first half of 1855 acquainting himself with the various curricula and disciplines of Catholic seminaries. He did not like a lot of what he saw.

[35] Snead-Cox, I. 18.

Strict discipline was often lacking—except at St. Sulpice in Paris, which he came to regard as a sort of model. He arrived at St. Edmund's without any experience, priestly or educational, but with some clearly held opinions about the proper nature of Catholic seminaries. He was by then twenty-three years old. It was not surprising that his appointment enkindled suspicions from the start. Those at the seminary, and in the Chapter of Westminster, who were anyway anxiously anticipating some infusion of Wiseman's 'Romanizing' policy, regarded Vaughan as the agent of it. Vaughan did not start well: he tried to get rid of Ward, then Professor of Dogmatic Theology. When he joined the Oblates in 1857, the suspicions were heightened, and Vaughan's position at St. Edmund's became an important part of the most notorious English Catholic dispute of the century. In 1861, the Holy See ruled that the position of Vaughan and the other Oblates at the seminary was a contravention of the Decrees of the Council of Trent, and Vaughan moved to St. Mary of the Angels in Bayswater, to join Manning. The experience had persuaded him that the existing Catholic practice in England, of educating lay and ecclesiastical students together, was inappropriate.

His mind turned to overseas missions. In 1863 he founded a Missionary Society and departed to the Americas on a fund-raising expedition. Had it not been for the American Civil War he would have gone straight to the United States. Instead he took a paddle-steamer for Panama, in December, hoping to push north and head for the California gold fields and the prospects of rich donations. In Panama, where the liberal government had passed a series of anti-clerical laws, he was arrested for saying Mass without a licence, and hurriedly left the country before proceedings could begin against him. He stayed in California for five months, overcoming the initial hostility of the Catholic Archbishop of San Francisco, raised subscriptions for his proposed missionary College in London, and encouraged devotions in the Sacred Heart among the astonished miners of the gold-rush shanty towns. He went next to Peru, to Lima, where the government stopped his collections, and then on to Santiago in Chile. There he had his main success, and with government approval raised large sums. He found it the most Catholic of the South American cities he visited—a feature which he attributed to the practice of holding regular Retreats. In March 1865, he began the voyage round Cape Horn in a British naval vessel, bound for Rio de Janeiro, intending then to go north to Pernambuco—a province still rich on the profits of sugar. But in Rio he heard of the death of Wiseman, and then, in June, of Manning's appointment to Westminster. He was recalled to England by Manning, and, giving up the proposed visit to the north-east of Brazil, he sailed for England, arriving at the end of July. On his return Manning released him from his duties to the Oblates of St. Charles in order to allow him to set up his Missionary College. He had collected £11,000 on his journeys.

The foundation of a College to train missionaries for work overseas was one of the greatest achievements of Vaughan's life. It gave an example of Catholic activism to a Church which, despite the Roman direction imparted by Wiseman and Manning, was still very inward-looking, and it helped to inspire generations of Catholic young men with noble vocations to a wider service. Vaughan had initially imagined he would himself become a missionary. Almost from the first perception of his priestly vocation, he sensed a 'haunting wish to get away from civilization altogether'.[36] This, initially, he interpreted as a call to work in Wales. On retreat at Fiumicino near Rome, prior to his ordination, he had envisaged the privation of a life spent 'as a solitary priest at a seaside town in Wales'.[37] But as he travelled around Europe examining seminaries, before his return to England and St. Edmund's, his horizons were elevated. With the internal troubles at St. Edmund's these inclinations grew into certainties, and, advised by the Jesuits in Farm Street,[38] he decided to found a College to train men for missionary work overseas. The example of the great Protestant Missionary Societies was important in this re-orientation of his priorities. First, he thought of training men for Africa: 'the feeling became so strong that he notes in his diary how, on one occasion, meeting a negro on the streets, he felt an almost irresistible longing

---

[36] Snead-Cox, I. 104.
[37] Ibid. I. 35.
[38] McCormack, 62.

to go and embrace him'.[39] Later, he thought of Japan as a possible scene for the work. Manning, whose advice he naturally sought, was cautious: the needs of the Church in England were pressing enough. A year later, in 1860, he discussed his plans with Wiseman as the two were on a drive together in the Isle of Wight. This proved a more encouraging exchange. Then, near to death once more through terrible ill-health, and laid up at Bayswater, he read the lives of St. Francis Xavier and St. Peter Claver. In Rome, during the first half of 1862 he prayed for direction and felt a sense of confirmation: he should definitely found a College for missionary preparation. Hence the expedition to raise funds to North and South America. On returning to England, in the second half of 1865, he purchased Holcombe House at Mill Hill, near London, and St. Joseph's Missionary Society set up its College there on 1 March 1866.

The teaching staff at first comprised himself and Fr. Bayley, a brother Oblate. There were twelve students. The College was extremely poor; there was no heating in the capacious building, and the community ate tins of preserved meat—in those days the food of the poor—in order to avoid employing a cook or using fuel in preparation. His health so deteriorated that Lady Herbert of Lea stepped in and had Vaughan removed to the relative affluence and warmth of Manning's house in Westminster. After three months there he recovered. Lady Herbert's patronage of the College was both financial and actual—she did a great deal of work around the place, becoming known, affectionately, as 'the Mother of the Mill'. There was also to hand, as her assistant, Miss Hanmer, who had been one of Florence Nightingale's nurses in the Crimea. From a cottage in the grounds, called 'The Rosary', she dispensed help to the aspirant missionaries and their teachers. The foundation-stone of the College buildings was laid by Manning in 1869, and the main residential part of St. Joseph's was opened in 1871—free of debt, an enormous tribute to Vaughan's enterprise. The community then numbered thirty-four. The Missionaries were to be Apostles of Ultramontanism. 'Our missioners will go out as Roman as any

Roman and as specially devoted to the Pope', Vaughan wrote
to Lady Herbert of Lea; 'In England a strong Papal adherence
is growing up. The same must be weaved into all our work in
pagan lands and in the Colonies.'[40] It was not to 'pagan lands'
or to the Colonies, however, that the Pope directed the first of
Vaughan's missionaries—but to the USA. They were to work
among the black population. In November 1871, Vaughan
himself sailed to Baltimore with the first band of priests;
thereafter he toured the Southern states to examine the social
and religious condition of black society for himself—and was
outraged by what he saw. In Memphis he observed 'Negroes
regarded even by priests as so many dogs'.[41] He criticized the
racial discrimination widely practiced in the Churches. Fired
with a renewed sense of the importance of the work he returned, via Canada, to England. St. Joseph's extended its work
as new areas were allocated by the Holy See over the following years—years during which, though by then Bishop of
Salford, Vaughan continued as Superior-General of the
Society. Men from Mill Hill were then despatched to Madras,
to North Borneo, to the New Zealand Maoris, to the Punjab,
Uganda, Congo, and the Philippines. In 1877 the St. Joseph's
missionary sisters were instituted. It was a very impressive
achievement.

Vaughan's time was not exclusively directed to this work.
In 1868 he had purchased *The Tablet*, determined that
England should have a reliable—Ultramontane—Catholic
paper. His experience of America had showed him the potential power of the press. *The Tablet* was no longer the pro-Irish
and Liberal journal fashioned by Lucas. Under John Wallis's
editorship from 1855 it had become Tory in politics and
markedly hostile to the claims of Irish Catholic Liberalism—
and that actually meant to the claims of Cardinal Cullen and
the Irish Hierarchy, all of whom were, by 1868, united in
the National Association of Ireland behind a union with the
Gladstonian Liberals. Manning had himself helped to bring
about the co-operation of the various parties. Vaughan's first
task, on assuming control of *The Tablet*, was to preserve its
anti-Liberalism whilst at the same time swinging the paper

[40] *Letters*, 89 (April 1868).   [41] Snead-Cox, I. 170.

behind Irish reforms in sympathy with Manning. This he achieved quite smoothly, and the paper became a strong advocate of the Disestablishment of the Irish Protestant Church. Although he had a lay editor, Vaughan spent at least one day a week in London working on editorial policy; and although he had no previous experience of journalism, his work was very successful. In 1878 he acquired the *Dublin Review* as well.

When Dr William Turner died, in 1872, Vaughan had been suggested by Manning as the successor in the Bishopric of Salford. It was, in its way, a controversial choice, since Vaughan was virtually unknown in the powerful Catholic Church of the North of England, with its line of Ushaw and Stonyhurst ecclesiastics. But Manning's influence prevailed, and for the next twenty years Vaughan was in Lancashire. 'This is the grandest place in England for popular energy and piety' he declared at once.[42] Though geographically small the diocese was important, comprising, as it did, Manchester and the industrial heartlands· of the north-west. It was heavily urban and overwhelmingly working-class. It was a place ideally suited for just the gifts Vaughan could bring: administrative skill, financial enterprise, and energetic construction. He began with the same priority that Wiseman and Manning had laid before their episcopal labours: the training of the clergy. But instead of seeking to create a regular Tridentine diocesan seminary, Vaughan decided to experiment with a small pastoral centre, where newly ordained priests could study before going out to the parishes. His appeal for money was successful, and the pastoral seminary was built next to the cathedral in 1874. In later years Vaughan came to regard this work as among his failures—the seminary did not survive. While it lasted, however, over sixty priests were given a specialist training not found elsewhere in the English Church. The expansionist work of his predecessor was maintained by Vaughan, who brought to it the additional capacity of successful—indeed astonishing—fund-raising. The new schools, the pastoral seminary, the Rescue work which came to dominate his interests, and the creation of new parishes: debts began to

[42] Snead-Cox, I. 251.

accumulate on a scale fast exceeding those of Bishop Turner's time. Vaughan was determined to get both the clergy and the laity to pay them off; and he succeeded. Diocesan synods became annual events, rather than every seven years, and were used to co-ordinate efforts for financial enterprise. It was depressing work, but without it there could be no Catholic renewal. 'The labour is great, the anxiety is continual, the results flatter neither vanity nor the senses,' Vaughan wrote.[43] At each synod, a 'Board of Temporal Administration' was appointed to advise on financial issues. The property of the parishes was vested in diocesan trustees. The debts of St. John's Cathedral, built in 1844, were paid off and the building consecrated in 1890. Forty new parishes were created during Vaughan's time as Bishop,[44] each one with a time-limit to achieve financial security.

When Vaughan arrived in Lancashire, he found that there already existed a good system of Catholic primary schools, founded by Bishop Turner. His main educational priority, therefore, lay in the area of secondary education—one traditionally dominated by the religious orders. Vaughan was determined to break their monopoly, and, in practical terms, this meant taking on the Jesuits of Stonyhurst. The Xaverian Brothers, who also conducted grammar schools, were less of a threat to his diocesan plans, since they had been invited to establish their secondary schools by Turner, and had a good working relationship with the diocese. The Jesuits were another matter. Formal relations were good; but Vaughan was concerned about the whole future of the diocese—about vocations to the priesthood. In an area where the secondary education was largely in the hands of a religious order, boys naturally tended to express their vocational preference within the order which had educated them. Vaughan feared a diocese in which the ordinary secular priesthood was in a minority. It was this consideration which underlay his conflict with the Jesuits. The immediate occasion was not of his making, however. In 1875 the Jesuits opened a secondary school in Manchester without his consent—claiming to exercise an

---

[43] Ibid. I. 310.
[44] Bolton, *Salford Diocese and its Catholic Past*, 132.

established privilege originally granted by the Holy See. There followed a protracted dispute between Fr. Peter Gallwey, the Provincial of the Jesuits, and Vaughan, precipitating the usual appeals to Rome. The issue became a central part of Manning's wider attempt at a redefinition of the relationship between the dioceses and the orders—leading to *Romanos Pontifices* in 1881. Advised by Manning, Vaughan proceeded to Rome in April 1875, to argue his case against the Jesuits at Propaganda. The opening of the Manchester School he regarded as 'a grave act of disobedience and insubordination'.[45] The Pope at first supposed that Manchester and Salford were rival cities, miles apart; Cardinal Franchi, at Propaganda, who was rather better informed, sought an accommodation which avoided raising matters of principle—an objective which taxed his diplomatic skills since Vaughan was raising the whole question precisely in order to settle a point of principle. As if to outflank the Jesuits spiritually, Vaughan said mass over the relics of St. Ignatius Loyola, founder of the Jesuits, in the Gesù, and then despatched a letter to the General of the Order demanding the closure of the school in Manchester. The General, whose sense of accommodation was as Roman as the Cardinal Prefect's, was prepared to arrange the closure of the school, but only on terms that did not prejudice the Jesuits' educational claims. This was, happily, eventually achieved, and on his return to England Vaughan proceeded to Stonyhurst and went on Retreat with the Jesuits. In the following year, 1876, Vaughan founded a secondary school of his own—the commercial academy of St. Bede's. It was conducted by the secular clergy. In 1877 the Salford Aquarium, which was situated next to St. Bede's, came on to the market, and Vaughan felt obliged to purchase it rather than see the site developed (as he had reason to believe) as a music hall and tea gardens. 'This would have ruined St. Bede's', he wrote to Lady Herbert.[46] After an unsuccessful attempt to maintain the Aquarium, Vaughan eventually incorporated the buildings into those of the College, and opened up the main rooms for public lectures of an improving and Catholic nature—principally for attracting Protestants to the faith. 'It was a letting

---

[45] Snead-Cox, I. 286.   [46] *Letters*, 291 (Sept. 1877).

down the net for them in a way we have not hitherto tried', he wrote.[47] Vaughan's other great educational work at Salford was the establishment, in 1884, of the Voluntary Schools Association. The local associations, with Manning's co-operation, were before long recognized as representing the general mind of the Catholic Church on educational issues. At first very limited in its demands, the Association had, by the time Vaughan moved to Westminster in 1892, become a vehicle for claiming equality with the Board Schools.

It was Vaughan's perception of the evils of the slums which became the major preoccupation of his work at Salford. His diagnosis was conventional: like Manning, his consciousness of social conditions developed at about the same pace as that of the intelligentsia in general. He saw the inappropriateness of some of the practices of classical Political Economy to social need, while not overthrowing the presuppositions of *laissez-faire* theory, and he saw, above all, the correlation between environment and moral behaviour. He differed from Manning in emphasis. Vaughan was more concerned with the pastoral aspects of a poor environment—with 'leakage' from the faith, especially by children. It cannot be said, however, that he neglected to point to the urgent need of housing and sanitary reform. What he envisaged was a division of labour. Catholics would join with others to seek better social conditions by the ordinary means available to citizens; and clergy, for their part, must emphasize the eternal hazards in the slums—the loss of faith consequent upon the break-up of families or the immorality sometimes inseparable from cramped living conditions. Together with his growing horror of the death rate among the working classes, from environmental causes, the Rescue work of the Salford years came to be his most urgent priority.

In 1884 he called a meeting of the Salford Chapter and set up a board of inquiry to determine the exact dimensions of the problem. The Committee was required to procure statistics of children who were lost to the faith either through the neglect or the death of their parents, or through proselytism by Protestant agencies or institutions, or through the

---

[47] Ibid. 305 (April 1879).

workhouses. They reported in June 1885, urging a full census in each Catholic parish of the diocese. This was duly held. It was an enormous undertaking for the clergy, but one which gave them an analytical familiarity with the social conditions of their flocks which had a lasting impression, and which fired very many with a sense of social activism. During 1886, as the returns came in, it became clear that the facts were as horrifying as Vaughan had perceived. About three-quarters of the 100,000 Catholics in Manchester and Salford were investigated: there were estimated to be some 8,445 children in danger and 2,653 in extreme danger. In November, as a result of the findings, Vaughan published *The Loss of Our Children*, a paper in which he defined the problem, and founded the Catholic Protection and Rescue Society. The main targets for assault by organized Catholic opinion were the Protestant philanthropic bodies, whose aid to the destitute was combined with proselytism, and the workhouses, where, despite good intentions and legal protection, Catholic children lost their faith in large numbers due to the antipathetic religious atmosphere. 'We are answerable for the souls of our brethren while we have power to save them', Vaughan declared.[48] The laity were mobilized. Indeed, it was one of Vaughan's greatest achievements that he called Catholic lay action into existence for this religious and social crusade. By the time he left Salford, two thousand laymen were involved in the Rescue work.[49] A network of vigilance committees was established, and money was collected for Catholic institutions to take care of the destitute. Vaughan gave his own episcopal income for the work. He set aside one night each week to entertain police officers, Poor Law guardians, and philanthropic workers—people whose expertise or experience could help the Rescue work. He introduced the Brothers of Charity, and the Sisters of Charity, from Ghent to set up homes for boys and girls. By 1890 the Society was conducting seven homes. Catholic children were withdrawn from the workhouses and placed in these institutions—which were inspected to enable them to receive grants from the poor rate. But the main costs of the Rescue work were met by contributions from the poor

---

[48] Snead-Cox, I. 412.   [49] McCormack, 208.

themselves, from the ordinary working-class parishioners of the Catholic churches of the diocese. On arrival as Archbishop in London, Vaughan continued the work there, too, building upon foundations already well-laid by Wiseman and Manning. In 1894 he organized a census in Westminster, and two years later, on the Salford model, created a Rescue Committee. In 1899 this was consolidated into the 'Crusade of Rescue'. The work was greatly assisted by a friendly arrangement made with Dr Barnardo, also in 1899, whereby Catholic children presented for entry to his homes should be transferred to Catholic institutions. Both in the foundation of institutions and in the creation of a lay climate of opinion calculated to educate itself on social aspects of the lives of the poor, Vaughan's Rescue work had an enormous significance.

In 1892 he left Lancashire for Westminster. 'My heart is still in Salford', he wrote.[50] He was sixty years old, still subject to severe illness, still impressed with the urgency of a ministry he must complete before a death he thought could not be far off. The appointment to succeed Manning was not controversial: it had been almost universally expected, and was, of course, Manning's own wish. When his name was placed first in the *terna* sent to Rome by the Chapter of Westminster it was endorsed by a meeting of all the bishops; the contrast with the heated exchanges and extended intrigues of 1865 was a great one. On arrival in London he had clear plans for his future work as Archbishop: a reversal of Manning's diocesan seminary policy, the creation of a Catholic Social Union, the activation of the laity by the clergy, and, above all, the foundation of a Cathedral in the metropolitan city. Within a year, in January 1893, he was created a cardinal by the Pope. His work at Westminster followed the schemes he had set himself, and this mostly meant more dedicated gathering of funds, and more of the sort of labour at which he was by now so expert—the stewardship of ecclesiastical interests and institutions. His success as Archbishop was precisely the achievement of the objectives he had laid down; essential work, quietly and effectively completed.

[50] Snead-Cox, II. 8.

St. Thomas's Seminary at Hammersmith, which Manning had once publicly referred to as the permanent memorial of his work at Westminster,[51] was closed down and the students transferred to Oscott near Birmingham—which now became the Central Seminary for a group of dioceses in the south and west of England. That was in 1893. Next, Manning's policy over universities was reversed. At a meeting of the Hierarchy in January 1895, it was agreed to petition Propaganda to allow the attendance of Catholics at the national Universities, and this was granted 'under certain conditions' in April.[52] Three bishops dissented. 'The consequence will be that the Bishops will present to the Catholic public a divided front', Vaughan reported to Cardinal Simeoni at Propaganda, early in 1896; 'it is a bad precedent, and will be the first time such a thing has taken place in England since the establishment of the Hierarchy.'[53] The laity had sent a petition to Propaganda in favour of the change in 1894, and in practice so many exemptions were being granted by individual bishops to allow particular Catholic young men to attend Oxford and Cambridge—in 1895 there were fifty at the two Universities —that the existing ban was beginning to look anomalous. Vaughan explained to Propaganda that the new policy was, anyway, hardly a departure from Manning's intentions. 'Cardinal Manning', he wrote, 'a year or two before his death, said to me that circumstances had changed, but that he was too old to change his attitude towards the Universities, but that the change would have to come after his death.'[54] In 1896 a Universities Board was set up to supervise arrangements for Catholic students at the national Universities.

Much of Vaughan's time at Westminster was taken up with the education question, with seeking to protect the Catholic Voluntary Schools by trying to work out a common defence of denominational education with the Anglicans, and by working to obtain such modifications to the 1870 Act as

[51] Ibid. II. 43.

[52] Westminster Dioc. Archives, ACTA, Low Week Meeting of the Bishops, 1895 V (23 April).

[53] Ibid. Vaughan Papers, 34/1. Draft Letter to the Cardinal Prefect of Propaganda, 28 Feb. 1896.

[54] Ibid. 402, Vaughan to the Cardinal Prefect, 19 May 1896.

would allow a more equitable allocation of funds from the local education rate to be made to the Catholic Schools. He accepted the Act of 1895 as at least a move in the right direction—it gave an increased subsidy and removed the rating of Voluntary school buildings—and saw the unfolding issue between the denominational schools and the Board schools as 'simply a question of Christianity or secularism'.[55] He welcomed the Act of 1902, which recognized the principle that both sorts of school should have an equal claim for maintenance costs, and regarded it as the sign that 'his last work was done'.[56] The Act, as he reported to Propaganda, was 'favourable to Christianity', secured only because the Conservative administration had won such a large electoral majority on the South African War policy. 'The general effect of the new law is to make Christian and Catholic Education a part of the law and Constitution of England', he wrote; 'In principle we have made a large and important advance.'[57]

The other great advance in his last years was the building of the cathedral of Westminster. This was to be a symbol of Catholic resurgence, a visible monument to the triumphalism of the Ultramontane Church, and also—though this proved a disappointment—a shrine for the relics of St. Edmund of England. In 1901 Vaughan procured St. Edmund's body from the Basilica of St. Sernin in Toulouse, but it turned out to be, though a saintly body, not actually St. Edmund's. Manning had purchased land for a cathedral in Carlisle Place, Westminster, in 1867, but had postponed work in order to collect funds for his educational programme. In 1883 the site of the Middlesex County Prison was purchased, to give a more accommodating plot, next to Manning's own house. Vaughan began to plan the cathedral as soon as he arrived in London. Some objected. The Catholic population was poor and small and already gave much for schools and charitable institutions, it was contended. Vaughan was unmoved. 'Churches are buildings, not merely *in* which, but *with* which, we worship God,' he said.[58] He wanted a large building, in the

---

[55] *Letters*, 429 (March 1897).
[56] Snead-Cox, II. 139.
[57] Westminster Dioc. Archives, Vaughan Papers, 230a, Draft Paper for the Cardinal Prefect of Propaganda, Jan. 1903.   [58] Snead-Cox, II. 327.

Roman basilica style, on the model of Constantine's Church of St. Peter in Rome, itself used as the model for the first Cathedral at Canterbury. There were two advantages of avoiding the gothic style. The new cathedral would not rival the ancient Abbey Church of Westminster; and the Roman style was less expensive—the shell could be completed leaving costly ornamentation to later generations. In the gothic style, on the other hand, decoration was actually part of the structure. So there came into existence, through the financial acumen of Vaughan, and the architectural genius of John F. Bentley, the splendid Byzantine cathedral with its austere vaults and its richly marbled side-chapels 'like bathrooms by Harrods' (as Roxburgh once remarked). Begun in 1895, the main structure was completed in eight years, despite delays caused when the bricklayers periodically took industrial action. Vaughan lived long enough to see his great cathedral roofed, though it remained unfinished and the building unconsecrated.

An issue which, for Vaughan, was both unnecessary and irritating, acquired a lot of publicity in the middle of his time at Westminster. Between 1894 and 1897 the old schemes of the Association for the Promotion of the Unity of Christendom were revived, despite the censure of its attitudes and assumptions by the Holy See in 1865. This time it was the Anglicans who initiated the ideal of reunion of Catholicism and Anglicanism—it was the wish of Lord Halifax, 'a true son of the Oxford Tractarians',[59] President of the English Church Union, the agency and theological clearing-house of the 'Anglo-Catholic' wing of the State Church. In a series of conversations with the Abbé Fernand Portal both men had persuaded themselves that the differences between the two churches were about inessentials. Both, as it turned out, spoke for a very narrow section of their own co-religionists. But just as Ambrose Phillipps de Lisle had convinced Wiseman, who had in turn convinced Pius IX, that a substantial portion of the Church of England was ready to return to Rome, so Portal and his sympathizers in Rome converted Leo XIII to the

[59] Bernard and Margaret Pawley, *Rome and Canterbury through Four Centuries. A Study of the Relations between the Church of Rome and the Anglican Churches, 1530–1981*, London 1981, 222.

belief that Anglicanism was at the point of surrender. 'I hear they are on the point of coming over', Leo told Vaughan[60]— who had to bear the onus of seeming to be unresponsive and unopen to the daring vision of a wider movement of opinion. Abbot Gasquet, with realism that was like Vaughan's (whose opinions he was representing in Rome on the question) was lectured by Leo on 'how the whole nation was being drawn to Catholicism'.[61] Vaughan was additionally offended by Portal himself, who, on a visit to England under the auspices of Halifax in 1894, during which there were excited conversations with 'Anglo-Catholic' priests, had omitted to call on him. In 1895 Vaughan set up a committee of Catholic divines to examine the case made out by the Reunionists—Gasquet, Canon Moyes, and Fr. David Fleming served on it. Dom Aidan Gasquet had become Prior of Downside in 1878 and was to become President of the English Benedictine Congregation in 1900. Distinguished as an historian, he was admirably suited to the work now entrusted to him. When, in July of the following year, the Holy See set up its own International Commission to examine the validity of Anglican Orders—which was by then recognized as the central issue—the members of Vaughan's Committee were all appointed. The persons also placed by Rome on the Commission were agreeable to Gasquet. 'One cannot fail to remark that there are none of the names of the French busybodies', he wrote in a private memorandum.[62] Vaughan himself did not wish to appear inflexible. He acknowledged that the mere existence of the 'Anglo-Catholic' party, with its yearnings for Catholic regularity—a movement of opinion without parallel among other European Protestants—was 'a Divine grace' which had been 'poured out over England'.[63] At the same time, in a speech to the Catholic Truth Society in Preston, he pointed out that the Catholic Church was always ready to adapt itself: 'the Church is free for the sake of some greater good to admit changes and modifications in her discipline and legislation which concern times and circumstances'. But on essentials

---

[60] Snead-Cox, II. 177.
[61] Ibid. II. 179.
[62] Downside Archives, Gasquet Papers, 942(2), 1896 (February).
[63] H. E. Vaughan, *The Reunion of Christendom*, London 1897, 8.

there could be no change; 'no question of Re-union can be seriously entertained without a recognition of the principle and the fact of Unity'.[64] He added: 'Anglicans are more widely separated in doctrine from one another within their own Church than they are separated from the Nonconformists who are without'. There was a lesson to be drawn: 'Who ventures to point to the Anglican establishment as exhibiting a visible mark of Divine Unity?'[65] For the Anglicans, he concluded decisively, there was but one proper course—'a gradual submission'.[66] The Cardinals of the Holy Office had arrived at the same conclusion. In July 1896, on the Feast of Our Lady of Mount Carmel, they unanimously declared Anglican Orders invalid, and in September this was published in the Bull *Apostolicae Curae*, drafted by Merry del Val and Gasquet. Pronouncements against the Anglican ordinal made by Julius III and Paul IV were cited. 'It thus becomes quite obvious that the controversy which has been recently revived had already long ago been settled by the judgement of the Apostolic See,' Leo XIII declared in the Bull, 'and the fact that one or two Catholic writers should have ventured to treat it as an open question is perhaps due to lack of sufficient knowledge of the aforesaid documents'.[67] Merry del Val was delighted. 'The way in which the Encyclical has been received is most satisfactory: surely it must do great good amongst the thoughtful and sincere', he wrote to Gasquet from Rome. 'Portal after the rap he has had is worse than ever', he added.[68] Vaughan, who now called belief in Reunion a 'new heresy', wrote to tell Gasquet that it was 'not even on the most distant horizon'.[69] Vaughan's view of the Church, and the whole tenor of Catholic leadership in England since the restoration of the Hierarchy, had been vindicated. It was a moment of great satisfaction for him.[70]

[64] Ibid. 19-20.
[65] Ibid. 25.   [66] Ibid. 33.
[67] *Apostolicae Curae*, London (CTS), 1967, 15.
[68] Downside Archives, Gasquet Papers, 942 (10A), Merry del Val to Gasquet, 10 July 1896.
[69] Ibid. (18), Vaughan to Gasquet, 6 Aug. 1896.
[70] Pawleys, 231. For an account of this episode, see J. J. Hughes, *Absolutely Null and Utterly Void. An account of the Papal Condemnation of Anglican Orders*, London 1968.

Conscious of the importance of marking the close of the century of revival, a committee of the bishops planned a public celebration of the thirteenth centenary of St. Augustine's arrival in Kent in 597, bearing the authority of the See of Rome to England.[71] It came to symbolize the advance and the success of the Catholic restoration of the nineteenth century. The field at Ebbsfleet where Augustine had landed—at a spot commemorated by Lord Granville with a stone cross in 1884—became the scene of three days of ceremonial in 1897. Cardinal Vaughan and the entire Hierarchy attended, together with representatives of Catholic dioceses overseas. The South Eastern Railway Company opened a special station on the line between Ramsgate and Minster, where it passed by Granville's cross. Civil dignitaries joined the procession before the great pontifical mass on Sunday, 12 September; they walked with eighty monks 'singing the same antiphon as had been chanted by St. Augustine'.[72]

As the century of Catholic revival moved towards its end, the life of Vaughan, too, was running out. Illness closed in with ever greater frequency; the life of dedicated attention to the stewardship of the English Church, and of faithful preservation of Catholic truth, became increasingly exhausting. With the education question successfully concluded in the Act of 1902, Vaughan felt that his work was done. By then, the burden of existence was a terrible trial for him. In the last restless months he moved from place to place, seeking somewhere to die in seclusion and repose—going first to Bad Nauheim, then to Derwent Hall to stay with Lord Edmund Talbot, and finally to his beloved College in Mill Hill. There he gazed frequently upon the site he had chosen for his grave. 'We are to be pleased', he wrote in his last days, 'not with our lower nature, which recoils, like Our Lord's, from suffering—but with our superior will that lives in the light and warmth of faith.'[73] So the last of the great Catholic prelates of Victorian England brought a triumphant era to an end. On 19 June

[71] Westminster Dioc. Archives, ACTA, Low Week Meeting of the Bishops, 1896, IV (14 April).
[72] *The Story of St. Augustine's, St. Ethelbert's and St. Benedict's, Ramsgate*, The Monastery Press, Ramsgate 1960, 12.
[73] Snead-Cox, II. 480.

1903, with a lucid mind and great fortitude, impressed by the frailty of human faith, tired in spirit and yet attaining an ultimate serenity, Vaughan was delivered into eternity. It was the Feast of the Sacred Heart.

Bibliography

Sources to which reference has been made

I. MANUSCRIPT SOURCES

Archives of the Sacred Congregation of Propaganda Fide, Rome. The series used are the *Scritture Riferite nei Congressi, Anglia.* There are thirty volumes for the nineteenth century, each with stamped folio numbering. They are of enormous bulk and of rather uneven and varying utility—there is more general and political material up to 1850, but after the restoration of the Hierarchy the letters and reports tend to relate to internal administrative concerns of the dioceses. Most of the items are in Italian.

Venerable English College Archives. It was the Talbot papers which were the most useful in this study. They are very extensive, in boxes, and are internally sorted into folders. There is a reliable cross-reference index. The few and rather disappointing number of letters from Manning may perhaps indicate the research ravages of E. S. Purcell, in composing his *Life* of the Cardinal in 1895. For a description of the archives, see Michael E. Williams, *The Venerable English College, Rome* (London 1979), Appendix 1, pp. 184–91.

Westminster Diocesan Archives. Papers consulted: the Wiseman Papers (especially the correspondence from the bishops, and Grant's letters from Rome in Box 137); the Vaughan Papers; and the Gradwell Papers. The archives are extremely well kept, and though the content is often patchy it is possible to acquire materials for a comprehensive view of the Church.

Archives of the English Benedictine Congregation, Downside Abbey. They are stored in the new library, and are sorted into general subjects—but often with little internal order under each head. The most useful for the present study were the Abbots' Papers (A(a)) and the Cardinal Gasquet collection. An excellent guide to the materials has been written by Dom Philip Jebb (*Downside Review*, vol. 93, no. 312, July 1975).

Clifton Diocesan Archives. These are now deposited at the Bristol Record Office. The enormous collection of Archbishop Errington's papers, and those of Bishop William Clifford, were consulted. There is no index to either, but they are sorted chronologically.

St. Dominic's Convent, Stone, Staffordshire. The papers of Archbishop Ullathorne are preserved here in the convent where he is buried. As well as a random selection of his letters, there is also a full collection of Ullathorne's drafts for his various published writings. The papers of Mother Margaret Hallahan supply some useful information on Ullathorne.

Stonyhurst College. The archives contain letters and memoranda relating to the English Province of the Society of Jesus, as well as to the College itself. Particularly helpful, despite its partisan flavour, is Glover's *Excerpts*—an extensive MS 'collection of notes, memoirs, and Documents, respecting the re-establishment of the English Province of the Society of Jesus', much of it drawing on materials from Jesuit sources in Rome.

Ushaw College. Here there are kept the other half of the surviving Wiseman Papers; some in files, some in bound volumes. There is a good index, but the letters are not as useful as the ones at Westminster, since they are less concerned with general Catholic issues.

English Province of the Society of Jesus Archives, Farm Street, London. This extremely well kept collection contains bound volumes of 'Letters of Bishops and Cardinals', covering the whole of the century, as well, of course, as the huge number of materials—not used in this study—relating to the internal history of the Society.

Birmingham Diocesan Archives, at Cathedral House in Birmingham. There are three published Reports on the contents of the archives, which provide a comprehensive and accurate index to the letters and papers. These concern most aspects of the affairs of the District and Diocese, as well as the business of individual bishops. A very extensive collection.

Note: for information about the *Manning Papers*, which were not made available for this work, see chapter 6, p. 246 footnote 9.

II. *JOURNALS*

Ampleforth Journal
Bulwark or Reformation Journal (1851–2)
Catholic Directory and Ecclesiastical Register
Downside Review
Hansard's Parliamentary Debates
Journal of Ecclesiastical History
Recusant History
The Dublin Review [*Wiseman Review* after 1961]
The Month
The Rambler [*Home and Foreign Review* after 1862]
The Tablet
The Times
Transactions of the Royal Historical Society
Victorian Studies

III. *PRINTED BOOKS*

Acton, Lord, *Selections from the Correspondence of the First Lord Acton*, ed. J. N. Figgis and R. V. Laurence, London 1917.
—— *Essays on Church and State*, London (ed. Douglas Woodruff), 1952.
—— *Lectures on Modern History*, London (Introduction by H. R. Trevor-Roper) 1960.
Addington, Raleigh, *The Idea of the Oratory*, London 1966.
—— *Faber, Poet and Priest. Selected Letters, 1833-1863*, London 1974.
Addison, W. G., *Religious Equality in Modern England, 1714-1914*, London 1944.
Ahlstrom, Sydney E., *A Religious History of the American People*, Yale 1972.
Allen, Louis, 'Letters of Phillipps de Lisle to Montalembert', in *Dublin Review* 228, no. 463 (1954).
Allies, M. H., *T. W. Allies*, London 1907.
Almond, Cuthbert, *The History of Ampleforth Abbey*, London 1903.
Altholz, Joseph, *The Liberal Catholic Movement in England*, Montreal 1962.
Amhurst, W. J., *The History of Catholic Emancipation and the Progress of the Catholic Church, 1771 to 1820*, London 1886.
Anson, P. F., *The Religious Orders and Congregations of Great Britain and Ireland*, London 1949.
Anstruther, G. E., *A Hundred Years of Catholic Progress*, London 1929.
Apostolicae Curae (Leo XIII, 1896), London CTS 1967.
Arnstein, Walker L., 'The Murphy Riots: A Victorian Dilemma', in *Victorian Studies*, XIX, no. 1 (1975).
—— *Protestant versus Catholic in Mid-Victorian England. Mr. Newdegate and the Nuns*, Columbia 1982.
Attwater, D., *The Catholic Church in Modern Wales*, London 1935.
Awful Disclosures of Maria Monk [1836], London, 1965 edn.

Bagshaw, E. G., *Mercy and Justice to the Poor*, London 1885.
Barmann, Lawrence, *Baron Friedrich von Hügel and the Modernist Crisis in England*, Cambridge 1972.
Barnes, A. S., *The Catholic Schools in England*, London 1926.
Bassett, Bernard, *Farm Street*, London 1948.
Bastable, J. D. (ed.), *Newman and Gladstone. Centennial Essays*, Dublin 1978.
Beck, G. A. (ed.), *The English Catholics 1850-1950*, London 1950.
Bedoyere, Michael de la, *The Life of Baron von Hügel*, London 1951.
Bellenger, D. T. J., 'The French Ecclesiastical Exiles in England, 1789-1815' (Cambridge Ph.D. thesis, 1978; Cambridge University Library).
Bennett, William, *Popery as Set Forth in Scripture: Its Guilt and Its Doom*, London 1850.
Birt, H. N., *History of Downside School*, London 1902.
Blakiston, Noel (ed.), *The Roman Question. Extracts from the Despatches of Odo Russell from Rome, 1858-1870*, London 1962.

Bolton, C. A., *Salford Diocese and its Catholic Past*, Manchester 1950.

Bossy, John, *The English Catholic Community, 1570-1850*, London 1975.

Bowden, T. W., *The Life and Letters of Frederick William Faber*, London 1869.

Brady, W. Maziere, *The Episcopal Succession in England, Scotland and Ireland, 1400 to 1875*, Rome 1876.

Brandon, Piers, *Hurrell Froude and the Oxford Movement*, London 1974.

Bricknell, W. S., *The Judgment of the Bishops upon Tractarian Theology*, Oxford 1845.

Brose, Olive, *Church and Parliament. The reshaping of the Church of England 1828-1860*, Stanford 1959.

Burke, Thomas, *Catholic History of Liverpool*, Liverpool 1910.

Butler, Charles, *Historical Account of the Laws Respecting Roman Catholics, and of the Laws passed for their Relief; with Observations on the Laws remaining in force against them*. London 1795.

—— *Historical Memoirs Respecting the English, Irish, and Scottish Catholics from the Reformation to the Present Time*, London 1819.

—— *A Letter on the Coronation Oath* [1825], London (second edn.) 1827.

—— *A Memoir of the Catholic Relief Bill Passed in 1829*, London 1829.

Butler, Cuthbert, *The Life and Times of Bishop Ullathorne, 1806-1889*, London 1926.

—— *The Vatican Council, 1869-1870*, London 1962.

Campion, Edmund (ed.), *Lord Acton and the First Vatican Council: A Journal*, Sydney 1975.

Chadwick, W. O., *The Victorian Church*, London 1966, 1970.

—— *Catholicism and History*, Cambridge 1978.

Chapman, Ronald, *Father Faber*, London 1961.

Chiniquy, Charles, *Fifty Years in the Church of Rome*, London, 1948 edn.

Chinnici, J. P., *The English Catholic Enlightenment: John Lingard and the Cisalpine Movement, 1780-1850*, Shepherdstown (West Virginia) 1980.

Clarke, Kenneth, *The Gothic Revival*, London, 1975 edn.

Cobbett, William, *A History of the Protestant "Reformation" in England and Ireland*, Dublin 1826.

Collingwood, C., *The Catholic Truth Society*, London 1965.

Columbanus (No. VI), *Unpublished Correspondence between the Rt. Rev. Dr Poynter and the Rev. Dr. O'Conor*, London 1813.

—— (No. VII), *The Gallican Liberties. Indispensable Securities for the Constitutional Government of the Irish Catholic Church*, London 1816.

Cross, Robert D., *The Emergence of Liberal Catholicism in America*, Cambridge, Mass. 1958.

Cwiekowski, F. J., 'The English Bishops and the First Vatican Council', in *Bibliothèque de la Revue d'Histoire Ecclésiastique*, Louvain 1971.

Denvir, John, *The Irish in Britain. From the Earliest Times to the Fall and Death of Parnell*, London 1892.

Dessain, C. S., *John Henry Newman*, London 1966.

Dignan, P. J., *A History of the Legal Incorporation of Catholic Church Property in the United States, 1784-1932*, New York 1935.

Dolan, J. P., *Catholic Revivalism. The American Experience, 1830-1900*, Notre Dame 1978.

Doyle, P. H., 'Bishop Goss of Liverpool and the importance of being English', in Stuart Mews (ed.), *Religion and National Identity. Studies in Church History*, 18 (1982).

Drane, F. R., *Life of Mother Margaret Mary Hallahan*, London, 2nd edn. 1929.

Duffy, Eamon, 'Ecclesiastical Democracy Detected', I (1779-87), II (1789-96), in *Recusant History*, 10 (Jan. and Oct. 1970).

—— (ed.), *Challoner and his Church. A Catholic Bishop in Georgian England*, London 1981.

Egan, Patrick K., *The Parish of Ballinasloe. Its History from the Earliest Times to the Present Day*, Dublin 1960.

Engels, Frederick, *The Condition of the Working Class in England* (trans. and ed. W. O. Henderson and W. H. Challoner), Oxford 1958.

Evennett, H. O., *The Catholic Schools of England and Wales*, Cambridge 1944.

Eyzaguirre, Jaime, *Historia de las instituciones políticas y sociales de Chile*, Santiago 1967.

Faber, Fredrick William, *All For Jesus: or, The Easy Ways of Divine Love*, London 1853.

Faber, G. S., *Letters on Tractarian Secession to Popery*, London 1846.

Ferrey, B., *Recollections of A. N. Welby Pugin*, London 1861.

Fitzpatrick, W. J., *The Life, Times, and Correspondence of the Right Rev. Dr. Doyle, Bishop of Kildare and Leighlin*, Dublin 1861.

Fothergill, Brian, 'Wiseman: The Man and his Mission', in *Wiseman Review*, 493 (1962).

—— *Nicholas Wiseman*, London 1963.

Fowler, J., *Richard Waldo Sibthorpe. A Biography*, London 1880.

Freemantle, Anne (ed.), *The Papal Encyclicals*, New York 1956.

Gasquet, Aidan Cardinal (ed.), *Lord Acton and his Circle*, London 1906.

—— *History of the Venerable English College in Rome*, London 1920.

—— 'Unpublished Letters of Cardinal Wiseman to Dr Manning', in *Dublin Review*, Oct.–Dec. 1921.

Gaunt, William, *The Pre-Raphaelite Tragedy*, London, 1975 edn.

Gilley, Sheridan, 'Protestant London, No-Popery and the Irish Poor', in *Recusant History*, 10 (1969-70), 11 (1971-2).

—— 'The Garibaldi Riots of 1862', in *Historical Journal*, XVI.4 (1973).
—— 'Supernaturalized Culture: Catholic Attitudes and Latin Lands, 1840–60', in Derek Baker (ed.), *The Materials, Sources and Methods of Ecclesiastical History. Studies in Church History*, 11 (1975).
—— 'Vulgar Piety and the Brompton Oratory, 1850-1860', in *Durham University Journal*, XLIII (1981).
Gillow, Joseph, *A Literary and Biographical History of the English Catholics*, London 1885.
Girouard, Mark, *The Return to Camelot. Chivalry and the English Gentleman*, London 1981.
Gladstone, W. E., *The Vatican Decrees in their bearing on Civil Allegiance: A Political Expostulation*, London 1874.
Gormann, W. G., *Converts to Rome. A biographical list of the more notable Converts to the Catholic Church in the United Kingdom during the last sixty years*, London (new edn.) 1910.
Gregorovius, Ferdinand, *The Roman Journals, 1852-1874*, ed. Friedrich Althaus, London 1911.
Gruber, J. W., *A Conscience in Conflict. The Life of St. George Jackson Mivart*, New York 1960.
Gruggen, G., and Keating, J., *Stonyhurst College*, London 1901.
Guy, R. E., *The Synods in English* [translation of the Decrees of the Synods of Westminster], Stratford 1886.
Gwynn, Denis, *The Struggle for Catholic Emancipation (1750-1829)*, London 1928.
—— *Cardinal Wiseman*, London 1929.
—— *The Second Spring, 1818-1852. A Study of the Catholic Revival in England*, London 1942.
—— *Lord Shrewsbury, Pugin, and the Catholic Revival*, London 1946.
—— *Father Dominic Barberi*, London 1947.
—— *Father Luigi Gentili and his Mission (1801-1848)*, Dublin 1951.

Haile, Martin, and Bonney, Edwin, *Life and Times of John Lingard, 1771-1851*, London 1912.
Harrison, Brian, *Drink and the Victorians. The Temperance Question in England, 1815-1872*, London 1971.
Healey, John, *Maynooth College. Its Centenary History*, Dublin 1895.
Heaney, John J., *The Modernist Crisis: von Hügel*, London 1969.
Hermann, Fr., *Catholicism in England. An Address delivered at the Catholic Congress at Malines (1863)*, London 1864.
Hickey, John, *Urban Catholicism*, London 1967.
Holmes, J. Derek, 'Newman and Mivart—Two Attitudes to a Nineteenth-Century Problem', in *Clergy Review*, L (1965).
—— 'Some unpublished passages from Cardinal Wiseman's correspondence', in *Downside Review*, 90 (1972).
—— 'Cardinal Raphael Merry del Val—an uncompromising Ultramontane', in *Catholic Historical Review*, LX (1974).
—— 'English Catholicism from Wiseman to Bourne', in *Clergy Review*, LXI (1976).

— *More Roman than Rome: English Catholicism in the Nineteenth Century*, London 1978.

Hughes, J. J., *Absolutely Null and Utterly Void. An Account of the Papal Condemnation of Anglican Orders*, London 1968.

Hughes, Philip, *The Catholic Question, 1688-1829*, London 1929.

Husenbeth, F. C., *A History of Sedgley Park School*, London 1856.

— *The Life of the Rt. Rev. Mgr. Weedall, D.D., President of St. Mary's College, Oscott*, London 1960.

— *The Life of the Right Rev. John Milner, D.D.*, Dublin 1862.

Jackman, S. W., *Nicholas Wiseman. A Victorian Prelate and his Writings*, Dublin 1977.

Kenny, Terence, *The Political Thought of John Henry Newman*, London 1957.

Lash, Nicholas, *Newman and Development. The Search for an Explanation in History*, London 1975.

Leetham, Claude, *Luigi Gentili. A Sower for the Second Spring*, London 1965.

— 'Gentili's Reports to Rome', in the *Wiseman Review*, 498 (1963-4).

Leslie, Shane, 'Irish Pages from the Postbags of Manning, Cullen and Gladstone', in *Dublin Review*, October 1919.

— *Henry Edward Manning. His Life and Labours*, London 1921.

Lesourd, Jean Alain, *Les Catholiques dans la société anglaise, 1765-1865*, Lille 1978.

Lilly, W. S., and Wallis, J. P., *A Manual of the Law specially affecting Catholics*, London 1893.

Lingard, John, *Observations on the Laws and Ordinances, which exist in Foreign States, relative to the religious concerns of their Roman Catholic Subjects. By a British Roman Catholic* [pub. anon.], London 1817.

— *History of England*, London 1819-30.

Lisle, Edwin De, *Pastoral Politics. A Reply to Dr. Bagshawe, Catholic Bishop of Nottingham*, London 1885.

Lucas, Edward, *The Life of Frederick Lucas M.P.*, London 1886.

Ludlow, John, *The Autobiography of a Christian Socialist*, ed. A. D. Murray, London 1981.

MacCaffrey, *History of the Catholic Church in the Nineteenth Century*, Dublin and St. Louis (Mo.), 2nd edn. 1910.

McClelland, V. A., *Cardinal Manning. His Public Life and Influence, 1865-1892*, London 1962.

— *English Roman Catholics and Higher Education, 1830-1903*, Oxford 1973.

McCormack, Arthur, *Cardinal Vaughan. The Life of the Third Archbishop of Westminster*, London 1966.

MacDougall, H. A., *The Acton-Newman Relations. The Dilemma of Christian Liberalism*, New York 1962.

McGrath, Fergal, *Newman's University. Idea and Reality*, Dublin 1951.

Machin, G. I. T., *The Catholic Question in English Politics, 1820 to 1830*, Oxford 1964.

— *Politics and the Churches in Great Britain, 1832 to 1868*, Oxford 1977.

MacHugh, James, *Father Gentili, Priest and Missionary*, Dublin 1958.

Maguire, J. F., *Father Mathew. A Biography*, London 1863.

Manning, H. E., Cardinal, *National Education. A Serman Preached in the Cathedral Church of Chichester by Henry Edward Manning, M.A.*, London 1838.

— *Ireland. A Letter to Earl Grey*, London 1868.

— *Caesarism and Ultramontanism*, London 1873.

— *Vatican Decrees in their bearing on Civil Allegiance*, London 1875.

— *The True Story of the Vatican Council*, London 1877.

— *Miscellanies*, London 1877.

— *The Catholic Church in Modern Society*, London 1880.

— *The Eternal Priesthood*, London 1883.

— *Is the Education Act of 1870 a Just Law?* London 1886.

— *The Future of the Primary Schools*, London 1886.

Martin, Brian, *John Henry Newman. His Life and Work*, London 1982.

Mathew, David, *Catholicism in England, 1535–1935*, London 1936.

— *Acton. The Formative Years*, London 1946.

May, J. Lewis, *Father Tyrrell and the Modernist Movement*, London (2nd edn.) 1938.

Maynard, Theodore, *The Story of American Catholicism*, New York 1960.

Milburn, David, *A History of Ushaw College*, Ushaw 1964.

Milburn, J. B., *The Restored Hierarchy, 1850–1910*, London 1911.

Milner, J., *The Case of Conscience Solved: or The Catholic Claims proved to be compatible with The Coronation Oath* [1801], London (2nd edn.) 1807.

— *An Elucidation of the Veto, in a threefold address to the Public, the Catholics, and the Advocates of Catholics in Parliament*, London 1810.

Morris, J., *Catholic England in Modern Times*, London 1892.

Newman, J. H., Cardinal, *Sermons Preached on Various Occasions*, London 1857.

— *An Essay in Aid of a Grammar of Assent*, London 1870.

— *Discussions and Arguments on Various Subjects*, London 1872.

— *A Letter Addressed to His Grace the Duke of Norfolk*, London 1875.

— *Lectures on the Present Position of Catholics in England, Addressed to the Brothers of the Oratory in the Summer of 1851*, London (new edn.) 1892.

— *Letters and Correspondence of John Henry Newman During his Life in the English Church*, ed. Anne Mozley, London 1898.

—— *The Idea of a University. Defined and Illustrated* [1852], London, 1907 edn.

—— *Apologia Pro Vita Sua* [1864], New York 1956 (Image Books edn.).

—— *Autobiographical Works*, ed. Henry Tristram, New York 1957.

—— *The Letters and Diaries of John Henry Newman*, ed. C. S. Dessain, London and Oxford, 1961–81.

—— *Loss and Gain. The Story of a Convert* [1848], London, 1962 edn.

Newsome, David, *The Parting of Friends. A Study of the Wilberforces and Henry Manning*, London 1966.

Norman, E. R., *The Catholic Church and Ireland in the Age of Rebellion, 1859–1873*, London 1965.

—— *Anti-Catholicism in Victorian England*, London 1968.

—— *The Conscience of the State in North America*, Cambridge 1968.

—— *Church and Society in England, 1770–1970*, Oxford 1976.

—— *Christianity in the Southern Hemisphere*, Oxford 1981.

O'Brien, C. C., *Parnell and his Party, 1880–90*, Oxford 1957.

O'Connell, Daniel, *Correspondence*, ed. W. J. Fitzpatrick, London 1888.

O'Meara, Kathleen, *Thomas Grant, First Bishop of Southwark*, London (2nd edn.) 1886.

O'Tuathaigh, M. A. G., 'The Irish in Nineteenth-Century Britain: Problems of Integration', in *Trans. of Royal Hist. Soc.*, Fifth Series, 31 (1981).

Patrick, J., 'Newman, Pugin and Gothic', in *Victorian Studies* (Winter, 1981).

Patrick Murphy on Popery in Ireland, or Confessionals, Abductions, Nunneries, Fenians and Orangemen [by G. H. Whalley], London 1865.

Pawley, Bernard and Margaret, *Rome and Canterbury through Four Centuries. A Study of the Relations between the Church of Rome and the Anglican Churches, 1530–1981*, London 1981.

Petre, M. D., *Modernism*, London 1918.

Pollen, John Hungerford, 'The Penal Clauses in the Emancipation Bill', in *The Month*, October 1908.

Pugin, A. Welby, *Contrasts*, London 1836.

—— *An Apology for the Revival of Christian Architecture*, London 1843.

—— *Church and State; Or Christian Liberty. An Earnest Address on the Establishment of the Hierarchy*, London [1850] 1875.

Purcell, E. S., *The Life of Cardinal Manning, Archbishop of Westminster*, London 1895.

—— *Life and Letters of Ambrose Phillipps de Lisle*, London 1900.

[Ramsgate] *The Story of St. Augustine's, St. Ethelbert's, and St. Benedict's, Ramsgate*, Ramsgate 1960.

Reynolds, E. E., *Three Cardinals*, London 1958.

Robo, Étienne, *The Story of a Catholic Parish: St. Joan's, Farnham*, Farnham 1938.

Roche, J. S., *A History of Prior Park College and its Founder, Bishop Baines*, London 1931.

Roe, W. G., *Lamennais in England. The Reception of Lamennais's Religious Ideas in England in the Nineteenth Century*, Oxford 1966.

Rowell, Geoffrey, *Hell and the Victorians. A study of the nineteenth-century theological controversies concerning eternal punishment and the after-life*, Oxford 1974.

St. Augustine's Abbey Church, Ramsgate. A Short Guide, Ramsgate 1968.

Schiefen, R. J., 'The Organization and Administration of Roman Catholic Dioceses in England and Wales in the mid-nineteenth century' (London University Ph.D. thesis, 1970).

—— 'The First Provincial Synod of Westminster (1852)', in *Annuarium Historiae Conciliorum* (1972).

—— 'Some Aspects of the Controversy between Cardinal Wiseman and the Westminster Chapter', in *Journal of Ecclesiastical History*, XXI, 2 (1970).

Smith, Sydney, *Works*, London (3rd edn.) 1845.

—— *Peter Plymley's Letters*, London, 1886 edn.

Snead-Cox, J. G., *The Life of Cardinal Vaughan*, London 1910.

Spearitt, Placid and Green, Bernard, *A History of the English Benedictine Congregation, 1558–1850*, Oxford 1978.

Strachey, Lytton, *Eminent Victorians* [1918], London, 1948 edn.

Sugg, Joyce, *A Saint for Birmingham?* [a Life of Newman], London CTS (n.d.).

Tayler, William Elfe, *Popery: Its Character and Its Crimes*, London 1847.

Throckmorton, Sir John, *Considerations arising from the Debates in Parliament on the Petition of the Irish Catholics*, London 1806.

Thureau-Dangin, Paul, *The English Catholic Revival in the Nineteenth Century*, London 1914.

Trappes-Lomax, Michael, *Pugin. A Medieval Victorian*, London 1932.

Trevor, Meriol, *Newman. The Pillar of the Cloud*, London 1962.

—— *Newman. Light in Winter*, London 1962.

Ullathorne, W. B., *Notes on the Education Question by the Right Rev. Bishop Ullathorne*, London 1857.

—— *A Pastoral Letter to the Faithful of the Diocese of Birmingham, by William Bernard Ullathorne*, Birmingham 1870.

—— *History of the Restoration of the Catholic Hierarchy in England*, London 1871.

—— *The Döllingerites, Mr Gladstone, and Apostates from the Faith*, London 1875.

—— *Letters*, ed. by the nuns of St. Dominic's Convent, Stone; London 1892.

—— *From Cabin-Boy to Archbishop. The Autobiography of Archbishop Ullathorne* [1891], London, 1941 edn.

Vaughan, Herbert Cardinal, *Popular Education in England. The Conscience Clause, the Rating Clause, and the Secular Current*, London 1868.

—— *Address on the Re-dedication of Catholic England to Blessed Peter, by Herbert Cardinal Vaughan*, London 1893.

—— *The Reunion of Christendom*, London 1897.

—— *The Young Priest. Conferences on the Apostolic Life* (ed. J. S. Vaughan), London 1904.

—— *Letters of Herbert Cardinal Vaughan to Lady Herbert of Lea, 1867 to 1903*, ed. Shane Leslie, London 1942.

Ward, Bernard, *History of St. Edmund's College, Old Hall*, London 1893.

—— *The Eve of Catholic Emancipation*, London 1911.

—— *The Sequel to Catholic Emancipation*, London 1915.

Ward, Wilfrid, *The Life and Times of Cardinal Wiseman*, London 1897.

—— *William George Ward and the Catholic Revival*, London (2nd edn.) 1912.

—— *The Life of John Henry, Cardinal Newman*, London 1912.

Watkin, David, *The Triumph of the Classical. Cambridge Architecture, 1804–1834*, Cambridge 1977.

Watkin, E. I., *Roman Catholicism in England, From the Reformation to 1950*, London 1957.

Weaver, M. J., (ed.), *Letters from a 'Modernist'. The Letters of George Tyrrell to Wilfrid Ward, 1893–1908*, London 1981.

Whateley, Richard, *Essays on the Errors of Romanism* (Third Series), London 1856.

White, Joseph Blanco, *Practical and Internal Evidence Against Catholicism*, London (revised edn.) 1826.

Williams, J. Anthony, *Bath and Rome: the Living Link*, Bath 1963.

Williams, Michael E., *The Venerable English College, Rome. A History, 1579–1979*, London 1979.

Wilson, Anselm, *Life of Bishop Hedley*, London 1930.

Winwar, Frances, *The Rossettis and their Circle*, London 1934.

Wiseman, Nicolas, Cardinal, *Twelve Lectures on the Connexion between Science and Revealed Religion delivered in Rome by Nicholas Wiseman, D.D.*, London 1836.

—— *A Letter Respectfully Addressed to the Rev. J. H. Newman*, London (third edn.) 1841.

—— *Words of Peace and Justice addressed to the Catholic Clergy and Laity of the London District on the Subject of Diplomatic Relations with the Holy See, by the Rt. Rev. Nicholas Wiseman D.D.*, London 1848.

—— *An Appeal to the Reason and Good Feeling of the English People on the Subject of the Catholic Hierarchy, by Cardinal Wiseman*, London 1850.

—— *The Social and Intellectual State of England, Compared with its Moral Condition. A Sermon delivered in St. John's Catholic Church,*

Salford, on Sunday, July 28th 1850, by the Right Rev. N. Wiseman, D.D., London 1850.

—— *Three Lectures on the Catholic Hierarchy by Cardinal Wiseman*, London 1850.

—— *Essays on Various Subjects by His Eminence Cardinal Wiseman*, London 1853.

—— *Recollections of the Last Four Popes and of Rome in their Times, by H. E. Cardinal Wiseman*, London (revised edn.) 1859.

—— *The Sermons, Lectures and Speeches delivered by His Eminence Cardinal Wiseman, Archbishop of Westminster, during his Tour of Ireland in August and September, 1858*, Boston 1859.

—— *Pastoral Letter of His Eminence the Cardinal Archbishop of Westminster enjoining a collection throughout the diocese for His Holiness the Pope*, London 1860.

—— *The Religious and Social Position of the Catholics in England. An Address Delivered to the Catholic Congress of Malines, August 21, 1863, by H. E. Cardinal Wiseman*, London 1864.

—— *Pastoral Letter of H. E. Cardinal Wiseman enjoining the Collection for the building of Churches and Schools in the Archdiocese*, London 1864.

Young, Urban, *Life of Father Ignatius Spencer*, London 1933.

—— *Dominic Barberi in England. A new series of letters*, London 1935.

Index